Syringe Exchange Programs
and the Opioid Epidemic

Also of Interest and from McFarland

Climate Change and Disaster Resilience: Challenges, Actions and Innovations in Urban Planning, edited by Joaquin Jay Gonzalez III, Roger L. Kemp and Alan R. Roper (2022) • *Keeping Schools Safe: Case Studies and Insights,* edited by Joaquin Jay Gonzalez III and Roger L. Kemp (2022) • *Brownfields Redevelopment: Case Studies and Concepts in Community Revitalization,* edited by Joaquin Jay Gonzalez III, Tad McGalliard and Ignacio Dayrit (2021) • *Cities and Homelessness: Essays and Case Studies on Practices, Innovations and Challenges,* edited by Joaquin Jay Gonzalez III and Mickey P. McGee (2021) • *Senior Care and Services: Essays and Case Studies on Practices, Innovations and Challenges,* edited by Joaquin Jay Gonzalez III, Roger L. Kemp and Willie Lee Brit (2020) • *Veteran Care and Services: Essays and Case Studies on Practices, Innovations and Challenges,* edited by Joaquin Jay Gonzalez III, Mickey P. McGee and Roger L. Kemp (2020) • *Legal Marijuana: Perspectives on Public Benefits, Risks and Policy Approaches,* edited by Joaquin Jay Gonzalez III and Mickey P. McGee (2019) • *Cybersecurity: Current Writings on Threats and Protection,* edited by Joaquin Jay Gonzalez III and Roger L. Kemp (2019) • *Eminent Domain and Economic Growth: Perspectives on Benefits, Harms and New Trends,* edited by Joaquin Jay Gonzalez III, Roger L. Kemp and Jonathan Rosenthal (2018) • *Small Town Economic Development: Reports on Growth Strategies in Practice,* edited by Joaquin Jay Gonzalez III, Roger L. Kemp and Jonathan Rosenthal (2017) • *Privatization in Practice: Reports on Trends, Cases and Debates in Public Service by Business and Nonprofits,* edited by Joaquin Jay Gonzalez III and Roger L. Kemp (2016) • *Immigration and America's Cities: A Handbook on Evolving Services,* edited by Joaquin Jay Gonzalez III and Roger L. Kemp (2016) • *Corruption and American Cities: Essays and Case Studies in Ethical Accountability,* edited by Joaquin Jay Gonzalez III and Roger L. Kemp (2016)

Syringe Exchange Programs and the Opioid Epidemic

Government and Nonprofit Practices and Policies

Edited by JOAQUIN JAY GONZALEZ III
and MICKEY P. McGEE

McFarland & Company, Inc., Publishers
Jefferson, North Carolina

ISBN (print) 978-1-4766-7311-0
ISBN (ebook) 978-1-4766-4110-2

LIBRARY OF CONGRESS AND BRITISH LIBRARY
CATALOGUING DATA ARE AVAILABLE

Library of Congress Control Number 2021061136

© 2022 Joaquin Jay Gonzalez III and Mickey P. McGee. All rights reserved

No part of this book may be reproduced or transmitted in any form or by any means, electronic or mechanical, including photocopying or recording, or by any information storage and retrieval system, without permission in writing from the publisher.

Front cover image © 2020 Abert/Shutterstock

Printed in the United States of America

*McFarland & Company, Inc., Publishers
Box 611, Jefferson, North Carolina 28640
www.mcfarlandpub.com*

Jay and Mick dedicate this book to those suffering from pain, suffering, and opioid addiction as well as their families, friends, and caregivers.

Acknowledgments

We are grateful for the support of the Mayor George Christopher Professorship at Golden Gate University as well as GGU's Pi Alpha Alpha Chapter and ICMA Student Chapter. We appreciate the encouragement from Dean Amy McLellan and our wonderful colleagues and students at the Edward S. Ageno School of Business, the Department of Public Administration, the Executive MPA Program, and the Doctor of Business Administration Program.

Our heartfelt "thank you!" goes to the contributors listed in the back section and the individuals, organizations, and publishers below for granting permission to reprint the material in this volume and the research assistance. They all expressed support for practical research and information sharing that benefits our citizens, communities, and cities.

American Society for Public Administration
Brenda J. Bond-Fortier
California Department of Public Health
Centers for Disease Control and Prevention
City and County of San Francisco
Coral H. Gonzalez
Don C. Des Jarlais
Elise B. Gonzalez
Golden Gate University Library
H. Daniel Xu
Hazelden Betty Ford Foundation
International City/County Management Association
Jaime Teeter Householder
Jenna Tyler
Karen Garrett
Kaiser Health News
Mark Kennedy
Michelle Hong-Gonzalez
National Association of County and City Health Officials
National Institute on Drug Abuse
National League of Cities
New York State Department of Health
PA Times
Paul C. Prevey
PM Magazine
San Francisco AIDS Foundation
San Francisco Department of Public Health
San Francisco Health Commission
Sarah Sweeney
Substance Abuse and Mental Health Services Administration
theconversation.com
U.S. Centers for Disease Control and Prevention
U.S. Department of Health and Human Services
U.S. Drug Enforcement Agency
U.S. Environmental Protection Agency
U.S. Food and Drug Administration
U.S. Substance Abuse and Mental Health Services Administration
University of San Francisco Library
Utah Department of Health

Table of Contents

Acknowledgments   vii
Preface   1

Part I. The Opioid Epidemic

1. Opioid Epidemic Causing Rise in Hepatitis C Infections and Other Serious Illnesses
   THOMAS J. STOPKA   7

2. Syringe Services Programs (SSPs) Fact Sheet
   CENTERS FOR DISEASE CONTROL AND PREVENTION   10

3. An Ethical Dilemma for Doctors: When Is It OK to Prescribe Opioids?
   TRAVIS N. RIEDER   13

4. The Opioid Epidemic Is Finally a National Emergency—Eight Years Too Late
   ERIN WINSTANLEY   16

5. As the Opioid Epidemic Continues, the Holidays Bring Need to Support Those in Grief
   EMILY B. CAMPBELL   19

6. Keeping Away from Criminalization
   SARAH SWEENEY   21

7. Stepping Up, Then Stepping Back
   BRENDA BOND-FORTIER   23

8. Needle Exchanges Find New Champions Among Republicans
   VICTORIA KNIGHT   25

Part II. Syringe Use and Infection Risks
• *A. HIV* •

9. Syringe-Exchange Programs Are Part of Effective HIV Prevention
   NATIONAL INSTITUTE ON DRUG ABUSE   31

10. Needle Exchanges Can Now Get Federal Funding
    ANNA GORMAN   36

11. Trump Pledges to End HIV Transmission by 2030. Doable, But Daunting
   CARMEN HEREDIA RODRIGUEZ ... 39

12. The Unexpected Public Health Emergency
   JENNA TYLER ... 43

13. An Addiction Researcher Shares 6 Strategies to Address the Opioid Epidemic
   NABILA EL-BASSEL ... 46

14. Why Are HIV Survival Rates Lower in the Deep South Than the Rest of the U.S.?
   SUSAN REIF and CAROLYN MCALLASTER ... 49

15. Should You Be Tested for HIV? Why June 27 Is a Good Day to Do It
   JODI SUTHERLAND ... 52

16. Violence Against Women Is Overlooked in Its Role in Opioid Epidemic
   NABILA EL-BASSEL ... 54

17. Fighting HIV in Miami, One Dirty Needle at a Time
   AMY DRISCOLL ... 57

• **B. Hepatitis C** •

18. Addressing Increases in Hepatitis C Infections Linked to the Opioid Epidemic
   DON C. DES JARLAIS ... 63

19. Hepatitis C and Injection Drug Use
   U.S. DEPARTMENT OF HEALTH AND HUMAN SERVICES ... 65

20. A "Safe" Space to Shoot Up: Worth a Try?
   STEPHANIE O'NEILL ... 68

21. Treating the New Hep C Generation on Their Turf
   PAULINE BARTOLONE ... 71

Part III. Practices, Programs, and Policies of Governments and Nonprofits

• **A. Federal** •

22. New Rules for Safe and Secure Prescription Drug Disposal Options
   U.S. DRUG ENFORCEMENT ADMINISTRATION ... 75

23. Safely Using Sharps (Needles and Syringes) at Home, at Work and on Travel
   U.S. FOOD AND DRUG ADMINISTRATION ... 77

24. HRSA Implementation Guidance of Syringe Services Programs
   U.S. DEPARTMENT OF HEALTH AND HUMAN SERVICES ... 83

25. Implementation Guidance for Syringe Services Programs
    U.S. Department of Health and Human Services — 85

26. Injection Drug Use
    Centers for Disease Control and Prevention — 89

27. Syringe Services Programs (SSPs) FAQs
    Centers for Disease Control and Prevention — 92

28. The Safety and Effectiveness of Syringe Services Programs
    Centers for Disease Control and Prevention — 96

29. CDC's Role in Safe Injection Practices
    Centers for Disease Control and Prevention — 102

30. CDC Program Guidance for Syringe Services Programs
    Centers for Disease Control and Prevention — 105

31. Medical Waste
    U.S. Environmental Protection Agency — 112

32. Opioid Overdose Reversal with Naloxone
    National Institute on Drug Abuse — 115

• B. State •

33. Syringe Exchange Programs in California: An Overview
    California Department of Public Health — 118

34. California Legal Code Related to Access to Sterile Needles and Syringes
    California Department of Public Health — 122

35. Florida Is the Latest Republican-Led State to Adopt Clean Needle Exchanges
    Sammy Mack — 125

36. Syringe Exchange in Southern Indiana to Respond to an Increase in HIV Cases
    Jeannie D. DiClementi — 128

37. HIV, STDs, and Hepatitis C
    New York State Department of Health — 131

38. Utah Syringe Exchange Program
    Utah Department of Health — 135

39. Arizona Declares Opioid Emergency, but Signals Are Mixed Over Best Response
    Will Stone — 142

40. Unable to Arrest Opioid Epidemic, Red States Warm to Needle Exchanges
    Shefali Luthra — 145

• C. County and City •

41. The Competing Views and a Way Forward
    ELISSA VELEZ *and* MICKEY P. MCGEE — 149

42. Harm Reduction Services in San Francisco: Executive Summary
    SAN FRANCISCO DEPARTMENT OF PUBLIC HEALTH — 155

43. Syringe Access and Disposal Programs in San Francisco
    SAN FRANCISCO DEPARTMENT OF PUBLIC HEALTH — 159

44. Syringe Disposal Practices of Intravenous Drug Users in Monterey County
    JAIME TEETER HOUSEHOLDER *and* MICKEY P. MCGEE — 163

45. How Did Ohio Local Government Leaders Dramatically Reduce Opioid Deaths?
    GERALD YOUNG — 170

46. How Lowell Is Fighting the Opioid Crisis
    AUDREY FRAIZER — 172

47. How One City Went "All In" to Fight the Opioid Epidemic
    INTERNATIONAL CITY/COUNTY MANAGEMENT ASSOCIATION — 175

48. The High Cost of Opioid Abuse in Your Community
    MARTY HARDING — 178

49. Boston's Heroin Users Will Soon Get a Safer Place to Be High
    MARTHA BEBINGER — 181

50. In Boston's "Safe Space," Surprising Insights into Drug Highs
    MARTHA BEBINGER — 184

51. What's Next for "Safe Injection" Sites in Philadelphia?
    ELANA GORDON — 186

52. "Crackhouse" or "Safehouse"?
    NINA FELDMAN — 188

• D. Nonprofits and Associations •

53. Offering Syringes Along with Prayers, Churches Help IV Drug Users
    TAYLOR SISK — 191

54. San Francisco AIDS Foundation's Syringe Access Services Evaluation Results
    ELISSA VELEZ *and* MICKEY P. MCGEE — 194

55. Leading the Fight Against the Opioid Crisis
    GEOFF BECKWITH — 204

56. Statement of Policy: Opioid Epidemic
    NATIONAL ASSOCIATION OF COUNTY AND CITY HEALTH OFFICIALS ... 209

57. Statement of Policy: Syringe Services Programs
    NATIONAL ASSOCIATION OF COUNTY AND CITY HEALTH OFFICIALS ... 218

Part IV. The Future

58. Some Good News on Opioid Epidemic: Treatment Options Are Expanding
    WILLIAM GREENE *and* LISA J. MERLO ... 225

59. Sterile Needles Can Stop the Spread of Disease in Prisons—Here's How
    JACK WALLACE ... 229

60. Meth vs. Opioids: America Has Two Drug Epidemics, but Focuses on One
    APRIL DEMBOSKY ... 232

61. Big Data for Big Disease
    H. DANIEL XU ... 235

62. Chittenden County's Hub and Spoke Model for Combatting Opioid Deaths
    PAUL C. PREVEY ... 237

Appendices

Appendix A. Glossary of Syringe Exchange and Opioid Terms, Abbreviations and Acronyms
    JOAQUIN JAY GONZALEZ III ... 243

Appendix B: Syringe Exchange Programs (2019): North American Syringe Exchange Network
    CENTERS FOR DISEASE CONTROL AND PREVENTION ... 251

Appendix C. Adopting a Harm Reduction Policy for Substance Abuse, STD and HIV
    SAN FRANCISCO HEALTH COMMISSION RESOLUTION NO. 10-00 ... 252

Appendix D. Press Release: Mayor Mark Farrell Announces Innovative Program to Fight Opioid Crisis on San Francisco Streets
    CITY AND COUNTY OF SAN FRANCISCO, OFFICE OF THE MAYOR ... 253

Appendix E. Executive Summary: Secure and Responsible Drug Disposal Act of 2010
    FEDERAL REGISTER ... 255

About the Contributors ... 265

Index ... 269

Preface

Syringe Exchange Programs and Safe Injection Services are outside-the-box interventions increasingly being used by governments, nonprofits, and citizens to combat a very serious issue that is percolating in tandem with America's burgeoning opioid epidemic and lingering COVID-19 pandemic. Because of the focus on the bigger picture, people who inject drugs (PWID) are often hidden and marginalized. And yet, according to the U.S. Centers for Disease Control and Prevention, there are close to a million Americans who inject a drug annually.

The increase in substance use has resulted in parallel increases in injection drug use across the U.S. The most commonly misused injected drug ranges from stimulants to painkillers—more specifically, heroin and fentanyl, but may include amphetamines, buprenorphine, benzodiazepines, barbiturates, cocaine, and methamphetamine. The increase has caused not only large increases in opioid deaths, but also thousands of viral hepatitis infections and is threatening progress made in HIV treatment and prevention.

The numbers reported by the U.S. Department of Health and Human Services are staggering:

- **130+**: People died every day from opioid-related drug overdoses
- **47,600**: People died from overdosing on opioids
- **81,000**: People used heroin for the first time
- **2 million**: People misused prescription opioids for the first time
- **10.3 million**: People misused prescription opioids in 2018
- **2 million**: People had an opioid use disorder in 2018
- **808,000**: People used heroin in 2018
- **15,349**: Deaths attributed to overdosing on heroin (in 12-month period ending February 2019)
- **32,656**: Deaths attributed to overdosing on synthetic opioids other than methadone (in 12-month period ending February 2019)

That is why an innovative solution is needed. According to the American Civil Liberties Union, Syringe Exchange Programs (also known as Needle Exchange Programs), when placed alongside other approaches, have helped mitigate the opioid epidemic by:

- Decreasing drug activity in the community
- Decreasing risky sexual activity by IV users
- Offering participants access to substance use disorder education
- Offering participants access to testing and treatment for IV-drug related diseases
- Decreasing rates of new HIV and hepatitis infection

- Offering participants first-line drug counseling
- Offering participants referrals to substance use disorder treatment
- Protecting law enforcement, first responders, and health care workers from accidental infection due to accidental needle pricks
- Decreasing overall financial burden on society for the treatment of infectious diseases and substance use disorders

Still, not everyone is convinced that an outside-the-box approach is necessary. This book elaborates on the discussion and debates, outlines policies and programs, as well as shares gripping stories of real people and their painful struggles.

Part I

The Opioid Epidemic

Part I provides eight colorful introductory essays discussing the intersection between the opioid epidemic and syringe exchange programs. The United States is in the epicenter of a skyrocketing eruption of addictions, overdoses and deaths from intravenous injections as well as the growing number of hepatitis C infections caused by this opioid epidemic. Collected essays include descriptions and facts on syringe services and programs, and the ethical dilemmas faced by doctors on prescribing opioids to patients. A debate is presented on the two public health crises that exist on how the medical community should address the challenges of the opioid epidemic.

The question is asked whether to trade one crisis, the opioid crisis, for another, a pain crisis. Attention-getting statistics are provided such as: "As the President's Commission on Combating Drug Addiction and the Opioid Crisis has described it, in the scale of deaths, it's like the September 11 terrorist attacks happening every three weeks." The enormity of the crisis is brought to our attention hopefully in time to save countless lives. Other topics addressed in Part I include: descriptions of diversion programs to tackle drug addictions at the root causes; how law enforcement agencies are working in collaborative partnerships with communities to reduce drug overdose deaths; and efforts to legalize of syringe exchange services.

Part II

Syringe Use and Infection Risks

Part II delves in the major infection risks—HIV and hepatitis C—associated with persons who inject drugs and why Syringe Exchange Programs (or Syringe Service Programs) are necessary for treatment and prevention. What are Syringe Service Programs (SSPs)? Are they legal? Do SSPs help people stop using drugs? Do SSPs reduce infections? Do SSPs cause more needles in public places? Do they lead to more crime and/or drug use? Are they cost effective? Do they reduce drug use and drug overdoses?

Assembled essays answer these questions while also describing and evaluating various topics on: syringe use and HIV and hepatitis C infection risks; the range of syringe exchange services which contribute effective HIV prevention and deaths; recent lifting of government bans on needle exchange services which would ultimately reduce infectious diseases by preventing intravenous transmission via "dirty needles." Essays include President Trump's pledge to end HIV transmission by 2030; proposed strategies to curb the opioid epidemic with recommendations such as making Naloxone available to all, integrating drug treatment into primary health care and increasing Medicare coverage for drug treatment in all states; why the Deep South has the highest rates of HIV diagnoses in the U.S.; and whether and why you should be tested for HIV today. Essays focused on hepatitis C address the increase in infections linked to the opioid epidemic, a review from the U.S. Department of Health and Human Services on frequently asked questions regarding hepatitis C and injection drug use, the pros and cons for providing safe injection sites and whether providing "a safe space to shoot up" is worth trying. The final essay concerns the treatment of hepatitis C for younger drug users as programs are focused more on the baby boomer generation who account for three-quarters of chronic diseases.

Part III

Practices, Programs, and Policies of Governments and Nonprofits

We gathered articles and essays on the best practices, programs and policies on syringe exchange and safe injection approaches being promoted and used by federal, state, local and nonprofit agencies and include chapters from:

- Federal agencies: Drug Enforcement Administration, Food and Drug Administration, U.S. Department of Health and Human Services, Centers for Disease Control and Prevention, Environmental Protection Agency National Institute on Drug Abuse;
- State examples from California, Florida, Indiana, New York State, Utah, Arizona, Ohio;
- County and City: City and County of San Francisco; Monterey County, California; Lowell, Worcester, Boston, Massachusetts; Philadelphia, Pennsylvania; and
- Nonprofits and associations: Radiant Church of North Carolina, San Francisco AIDS Foundation, Massachusetts Municipal Association, National Association of County and City Health Officials.

The federal agency section focuses on drugs—the safe and secure prescription and disposal options; injection drug use; opioid overdose reversal with Naloxone—and on syringes—safety aspects, service programs and medical waste processes and procedures. The states section provides overviews and examinations or several state syringe programs and include information collected from California, Florida, Indiana, New York, Utah and Arizona. Several essays highlight a shift in thinking by policy makers on the funding and adoption of syringe exchange services and programs, especially in the red states of the U.S. The county and city section describes the high degree of complexity involved in managing the very real problem of the opioid epidemic in their communities. Local governments face competing views from the communities they serve on how to reduce opioid overdose deaths and provide safe places for intravenous drug users. The nonprofit and associations section contains several essays on how they are working to provide programs and services to help intravenous drug users.

Part IV

The Future

We conclude with reflective essays on the shifts in public policy regarding medical cost coverage for drug addiction, clean syringe services reforms, the "other epidemic" in America, methamphetamines, and a final essay on the potential for big data and data analysis to help create solutions to end the opioid epidemic and hopefully PWID (people who inject drugs) issues as well.

Appendices

The appendices yield important citizen resources and documents on syringe exchange programs and the opioid epidemic, including a comprehensive Glossary of Syringe Exchange and Opioid Terms, Abbreviations and Acronyms; CDC's Syringe Exchange Programs (2019): North American Syringe Exchange Network listing; the San Francisco Health Commission resolution Adopting a Harm Reduction Policy for Substance Abuse, STD and HIV; the press release from the San Francisco Mayor's Office on an Innovative Program to Fight Opioid Crisis on San Francisco Streets; and the executive summary of the landmark Secure and Responsible Drug Disposal Act of 2010.

Part I

The Opioid Epidemic

1. Opioid Epidemic Causing Rise in Hepatitis C Infections and Other Serious Illnesses*

THOMAS J. STOPKA

Many Americans now know that, over the past decade, opioid addiction and deaths from opioid overdose in the U.S. have skyrocketed.

But we don't hear as often about the other epidemics intertwined with this public health crisis. In rural Scott County, Indiana, for example, prescription opioid injections have been linked to overlapping outbreaks of HIV and the hepatitis C virus.

This is a "syndemic": multiple diseases feeding off of one another, compounding a community's health burdens.

Syndemic theory—first introduced by medical anthropologist Merrill Singer more than a decade ago—explains how epidemics interact with one another. The interplay of these diseases increases the risk for a number of infections, like sexually transmitted infections and HIV.

There are many interrelated epidemics within the "opioid syndemic." Together, they make up perhaps the biggest public health challenge in the U.S. since the advent of the AIDS epidemic.

What We Need to Know

Before we can tackle this challenge, we need to understand where the opioid syndemic is most intense.

In the U.S., we have many public health surveillance systems that assess changes across geography and time. For example, AIDSVu, an online interactive map, tracks HIV data across U.S. counties. In some regions, the data maps across ZIP Codes and census tracts.

Systems such as these help us compare disease outcomes across different places and demographic groups. However, when it comes to the opioid syndemic, we need to do more to identify local hotspots. Hotspots are places where outbreaks cluster together in a

---

*Originally published as Thomas J. Stopka, "Opioid Epidemic Causing Rise in Hepatitis C Infections and Other Serious Illnesses," *The Conversation*, https://theconversation.com/opioid-epidemic-causing-rise-in-hepatitis-c-infections-and-other-serious-illnesses-82040 (September 25, 2017). Reprinted with permission of the publisher.

statistically significant way, in adjacent neighborhoods or communities with elevated disease rates.

Scientists like myself have started using a range of geospatial and statistical approaches to improve our understanding of the opioid syndemic. These tools allow us to find patterns in data on related health issues. We can also determine which characteristics of an individual, community or social network—such as syringe sharing and unsafe sex—are associated with hotspots.

These analyses can help public health departments and clinicians target local responses where they are most needed, when they are most needed and with the local subpopulations that most need them.

Finding Hotspots

In Massachusetts, where I am based, opioid overdose deaths quintupled over the past 15 years. The state Senate and Governor Charlie Baker have established a new legislative mandate to systematically assess the key factors associated with the opioid syndemic.

There are many health issues associated with opioid use, including HIV, hepatitis C, STIs, soft tissue infections, mental illness and neonatal abstinence syndrome, which is related to exposure to drugs in the womb. For example, hepatitis C infections nationwide have nearly tripled since 2010.

Working alongside local and state public health departments, academic institutions and community-based agencies, we study the distribution of these health issues across Massachusetts and beyond. Our "risk maps" help us better understand the geographic distribution of opioid syndemic illnesses over time.

We measure risks by the burden of disease (e.g., the number of fatal overdoses) and rates (e.g., the number of hepatitis C infections per 100,000 people) across local communities. We also measure and map risk behaviors—such as syringe sharing, unsafe sex and doctor shopping—through surveys with health care professionals and people in the throes of addiction.

We have identified a number of hotspots tied to the opioid syndemic. For example, some hotspots for prescription opioids appear to overlap with drug overdoses.

We've identified cities and towns with significant clusters of hepatitis C and HIV. Springfield, Boston, Fall River, New Bedford and parts of Cape Cod, for instance, have notable overlapping hotspots for opioid overdose deaths, hepatitis C and HIV.

Among youth and young adults, we've also noted an increase in infectious endocarditis, an infection of the heart valve often caused by reuse and sharing of contaminated syringes.

How Hotspot Mapping Can Help

Mapping the opioid syndemic and related hotspots, we can better inform public health policy decisions, as well as clinical decisions for health care workers.

Such analyses can help to pinpoint the locations, communities and specific behaviors that could most benefit from interventions. For example, peer navigators who have "been there and done that" could visit overlapping hotspots and make it easier for high-risk populations to access sterile syringes, condoms, hepatitis C treatment and naloxone, the overdose reversal drug.

Additional programs could focus on educating medical providers, pharmacists and patients in hotspots, to improve opioid prescribing practices and increase disease testing rates.

Released inmates have some of the highest risks for opioid overdose. Corrections facilities could try to improve their transitions back into local hotspot communities, by facilitating direct referrals to drug treatment programs and job training programs.

Of course, it will take continued collaboration and enhanced funding from governments and foundations to see these efforts forward. But there is no better time than the present to address one of our nation's largest health crises.

2. Syringe Services Programs (SSPs) Fact Sheet*

CENTERS FOR DISEASE CONTROL AND PREVENTION

- The opioid crisis is fueling a dramatic increase in infectious diseases associated with injection drug use.
- Reports of acute hepatitis C virus (HCV) cases rose 3.5-fold from 2010 to 2016.[1]
- The majority of new HCV infections are due to injection drug use.
- Over 2,500 new HIV infections occur each year among people who inject drugs (PWID).[2]
- Syringe Services Programs (SSPs) reduce HIV and HCV infections and are an effective component of comprehensive community-based prevention and intervention programs that provide additional services. These include vaccination, testing, linkage to infectious disease care and substance use treatment, and access to and disposal of syringes and injection equipment.

Helps Prevent Transmission of Blood-Borne Infections

For people who inject drugs, the best way to reduce the risk of acquiring and transmitting disease through injection drug use is to stop injecting drugs. For people who do not stop injecting drugs, using sterile injection equipment for each injection can reduce the risk of acquiring and transmitting infections and prevent outbreaks.

SSPs are associated with an estimated 50% reduction in HIV and HCV incidence.[3] When combined with medications that treat opioid dependence (also known as medication-assisted treatment), HCV and HIV transmission is reduced by over two-thirds.[4]

SSPs serve as a bridge to other health services, including HCV and HIV testing and treatment and medication-assisted treatment for opioid use disorder.[5]

Helps Stop Substance Use

The majority of SSPs offer referrals to medication-assisted treatment,[6] and new users of SSPs are five times more likely to enter drug treatment and three times more likely to stop using drugs than those who don't use the programs.

---

*Public document originally published as Centers for Disease Control and Prevention, "Syringe Services Programs (SSPs) Fact Sheet," https://www.cdc.gov/ssp/syringe-services-programs-factsheet.html#stop-substance (May 23, 2019).

SSPs prevent overdose deaths by teaching people who inject drugs how to prevent overdose and how to recognize, respond to, and reverse a drug overdose by providing training on how to use naloxone, a medication used to reverse overdose. Many SSPs provide "overdose prevention kits" containing naloxone to people who inject drugs.[7-12]

Helps Support Public Safety

SSPs have partnered with law enforcement, providing naloxone to local police departments to help them respond and prevent death when someone has overdosed.[13]

SSPs also protect first responders and the public by providing safe needle disposal and reducing the presence of discarded needles in the community.[14-19]

In 2015, CDC's National HIV Behavioral Surveillance System found that the more syringes SSPs distributed per the number of people who inject drugs in a geographic region, the more likely the people who inject drugs in that region were to dispose of used syringes safely.[20]

Studies in Baltimore[21] and New York City[22] have also found no difference in crime rates between areas with and areas without SSPs.

Notes

1. Centers for Disease Control and Prevention. Surveillance for Viral Hepatitis—United States, [PDF—1.5 MB, 75 pages].

2. Centers for Disease Control and Prevention. Estimated HIV incidence and prevalence in the United States, 2010–2015. HIV Surveillance Supplemental Report. 2018; 23(No. 1) [PDF—2 MB, 77 pages]. Published March 2018.

3. Platt, L., Minozzi, S., Reed, J., et al. Needle syringe programs and opioid substitution therapy for preventing hepatitis C transmission in people who inject drugs. *Cochrane Database Syst* Rev. 2017;9:CD012021. doi:10.1002/14651858.CD012021.pub2.

4. Fernandes, R.M., Cary, M., Duarte, G., et al. Effectiveness of needle and syringe programs in people who inject drugs—An overview of systematic reviews. *BMC Public Health*. 2017;17(1):309. doi:10.1186/s12889-017-4210-2.

5. HIV and Injection Drug Use—Vital Signs—CDC. Centers for Disease Control and Prevention. Published December 2016.

6. Des Jarlais, D.C., Nugent, A., Solberg, A., Feelemyer, J., Mermin, J., Holtzman, D. Syringe service programs for persons who inject drugs in urban, suburban, and rural areas—United States, 2013. *MMWR Morb Mortal Wkly Rep*. 2015;64(48):1337–1341. doi:10.15585/ mmwr.mm6448a3.

7. Seal, K.H., Thawley, R., Gee, L. Naloxone distribution and cardiopulmonary resuscitation training for injection drug users to prevent heroin overdose death: A pilot intervention study. *J Urban Health*. 2005;82(2):303–311. doi:10.1093/jurban/jti053.

8. Galea, S., Worthington, N., Piper, T.M., Nandi, V.V., Curtis, M., Rosenthal, D.M. Provision of naloxone to injection drug users as an overdose prevention strategy: Early evidence from a pilot study in New York City. *Addict Behav*. 2006;31(5):907–912. doi:10.1016/j. addbeh.2005.07.020.

9. Tobin, K.E.,, Sherman S.G., Beilenson, P., Welsh, C., Latkin, C.A. Evaluation of the Staying Alive program: Training injection drug users to properly administer naloxone and save lives. *Int J Drug Policy*. 2009;20(2):131–136. doi:10.1016/j.drugpo.2008.03.002.

10. Doe-Simkins, M., Walley, A.Y., Epstein, A., Moyer, P. Saved by the nose: Bystander-administered intranasal naloxone hydrochloride for opioid overdose. *Am J Public Health*. 2009;99(5):788–791. doi:10.2105/ajph.2008.146647.

11. Bennett, A.S., Bell, A., Tomedi, L., Hulsey, E.G., Kral, A.H. Characteristics of an overdose prevention, response, and naloxone distribution program in Pittsburgh and Allegheny County, Pennsylvania. *J Urban Health*. 2011;88(6):1020–1030. doi:10.1007/s11524-011-9600-7.

12. Leece, P.N., Hopkins, S., Marshall, C., Orkin, A., Gassanov, M.A., Shahin, R.M. Development and implementation of an opioid overdose prevention and response program in Toronto, Ontario. *Can J Public Health*. 2013;104(3):e200–204.

13. Childs, R. Law enforcement and naloxone utilization in the United States. FDA website[PDF—1 MB, 24 pages].

14. Tookes, H.E., Kral, A.H., Wenger, L.D., et al. A comparison of syringe disposal practices among injection drug users in a city with versus a city without needle and syringe programs. *Drug Alcohol Depend.* 2012;123(1–3):255–259. doi:10.1016/j.drugalcdep.2011.12.001.

15. Riley, E.D., Kral, A.H., Stopka, T.J., Garfein, R.S., Reuckhaus, P., Bluthenthal, R.N. Access to sterile syringes through San Francisco pharmacies and the association with HIV risk behavior among injection drug users. *J Urban Health.* 2010;87(4):534–542. doi:10.1007/s11524-010-9468-y.

16. Klein, S.J., Candelas, A.R., Cooper, JG, et al. Increasing safe syringe collection sites in New York State. Public Health Rep. 2008;123(4):433–440. doi:10.1177/003335490812300404.

17. de Montigny, L., Vernez, Moudon A,, Leigh, B., Kim, S.Y. Assessing a drop box program: a spatial analysis of discarded needles. *Int J Drug Policy.* 2010; 21(3):208–214. doi:10.1016/j.drugpo.2009.07.003.

18. Doherty, M.C., Junge, B., Rathouz, P., Garfein, R.S., Riley, E., Vlahov, D. The effect of a needle exchange program on numbers of discarded needles: a 2-year follow-up. *Am J Public Health.* 2000;90(6):936–939.

19. Bluthenthal, R.N., Anderson, R., Flynn, N.M., Kral, A.H. Higher syringe coverage is associated with lower odds of HIV risk and does not increase unsafe syringe disposal among syringe exchange program clients. *Drug Alcohol Depend.* 2007;89(2–3):214–222.

20. Centers for Disease Control and Prevention. HIV Infection, Risk, Prevention, and Testing Behaviors among Persons Who Inject Drugs—National HIV Behavioral Surveillance: Injection Drug Use, 20 U.S. Cities, 2015. HIV Surveillance Special Report 18. Revised edition [PDF—2 MB, 38 pages]. Published May 2018. Accessed July 30, 2018.

21. Marx, M.A., Crape, B., Brookmeyer, R.S., et al. Trends in crime and the introduction of a needle exchange program. *Am J Public Health.* 2000;90(12),1933–1936.

22. Galea, S., Ahern, J., Fuller, C., Freudenberg, N., Vlahov, D. Needle exchange programs and experience of violence in an inner city neighborhood. *J Acquir Immune Defic Syndr.* 2001;28(3), 282–288.

3. An Ethical Dilemma for Doctors

When Is It OK to Prescribe Opioids?*

Travis N. Rieder

America's opioid crisis is getting worse. The role of prescription opioids has both the medical establishment and the government justifiably worried.

In response, the National Academies of Science, Engineering and Medicine released an official report. And, on September 21, 2017, the National Academy of Medicine released a special publication calling clinicians to help combat the crisis.

As a bioethicist working on the ethical and policy issues regarding prescription opioids, I am grateful to the National Academy of Medicine for inviting me to serve on this publication's authorship team, and for taking seriously the ethical component of the prescription opioid crisis. The opioid epidemic is shot through with ethical challenges.

There are many discussions we could have, but I will here focus on just one of them: the issue of morally responsible prescribing. Should prescription opioids be used at all? And if so, how? The question is obviously important for clinicians, but the rest of us—patients—should understand what our doctors and nurses owe us regarding our care.

Two Public Health Crises

One of the central challenges of the opioid epidemic is figuring out how to respond without harming pain patients.

If opioids prevent significant suffering from pain, then the solution to the prescription opioid problem cannot simply be to stop using them. To do so would be to trade one crisis (an opioid crisis) for another (a pain crisis).

The data suggest, however, that pain patients' interests will not always run counter to the goal of curbing the opioid crisis. The evidence favoring opioid therapy for chronic, noncancer pain is very weak, and there's some evidence that opioid therapy can actually increase one's sensitivity to pain.

Opioid therapy also comes with significant costs—the risk of addiction and the potential for drowsiness, constipation, nausea and other side effects.

As a result, more of the medical community is realizing that opioids are simply not

---

*Originally published as Travis N. Rieder, "An Ethical Dilemma for Doctors: When Is It OK to Prescribe Opioids?," *The Conversation*, https://theconversation.com/an-ethical-dilemma-for-doctors-when-is-it-ok-to-prescribe-opioids-84114 (September 24, 2017). Reprinted with permission of the publisher.

good medications for chronic, noncancer pain. Getting patients off long-term opioid therapy may well improve their lives.

Should We Use Opioids at All?

It would be nice if we could simply stop using opioids. But the situation is rather more complicated than that.

Even if opioid therapy shouldn't be first-line (or even second-line) treatment for chronic pain, that doesn't mean that it won't work for anyone. Patients are individuals, not data points, and risks of opioid therapy—as well as the risks of not providing pain relief—are not the same for everyone.

This is important because debilitating chronic pain can lead to a life that seems not worth living, and sometimes even to suicide. In the face of life-destroying pain, if we run out of other options, it's not clear that we should avoid using a third-line treatment in the hopes of saving a life.

Those who have been on high doses of opioids for years or decades pose another serious challenge. Many of these patients are concerned about the backlash against opioids. Some believe that the opioids are saving their lives. Others may be terrified of going into withdrawal if their medication is taken away.

If we move away from opioid therapy too abruptly, physicians may abandon these patients or force them to taper before they are ready. Tapering, under the best of circumstances, is a long, uncomfortable process. If it's badly managed, it can be hell. The health care system created these patients, and we don't get to turn our backs on them now.

Finally, opioids are important medications for acute, surgical and post-traumatic pain. Such pain can require long-term treatment when a series of surgeries stretches out for months, or when a traumatic injury requires a long, painful recovery. In these cases, opioids often make life manageable.

Although calls to limit opioid prescriptions generally don't target these patients, we might reasonably worry about shifting attitudes. If medical culture becomes too opioid-phobic, who will prescribe for these patients?

Responsible Prescribing

Fighting the epidemic with nuance will require constant vigilance. In the new National Academy of Medicine publication, we suggest a number of ways that clinicians can work toward responsible prescribing and management of opioids.

In short, clinicians must prescribe opioids only when appropriate, employing nonopioid pain management strategies when indicated. Evidence supports the use of acetaminophen and ibuprofen, as well as physical therapy, exercise, acupuncture, meditation and yoga.

Clinicians must also be willing to manage any prescriptions they do write over the long term. And, at every stage, prescribers should collaborate with others as needed to ensure that patients receive the necessary care.

Although clinicians shouldn't be "anti-opioid," they should be justifiably wary of prescribing for chronic, noncancer pain. And when a prescription is appropriate, the clinician should not write for more than is needed.

Patients should go into opioid therapy with a rich understanding of the risks and benefits. They should also have a plan of care, including an "exit strategy" for getting off the medication.

A Role for Nonclinicians?

The suggestions above may seem straightforward, and perhaps even obvious. So it's important to point out that this work is time-consuming and sometimes—as in the case of high-risk patients—challenging. Counseling, advising and trying to avoid unnecessary opioid use is much more difficult than writing a quick prescription.

Although this difficult work is still the clinician's responsibility, the rest of us can make it easier for them to do their job well. After all, no one likes to experience unnecessary pain. Our expectation of powerful pain relief is part of the cultural backdrop of the epidemic.

That expectation is going to have to change. Moderate acute pain from injury, dental procedures or whatever may have yielded a prescription for Percocet or Vicodin in the past. And when we are the ones in pain, we might still prefer that doctors hand out such medication like candy. But the opioid epidemic is teaching us that we don't, in fact, want that to be clinicians' standard practice. We shouldn't demand exceptions for ourselves.

4. The Opioid Epidemic Is Finally a National Emergency— Eight Years Too Late*

Erin Winstanley

"It has been many long, hard, agonizing battles for the last few years and you fought like a warrior every step of the way. Addiction, however, won the war. To the person who doesn't understand addiction, she is just another statistic who chose to make a bad decision."

Despite working nearly two decades as an addiction scientist, I cannot read Kelsey Grace Endicott's mother's eulogy without crying. The opioid epidemic has turned those who lost their lives to addiction into statistics, while leaving their families in sorrow.

Overdose deaths in the U.S. have tripled since 2000, with 52,404 deaths in 2015 as the highest ever recorded. While the Centers for Disease Control and Prevention (CDC) has yet to release official statistics for 2016, early estimates put the number of deaths at as many as 65,000.

In a speech on October 26, 2017, President Trump declared the opioid epidemic a national emergency. Nearly a decade into this epidemic, this national emergency was declared at least eight years too late. Policymakers have missed opportunities to implement strategies scientifically demonstrated to reduce overdose deaths and help people recover.

His announcement was vague on details and did not specify how much money would be dedicated to reducing overdose deaths. The president restated many initiatives that have already been initiated and focused on supply-reduction efforts that, while important, do little for the millions of Americans who are struggled with opioid addiction. We have proven prevention and treatment services that we need to significantly expand, and states need the money to do this.

The Right Treatments

Declaring the opioid epidemic a national emergency expands the availability of federal funding; frees up public health workers to address the issue; and makes it possible to remove regulatory barriers to lifesaving medications.

---

*Originally published as Erin Winstanley, "The Opioid Epidemic Is Finally a National Emergency—Eight Years Too Late," *The Conversation*, https://theconversation.com/the-opioid-epidemic-is-finally-a-national-emergency-eight-years-too-late-82623 (August 27, 2017). Reprinted with permission of the publisher.

In a speech on May 11, Attorney General Jeff Sessions suggested that tools like "Just Say No" and Drug Abuse Resistance Education (DARE) can help fight the opioid epidemic.

However, addiction science has repeatedly proven that such drug prevention programs are ineffective. Some would argue that we are biologically wired to try new things, so education alone is not sufficient to prevent repeated drug use.

Prevention efforts are part of the solution, but we need more immediate solutions for people already ensnared by addiction. Naloxone, known by the brand name Narcan, is usually the only thing that can prevent death when someone has overdosed on opioids. Science has unequivocally demonstrated that naloxone can reverse an opioid overdose, if administered in time and in an adequate dose.

When patients with opioid use disorders are treated with FDA-approved medications like methadone and buprenorphine, they not only reduce their use of opioids but they are also less likely to overdose. When these drugs are used to treat addiction, they are referred to as medication-assisted treatment. Medication-assisted treatment helps many people, particularly early in recovery, when otherwise their brains seem to focus only on using more drugs. In fact, a National Institute on Drug Abuse study found that only about 7 percent of patients can stop using opioids without buprenorphine.

We need drugs like naloxone and buprenorphine to prevent deaths and help people recover from addiction. In the past few years, state governments have taken significant steps to remove regulatory barriers and expand community access to naloxone.

But policies are infrequently aligned with addiction science. In 2015, only 11 percent of people who needed addiction treatment received it. There are not enough medication-assisted treatment slots available: A recent study estimated that the U.S. was short 1.3 million treatment slots for medication-assisted treatment in 2012. Demand has only increased since then.

There is an entrenched belief that people choose to use drugs and that this choice reflects a moral failing. Even the director of the U.S. Department of Health and Human Resources—which cites medication-assisted treatment as part of its strategy—has been quoted saying: "If we're just substituting one opioid for another, we're not moving the dial much."

Moving Too Slowly

Early on, everyone believed that the epidemic was fueled by widely available prescription pain relievers. Books like *American Pain* by John Temple described "drug tourists" routinely traveling from states like Kentucky and West Virginia to Florida, where millions of prescription pills were dispensed at "pill mills."

Such overprescribing and doctor-shopping did contribute to the current epidemic. States have been successful at dispensing fewer prescription opioids, but this doesn't help the nearly 2.6 million Americans already addicted, or the 329,000 who report currently using heroin.

And, since 2014, it has become clear that the epidemic is no longer just about prescription opioids. In addition, heroin is frequently mixed or substituted with powerful synthetic opioids like fentanyl or carfentanil. They require far more of the overdose reversal drug naloxone than is routinely dispensed in communities.

Meanwhile, in poor and rural areas, community resources for public services are being exhausted by the costs of the epidemic.

Areas that have been disproportionately impacted by the epidemic, like West Virginia, have woefully inadequate access to harm-reduction services like syringe exchange programs and specialty addiction treatment. A clinic at our university that dispenses buprenorphine has more than 600 people on its waiting list. We will soon open a second clinic that will help reduce but not eliminate the waiting list.

A bill signed into law by President Obama, the 21st Century Cures Act, is making approximately $1 billion in funding available to help states combat the opioid epidemic. But, as Dr. Keith Humphreys at Stanford University has said: This is not enough. We likely need 50 times that, as Ohio spent $1 billion in 2016 on the opioid epidemic.

Fighting Back

It can be hard to grasp the devastation of the opioid epidemic. As the President's Commission on Combating Drug Addiction and the Opioid Crisis has described it, in the scale of deaths, it's like the September 11 terrorist attacks happening every three weeks. A national emergency would have been declared 10 years ago if such a disaster occurred every three weeks. And it can be even harder to imagine the emotional turmoil and the depth of sorrow felt by the families who've lost their daughters, sons, brothers, sisters, mothers and fathers.

I think it's fair to say that we all want a simple solution—something that we can wrap our arms around. Something that can be done in one legislative session. But that has not worked and it will not work, just as declaring a national emergency is not enough.

Addiction scientists know what needs to be done to turn the tide. While we may not understand every aspect of the epidemic and certainly need more research to understand these deaths of despair, we are eager to collaborate with communities to find empirically informed solutions, such as medication-assisted treatment. The President's Commission on Combating Drug Addiction and the Opioid Crisis consists of four politicians and one addiction scientist. It might help to start by asking an expert, rather than politicians, what should be done.

5. As the Opioid Epidemic Continues, the Holidays Bring Need to Support Those in Grief*

Emily B. Campbell

For all the warm memories and goodwill shared during the holiday season, for many it is a time of acute grief. The American opioid crisis is rightfully understood as the worst public health crisis in American history, killing over 70,000 people last year alone. Behind the statistics are the private, aching pains for loved ones lost.

As part of my research on grief in the American opioid epidemic, I attended over 30 community events, vigils and support group meetings, and interviewed 23 mothers whose children died of an opioid overdose. These experiences give me insights into how to care for those dealing with the loss of a loved one to addiction or overdose.

Be Quiet And Listen

For many who know someone who has lost a loved one, it can be hard to know what to say or how to respond. Conversely, for those who have lost a love one, the silence can be deafening.

If you want to be supportive, consider your relationship to the person and the deceased and find an opportunity to approach the person one-on-one. Here are some things to keep in mind:

1. Listen and affirm. Let the person know you are willing to lend an ear. If someone takes you up on your offer, stop what you are doing and listen. Put away your cellphone or other distractions and focus on your interaction with that person. Allow them to speak and listen, without jumping to offer advice or talk about yourself. Losing someone you love is painful. Letting people express their feelings without feeling judged or corrected can be very powerful. Simple phrases like "I hear you" offer validation.

2. Give the gift of time. Grief can be a very isolating experience, so spending time with others is important. One mother described being taken out to lunch by

---

*Originally published as Emily B. Campbell, "As the Opioid Epidemic Continues, the Holidays Bring Need to Support Those in Grief," *The Conversation*, https://theconversation.com/as-the-opioid-epidemic-continues-the-holidays-bring-need-to-support-those-in-grief-108592 (December 20, 2018). Reprinted with permission of the publisher.

her late son's friends on the one-year anniversary of his death. Their time together affirmed that her son was loved and missed by others and helped change an unbearable day into something else.

3. Names matter. One of the things that came up time and again from mothers who had lost their children to overdose was missing the sound of their child's name. One mother explained the change from hearing and saying her son's name many times a day to not hearing it spoken at all. For her, the difference between, "I'm sorry for the loss of your son" and "I'm sorry for the loss of Jim" is profound.

4. If you have a fond memory of the person, share it. Many describe the joy of hearing about their loved one from others that knew them. One mother shared a card that a former teacher had written to her after her son's death. They had not interacted for many years, and knowing her son was remembered by this person was deeply comforting.

5. A person is more than their cause of death. The often tragic and dramatic nature of a fatal overdose can sometimes overshadow the person's life. This is also true for alcohol-related deaths and suicide. It's important to remember that each person had a life history, a sense of humor and hope for the future. An entire life is not defined merely by how it ends.

6. If you can't say it, try writing. If you don't know how to approach the person or know what to say, consider writing an email or sending a card. This form of support can open up future conversations and does not put anyone directly on the spot. It can simply say, "Thinking of you this time of year. If you ever want to talk about Jim or just get a coffee, please let me know."

7. Grief is universal but takes many forms. The experience of grief varies widely. There is no time limit on grief, and for many, the grieving process is lifelong. For some, staying busy is curative, while for others, it can be hard to keep going. This is especially true during the holidays.

8. If you are grieving, you are not alone. There are support groups in person and online. Team Sharing is a national online and in-person platform and advocacy group for parents who have lost their children to overdose. Grief Recovery After Substance Passing (G.R.A.S.P.) provides a directory of in-person support meetings as well.

6. Keeping Away from Criminalization*

SARAH SWEENEY

In many cities across America, addiction is a very real issue that is impacting lives every second of every day. It tears families apart and tortures the human spirit, separating a person from themselves and those in their lives who would otherwise support them. Living and working in the Seattle area, this reality has become all too clear, especially as a service provider in the community. Just two weeks ago I was getting off the bus heading into the office and noticed a man firing up his crack pipe … it was 8 in the morning.

Situations such as these, and recognizing the increasing prevalence or visibility of drug use in public, are at the heart of this social issue. Drug addiction and homelessness bring to mind the question, "Which came first, the chicken or the egg?" Are drug addicts homeless, or are the homeless drug addicts? This question is too simple for such a complex collection of issues, and merely scratches the surface of such a large iceberg below the surface of vulnerability in our streets. It is very true that not all people who use or are addicted to drugs are homeless, nor are all those who are homeless using or addicted to drugs. These are simple stereotypes and stigmas created by those who do not understand the root causes of either issue.

In Seattle particularly, there have been efforts made to connect people to services and decrease the frequency of criminal convictions stemming from actions performed while intoxicated, for those addicted to illicit drugs. One such effort, the Law Enforcement Assisted Diversion (LEAD) program, has been shown to reduce the recidivism of low-level criminal offenders and instead offer a treatment based alternative. This program was additionally designed to decriminalize public drug use and prostitution, offering alternatives to those who would otherwise spend time behind bars and have on their record criminal charges that would affect their ability to obtain employment, housing and potentially other social service benefits available to them.

According a *Seattle Times* article, efforts at addressing these issues must focus on preventive measures that tackle drug addiction at the root causes. We must fund primary education and open doors to job training in order to sustain progress in low-barrier access to community resources that combat drug addiction. We must also minimize access to street thugs who provide these damaging drugs to vulnerable people on the streets.

---

*Originally published as Sarah Sweeney, "Keeping Away from Criminalization," *PA Times*, https://patimes.org/keeping-away-from-criminalization/ (September 25, 2019). Reprinted with permission of the publisher and author.

So How Did We Get Here?

Often times, those engaged in drug addiction are victims of trauma, have been exposed to substances as an infant, have lost job opportunities or have experienced the loss of housing or the breaking up of families at the hands of various social issues. Homelessness can also be tied to similar root causes, and many times not at the fault of the victim. Homelessness could be a side effect of unintended consequences of the market, disability, injury or fluctuations of life's events such as divorce and children aging out of foster care.

A big issue that has become fairly prevalent in regard to addiction is the over prescription of opioids by doctors. This has led to increased addiction rates and has acted as a gateway drug for harder substances such as heroin and cocaine to address chronic pain issues as detailed in this CDC report. Medical providers who are drawn in by financial rewards or kickbacks might look the other way when writing prescriptions for clients in search of narcotic drugs to feed their addiction. Many times, in the cases of patients who undergo serious medical interventions (such as surgeries) or older patients experiencing chronic pain, doctors willingly prescribe pain medications to treat the presenting problem. If not monitored closely, patients may become addicted and therefor turn to these harder drugs to meet the needs of their addiction, especially if their providers attempt to titrate their prescriptions.

Where Do We Go from Here?

To get ahead of the drug addiction trend in any of our communities, we must address the issue head on. Prioritizing funding for intervention programs, early childhood education and funding job training or employment opportunities, as well as decriminalizing drug related offenses is the key to a more successful future in our communities. There are so many vulnerable children and adults who are engaged in substance use and abuse systems, and without appropriate interventions we will never solve the problem. Without closer monitoring of narcotic prescription writing and titrating pain medication programs, we won't ever address the issue of chronic pain management. Clients are at risk of being left in the lurch of addiction and pain issues. We must act fast to ensure a successful future for those who are at greatest risk.

7. Stepping Up, Then Stepping Back*

BRENDA BOND-FORTIER

Most communities are struggling to get a handle on the recent opioid crisis. In some states, this crisis results in thousands of deaths each year. This is not a crisis of cities, nor it is a crisis within a specific economic or ethnic population. The opioid crisis is present in almost every community and has challenged public safety and public health professionals in new ways. There is no question that today's opioid crisis is a "wicked problem."

In previous decades, law enforcement would work with other law enforcement agencies to implement as much "law enforcement" as possible. These law enforcement tactics of the 1980s and 1990s will not work in addressing today's opioid crisis (they didn't really work then either). Militaristic, heavy-handed strategies which emphasize "lock 'em up" approaches are outdated and ineffective. As many suggest, the war on drugs turned out to be a flawed policy. Fortunately, sentiments by modern law enforcement leaders reflect this and open the conversation to non-traditional, comprehensive and holistic ways of getting at this problem. Fast forward several decades and we find the crisis to be as difficult as previous crises, but professionals in law enforcement are approaching crisis response and prevention in very different ways.

Some of the shifts in thinking have grown out of complete frustration as officers on the street are seeing the same individuals struggling with drug addiction. The criminal justice system has not been equipped to serve these individuals in sustainable ways, due in part to the limited treatment options. Drug Courts have been launched and there are indications that they are having a positive impact on addiction and crime. However, like treatment, there is a great need for more, and evidence-based practices are still underfunded and out of reach for many families and communities.

Despite these financial challenges, there are innovative approaches underway across many communities in their attempts to respond to the opioid crisis and prevent further abuse. Integration of research into practice is more of a mainstay in state and federal grants, and public service institutions are more aware of the need to adopt evidence-based practices.

Take for example one approach, adopted by the city of Lowell, Massachusetts. Funded by the U.S. Bureau of Justice Assistance Strategies for Policing Innovation, the program is designed as a collaborative community approach to reducing overdose deaths. The program was launched by the police department and fire departments, sparked by

---

*Originally published as Brenda Bond, "Stepping Up, Then Stepping Back," *PA Times*, https://patimes.org/stepping-up-then-stepping-back-the-dynamic-role-of-law-enforcement-in-tackling-the-opioid-crisis/ (June 4, 2018). Reprinted with permission of the publisher and author.

the interests of an officer and firefighter. The approach centers on an outreach strategy, reaching addicted individuals out in the community. An outreach team, consisting of a police officer, firefighter and treatment provider, conduct outreach visits with individuals who have experienced an overdose, quickly working to get the individual into treatment. Their outreach takes them to homes, shelters and homeless encampments.

The strategy was originally situated in the police department, with other agencies, including the City's Health Department, serving as partners. Under the leadership of the police department, federal grants funds were secured, and services strengthened. As the program evolved, mental health, ambulatory, and hospital services were brought into the fold. A memorandum of understanding was created to describe and delineate roles and responsibilities, and a formal evaluation was launched. As more individuals were being served, and as the program has evolved, the management of the program has been moved to the City Health Department. This allows the police to move away from management, to support. However, the police remain critical to the outreach efforts. In addition, each organizational representative is charged with increasing awareness of the program within their own agencies. This, along with the memorandum of understanding, facilitate an institutionalized and sustainable approach, so that this is not a "program" but rather a way of addressing their wicked community problem.

There are several key take-aways from this example, as it is applied to the current opioid crisis. First, as with many public safety challenges, the police often end up serving as the go-to agency in responding to emerging or evolving crises. This is natural as they are trained and equipped as first responders. They are first on the scene and must be prepared in emergency response, but then as conduits for service. However, the police can serve as facilitators, leading communities in the right direction. In this example, the police helped launch the approach, secure funding, but then appropriately shifted their role given the nature of the challenge. The shift does not take away their important engagement in the issue, but reinforces a comprehensive, collaborative approach. In turn, individuals and agencies build their capacity to collective address the current crisis—opioid addiction and related deaths. Importantly, this dynamic engagement also facilitates and supports future collaboration around unknown, but assured challenges ahead.

8. Needle Exchanges Find New Champions Among Republicans*

Victoria Knight

Once repellent to conservative politicians, needle exchanges are now being endorsed and legalized in Republican-controlled states.

At least four legislatures have considered bills to allow hypodermic needle exchanges, and two states, Georgia and Idaho, made them legal in 2019. In each of these states, the House and Senate are controlled by Republicans and the governor is a Republican.

Florida, Missouri, Iowa and Arizona have introduced bills this legislative session that would allow needle exchanges in their state. The measures were all sponsored or co-sponsored by Republicans.

As much as this has been a series of victories for public health officials who see how needle exchanges—also called syringe exchanges—stymie the spread of blood-transmitted diseases, it has been a triumph of public health policy research. For years, research has shown the benefit of needle exchanges, but now that the opioid epidemic and infectious diseases have affected their own communities, lawmakers are listening.

"The reality is maybe 10 or 15 years ago this wasn't where Georgia was," said Republican state Rep. Houston Gaines, the sponsor for Georgia's needle-exchange law. "But the medical and science community has shown that this works. My hope is as Republicans, we can always be willing to embrace programs and ideas if they're proven to work."

Republicans have not always held this mindset.

Needle-exchange programs, pioneered in Amsterdam in 1983, allow individuals to get sterile needles free of charge and safely dispose of dirty needles and syringes used for drug injection. The programs have been proved to reduce the risk of getting and transmitting HIV, viral hepatitis and other bloodborne infections through sharing needles.

Syringe exchange programs also give public health officials an opportunity to offer educational and medical services, such as referrals to substance use disorder programs and HIV or hepatitis testing.

Currently, 28 states and the District of Columbia allow needle exchanges.

---

*Originally published as Victoria Knight, "Needle Exchanges Find New Champions Among Republicans," *Kaiser Health News*, https://khn.org/news/needle-exchanges-find-new-champions-among-republicans/ (May 9, 2019). Reprinted with permission of the publisher. Kaiser Health News is a nonprofit news service covering health issues. It is an editorially independent program of the Kaiser Family Foundation that is not affiliated with Kaiser Permanente.

In 1988, Tacoma, Wash., established the nation's first exchange program and with it came Republican opposition. North Carolina Republican Sen. Jesse Helms led Congress in banning the use of federal funds for needle-exchange programs that year. An ultraconservative, Helms said allowing needle exchanges was the same as the government saying, "It's not only all right to use drugs, but we'll give you the needles."

Despite the federal government refusing to fund research on the exchange programs, public health evidence of their effectiveness started to stack up, as did the number of states allowing the programs.

Multiple studies found that exchanges reduced the spread of hepatitis B, hepatitis C and HIV. These programs could also be cost-effective; a 2014 study found that for every dollar invested in expanding a needle exchange, $6 could be saved in HIV treatment. Other research found that going to an exchange program led drug users to enroll in substance abuse treatment programs.

The tipping point for many Republicans, however, came in a 2015 HIV outbreak related to the injection-drug epidemic in Scott County, Ind., a strong GOP state. In a matter of months, more than 150 people were newly diagnosed with HIV in a rural county with 24,000 residents.

Mike Pence, then the governor and now the vice president, was initially opposed to needle-exchange programs. Two months after the HIV outbreak was detected, Pence declared a public health emergency and allowed a limited needle exchange in Scott County. (Pence's White House staff did not respond to several requests for comment.)

Asal Sayas, director of government affairs at amfAR, the Foundation for AIDS Research, said this was a critical moment for Republicans with rural constituents. "A lot of communities realized they were also vulnerable and had situations similar to Scott County, where there was minimal HIV care and no syringe exchange," said Sayas.

The syringe exchange in Scott County was effective, and it had a ripple effect.

An analysis by amfAR found that after Scott County's needle-exchange program, the number of exchange programs across the country spiked. The organization's most recent count is at 320.

Other Republican-leaning states also passed legislation allowing needle exchanges—Kentucky and Ohio in 2015, North Carolina in 2016 and Louisiana, North Dakota, Tennessee and Virginia in 2017.

Though critics said Pence waited too long to implement the program, the move has been hailed by conservative state lawmakers who in the ensuing years began supporting needle-exchange programs.

Attitudes among Republicans on the federal level are also shifting.

In December 2015, three congressional Republicans from states hit hard by the opioid crisis, Sen. Shelley Moore Capito of West Virginia and Senate Majority Leader Mitch McConnell and Rep. Hal Rogers, both of Kentucky, inserted language into an omnibus spending bill that partially repealed the federal funding ban. That provision allows federal dollars to be used for operating needle-exchange program operations, just not for the drug-injection devices themselves.

Following President Donald Trump's announcement that he wants to end the HIV epidemic, Secretary of Health and Human Services Alex Azar expressed his support for needle exchanges. "Syringe-services programs aren't necessarily the first thing that comes to mind when you think about a Republican health secretary, but we're in a battle between sickness and health, between life and death," Azar said at the National HIV

Prevention Conference in Washington in March. "The public health evidence for targeted interventions here is strong."

AmfAR's Sayas said it's important to remember how effective needle exchanges could be in achieving Trump's HIV goals. "The administration's plan targets 48 counties with high HIV diagnoses and seven states with a high rural burden of HIV," said Sayas. "In six of those seven rural states, needle exchanges are illegal. If we're serious about wanting this plan to work, we need to consider that."

Despite the movement among some Republicans to accept needle exchanges, 13 states still have laws that make them illegal. All of those have Republican governors and Republican-majority legislatures, except for Kansas, which has a Democratic governor.

Nine states have either no law that prohibits syringe programs or only locally permitted needle exchanges, which means that it is up to each city or county to decide whether to operate needle exchanges.

In states that have given localities control of needle-exchange programs, there has been some movement to shut down the programs. Charleston, W.Va., suspended its needle exchange in 2018 after law enforcement officers complained about needles littering the streets and the mayor joined the opposition. Two programs in Indiana shut down in 2017 because of local opposition, although one has since reopened through a nonprofit health center.

Republican Rep. Ed Clere was one of the authors of Indiana's needle-exchange legislation. He said local control of the needle exchanges often means decisions now play out among local conservative lawmakers.

"I don't want you to think that I don't like local approval. It's just the way the approval process works, it just tends to be very political," Clere said in an interview. "The people who make the decision, the commissioners, don't have medical or research background. Instead of talking about the research evidence, the discussion ends up being about needles on playgrounds or drug use, which is just not useful."

Part II

Syringe Use and Infection Risks

• *A. HIV* •

9. Syringe-Exchange Programs Are Part of Effective HIV Prevention*

NATIONAL INSTITUTE ON DRUG ABUSE

December 1 is World AIDS Day. There is much to celebrate in the scientific battle to understand and fight HIV. Antiretroviral therapy has made HIV a treatable and livable condition. Clinical trials are currently testing antibodies to the virus that may soon produce a vaccine. But even with increasing biomedical knowledge of the virus itself and how to counteract or clear it from the body, the first line of defense is prevention.

Decades of public health awareness about the dangers of unprotected sex have had an impact on reducing the spread of HIV, which is still mainly transmitted sexually; but in 2010, eight percent of new cases were a result of injection drug use. One of the best available strategies for reducing the spread of HIV among drug users is syringe-exchange programs (also called syringe service programs); their effectiveness has been proven through abundant research. When syringe exchange was finally implemented in southern Indiana last year, for instance, it was a major factor in bringing the HIV outbreak in Scott County under control. But while the science of how to prevent HIV transmission is solid, misconceptions about these programs have prevented wider implementation and limited their public health impact.

Critics charge that harm-reduction strategies like syringe exchange programs will increase drug use, but study after study, both in the U.S. and other countries, has shown that this is not the case. Such programs are also sometimes opposed philosophically, being viewed as a public endorsement of drug use. This view arises from a moral framing of addiction as opposed to a medical framing. When injecting heroin or prescription opioids is seen as a lapse of morals and willpower, any concession to this practice by dispensing clean syringes is seen as condoning an immoral and illegal behavior.

But few people inject opioids—including prescription pain relievers and heroin—unless they have an addiction, and the science is clear that addiction is a medical, not a moral issue. Because of severely compromised brain circuitry, the ability of a person with an addiction to exert control over their drug use is greatly diminished. Without

---

*Public document originally published as National Institute on Drug Abuse, "Syringe-Exchange Programs Are Part of Effective HIV Prevention," https://www.drugabuse.gov/publications/drugfacts/drug-use-viral-infections-hiv-hepatitis (July 2019).

treatment, the individual is usually unable to stop on their own; thus until they get help, they are at risk for a range of adverse and even life-threatening outcomes. Syringe exchange, as part of a comprehensive prevention program, minimizes the risks injection drug users will contract HIV or hepatitis C (HCV) infection or spread them to other people in the community.

Syringe exchange programs connect the population of injection drug users with healthcare, providing HIV screening and treatment and counseling, and, importantly they provide an opportunity for reaching out to people with addictions and encouraging them to engage in substance use disorder treatment. When an individual's substance use can be addressed, their risk of contracting HIV and other infectious diseases like HCV, or transmitting them to others in the community, is also lessened—the principle known as "treatment as prevention." Failure to implement programs that will reduce these risks is irresponsible from a public health perspective.

Thus the benefits from syringe exchange programs are multi-faceted, reducing the transmission of HIV, HCV, and other infectious diseases as well as increasing access to treatment for drug addiction. However, it requires a realistic mindset in our society's approach to drug use and addiction. Syringe exchange, by itself, may not reduce drug use. But denying injection drug users clean injection equipment does nothing to lessen or discourage their drug use—it only makes another public health crisis, such as another HIV outbreak and the undeterred expansion of HCV, more likely. Such crises do not only affect the individuals who contract the disease. According to the Centers for Disease Control and Prevention, lifetime treatment cost of a single case of HIV infection is $379,668; the costs of treating the patients who contracted HIV and HCV in Scott County over the next decades are expected to approach $90 million.

Unfortunately, recent research has shown that rural areas are very poorly served by syringe service programs compared to urban settings, even though about half of injection drug users are rural. A CDC report showed that the demographic shift among people who inject drugs toward more white and rural populations, who are more likely to engage in needle sharing in part because of limited access to syringe service programs, threatens to undo the recent gains made in reducing the number of new HIV diagnoses.

As we consider how far we've come in addressing HIV/AIDS, we should ensure that scientific evidence is guiding our efforts to achieving the first HIV-free generation. We must make sure that public health officials across the country know how effective harm-reduction strategies such as syringe service programs are and address lingering misconceptions that have hindered implementing them. As highlighted in the recent Surgeon General's report, Facing Addiction in America, how we respond to this crisis is a moral test for our country. We must be guided by the best available science to develop realistic solutions to reduce drug use, addiction, and associated health risks like HIV.

What's the Relationship Between Drug Use and Viral Infections?

People who engage in drug use or high-risk behaviors associated with drug use put themselves at risk for contracting or transmitting viral infections such as human immunodeficiency virus (HIV), acquired immune deficiency syndrome (AIDS), or hepatitis. This is because viruses spread through blood or other body fluids. It happens primarily in two ways: (1) when people inject drugs and share needles or other drug equipment and (2) when drugs impair judgment and people have unprotected sex with an infected partner. This can happen with both men and women.

Drug use and addiction have been inseparably linked with HIV/AIDS since AIDS was first identified as a disease. According to the CDC, one in 10 HIV diagnoses occur among people who inject drugs.[1] In 2016, injection drug use (IDU) contributed to nearly 20 percent of recorded HIV cases among men—more than 150,000 patients. Among females, 21 percent (about 50,000) of HIV cases were attributed to IDU.[2] Additionally, women who become infected with a virus can pass it to their baby during pregnancy, regardless of their drug use. They can also pass HIV to the baby through breastmilk.

What Is HIV/AIDS?

HIV stands for human immunodeficiency virus. This virus infects the body's immune cells, called CD4 cells (T cells), which are needed to fight infections. HIV lowers the number of these T cells in the immune system, making it harder for the body to fight off infections and disease. Acquired immune deficiency syndrome (AIDS), is the final stage of an HIV infection when the body is unable to fend off disease. A person with a healthy immune system has a T cell count between 500 and 1,600.

Being infected with HIV does not automatically mean that it will progress to AIDS. A patient is diagnosed with AIDS when identified with one or more infections and a T cell count of less than 200.

More than 1.1 million people in the United States live with an HIV infection, with an estimated 162,500 who are unaware of their condition.[3] While there are medicines that help prevent the transmission and spread of HIV and its progression to AIDS, there is no vaccine yet developed for the virus, and there is no cure.

What Is Hepatitis?

Hepatitis is an inflammation of the liver and can cause painful swelling and irritation, most often caused by a family of viruses: A, B, C, D, and E. Each has its own way of spreading to other people and needs its own treatment. Hepatitis B virus (HBV) and hepatitis C virus (HCV) can spread through sharing needles and other drug equipment. Infections can also be transmitted through risky sexual behaviors linked to drug use, though this is not common with HCV.

Hepatitis can lead to cirrhosis—scarring of the liver—resulting in loss of liver function. It can also lead to liver cancer. In fact, HBV and HCV infections are the major risk factors for liver cancer in the United State.[4]

There is a vaccine to prevent HBV infection and medicines to treat it. There are also medicines to treat HCV infection, but no vaccine. Some people recover from infection without treatment. Other people need to take medicine for the rest of their lives and be monitored for liver failure and cancer.

How Does Drug Use Affect Symptoms and Outcomes of a Viral Infection?

Drug use can worsen the progression of HIV and its symptoms, especially in the brain. Studies show that drugs can make it easier for HIV to enter the brain and cause greater nerve cell injury and problems with thinking, learning, and memory. Drug and alcohol use can also directly damage the liver, increasing risk for chronic liver disease and cancer among those infected with HBV or HCV.

How Can People Lessen the Spread of Viral Infections?

People can reduce the risk of getting or passing on a viral infection by:

- **Not using drugs.** This decreases the chance of engaging in unsafe behavior, such as sharing drug-use equipment and having unprotected sex, which can lead to these infections.
- **Never sharing drug equipment.** However, if you inject drugs, never share needles or injection equipment. Many communities have syringe services programs (SSPs) where you can get free sterile needles and syringes and safely dispose of used ones. They can also refer you to substance use disorder treatment services and help you get tested for HIV and hepatitis. Contact your local health department or North American Syringe Exchange Network (NASEN) to find an SSP. Also, some pharmacies may sell needles without a prescription.
- **Getting tested and treated for viral infection.** People who inject drugs should get tested for HIV, HBV, and HCV. Those who are infected may look and feel fine for years and may not even be aware of the infection. So, testing is needed to help prevent the spread of disease—whether or not you are among those most at risk or part of the general population. Get treatment if needed. Read more about HIV testing at the HIV.gov webpage, HIV Test Types.
- **Practicing safe sex every time.** People can reduce their chances of transmitting or getting HIV, HBV, and HCV by using a condom every time they have sex. This is true for those who use drugs and those in the general population.
- **Pre-exposure prophylaxis (PrEP) for HIV.** PrEP is when people who are at significant risk for contracting HIV take a daily dose of HIV medications to prevent them from getting the infection. Research has shown that PrEP has been effective in reducing the risk of HIV infection in people who inject drugs.
- **Post-exposure prophylaxis (PEP) for HIV.** PEP is when people take antiretroviral medicines to prevent becoming infected after being potentially exposed to HIV. According to the CDC, PEP should be used within 72 hours after a recent possible exposure and only be used in emergency situations. If you think you've recently been exposed to HIV during sex, through sharing needles, or sexual assault, talk to your health care provider or an emergency room doctor about PEP right away.
- **Getting vaccinated for HBV.** If you live in the same household, have sexual contact with or share needles with a person with HBV, then you should be vaccinated to prevent transmission. Read more about the vaccine on the CDC's webpage, Hepatitis B In-short.

- **Getting treatment for substance use disorder.** Talk with a counselor, doctor, or other health care provider about substance use disorder treatment, including medications if you have opioid use disorder. To find a treatment center near you, check out the locator tools on Substance Abuse and Mental Health Services Administration (SAMHSA) or www.hiv.gov, or call 1-800-662-HELP (4357).

Notes

1. Centers for Disease Control and Prevention (CDC). *HIV and Injection Drug Use.* 2017. https://www.cdc.gov/hiv/risk/idu.html.
2. Centers for Disease Control and Prevention (CDC). *HIV Surveillance Report: Diagnoses of HIV Infection in the United States and Dependent Areas.* 2017. https://www.cdc.gov/hiv/pdf/library/reports/surveillance/cdc-hiv-surveillance-report-2017-vol-29.pdf.
3. Centers for Disease Control and Prevention (CDC). *HIV in the United States: At a Glance.* 2017. https://www.cdc.gov/hiv/statistics/overview/ataglance.html.
4. Ly, K.N., Xing, J., Klevens, R.M., Jiles, R.B., Ward, J.W., Holmberg, S.D. The increasing burden of mortality from viral hepatitis in the United States between 1999 and 2007. *Ann Intern Med.* 2012;156(4):271–278. doi:10.7326/0003-4819-156-4-201202210-00004.

10. Needle Exchanges Can Now Get Federal Funding*

Anna Gorman

LOS ANGELES—At precisely 8:30 a.m. on a Tuesday morning, the doors to the needle exchange on Skid Row open and the daily procession of injection drug users begins.

Michael Poor, 47, is one of the first customers. He has used his last clean syringe. Poor, who is homeless and addicted to methamphetamines, says coming to the downtown exchange puts his mind at ease: clean needles lower his risk for HIV.

"It is a very needed service, not just in downtown but anywhere drugs are an issue," says Poor, a lanky, friendly man who is missing all of his teeth. "Thanks to needle exchange … I have stayed pretty healthy, which is a hard thing to do when you are injecting drugs."

Needle exchanges like the one Poor visits could receive a financial boost following a decision by Congress to lift a ban on federal funding. As abuse of prescription drugs and opiates continues to spread across the nation, more states are considering exchanges as a way to save lives.

Indiana, for instance, opened its first exchange after an HIV outbreak last year.

The change in federal policy, part of a spending bill approved in February 2016, allows funding only in areas where drug-related cases of hepatitis and HIV are rising or are likely to. State and city health departments will make that determination along with the federal Centers for Disease Control and Prevention, according to the legislation.

The money can be used to pay for staff and programs, but not for syringes.

"It is really an important and historic moment for us at syringe exchanges," said Mark Casanova, executive director of Homeless Health Care Los Angeles, which runs the syringe exchange on Skid Row, known as the Center for Harm Reduction. "But it doesn't go far enough."

Casanova said about a third of his $350,000 budget for the exchange program is spent on the 1.2 million syringes he hands out each year, and he will have to continue relying heavily on private donations to pay for them.

Despite the restrictions, lifting the ban underscores a growing recognition that needle exchange programs can help reduce the spread of infectious diseases, said Daniel Raymond, policy director for Harm Reduction Coalition.

---

*Originally published as Anna Gorman, "Needle Exchanges Can Now Get Federal Funding," *Kaiser Health News*, https://khn.org/news/needle-exchanges-can-now-get-federal-funding/ (February 17, 2016). Reprinted with permission of the publisher. Kaiser Health News is a nonprofit news service covering health issues. It is an editorially independent program of the Kaiser Family Foundation that is not affiliated with Kaiser Permanente. Blue Shield of California Foundation helps fund KHN coverage in California.

"This is a huge victory," said Raymond, whose national organization advocates and provides training for exchange programs. "It is in some way the last chapter of an era where syringe exchange was considered too volatile and too partisan [for policy makers] to come to a consensus."

Critics of needle programs counter that opening the door to federal funding could leave less money for treatment of people who want to get sober. The new law does not allot additional funds for the exchanges, but rather allows them to compete for existing drug program money.

"The dollars are precious these days," said Calvina Fay, executive director of Drug Free America Foundation, a drug policy and prevention organization. "When we have people wanting to get clean and standing in line waiting for a treatment bed ... the money could certainly be better spent."

Needle exchanges began at the height of the AIDS epidemic and today number roughly 200 around the United States, including about 40 in California.

Using clean syringes continues to be the safest way to prevent transmission among injection drug users, according to a 2012 CDC report, which said the percentage of injection drug users infected with HIV dropped by half from the mid–1990s to 2009.

"Syringe programs have really been concentrated in large cities and have done an excellent job of preventing HIV infection where they have been implemented, but we now really need to move to address the new injectors that we see in small towns and in rural areas, particularly in Appalachia," said Don Des Jarlais of the Icahn School of Medicine at Mount Sinai, who has spent 25 years studying the exchanges.

Des Jarlais said federal funding should enable existing centers to expand and new ones to open. "With the exception of a few states, there really has not been adequate funding of needle exchange programs in the U.S.," he said.

Libby Harrison, who manages the Cincinnati Exchange Project in Ohio, said it was "about damn time" for the change in federal policy.

"We've had the science on syringe exchange for almost 30 years. People and their politics getting in the way of science drives me crazy," said Harrison, whose exchange has two staff members and is open three days a week in a region that has been hit hard by drug abuse.

Inside the lobby of the Harm Reduction Center in Los Angeles, customers wait in a line marked with red tape on the floor. A poster on the wall reads in big letters, "Needle exchange saves lives."

At the front of the room, plastic bins are filled with syringes, sterile water ampoules, rubber bands, antibacterial ointment and alcohol swabs. An oversized, locked red bin sits nearby, and clients deposit dirty needles into it.

They don't need appointments, insurance or even identification. They simply answer a few questions, including whether they are homeless. When 26-year-old Eli Guerra walks up to the front counter, he tells the clerk he is out of needles. The clerk asks him what he uses now.

"Whatever I get my hands on," he replies.

Guerra, who uses heroin, has been coming to the needle exchange for about a year but says he hopes this will be one of his last visits.

"This ain't me, really," he says. "I am really trying to stop."

Chloe Blalock, program coordinator of the center, said she hopes federal funding will enable her to hire more people and expand services such as therapy, medical care, overdose prevention training and medication-assisted treatment. For now, she can afford to stay open only seven hours on weekdays and six on weekends.

"We should be open 24 hours," she said. "From a public health standpoint, you want to make sure people have what they need—or more than what they need—no matter what."

On a recent Tuesday, Dr. Rolando Tringale was at the center, teaching medical students about the health effects of drug use.

Tringale, who treats abscesses and wounds, explained why staffers hand out alcohol swabs. "This is an important part of harm reduction education, preventing skin-based infections," he said.

Diamond Mendoza, a self-described homeless man who is addicted to heroin, said that since coming to the exchange he has learned a lot about injecting drugs more safely. He wipes his skin with alcohol before puncturing it. He goes to see the doctor whenever he gets a wound or an abscess. And he always uses clean needles, he said.

"I don't have HIV because I am really careful," said Mendoza, who exchanged 40 needles on a recent morning.

Michael Poor said he has been using drugs since getting hooked on Vicodin, when he was a registered nurse. At first, Poor said, he couldn't get clean syringes and often reused and shared them.

"You had to use one that had been used 15 or 20 times," he said.

He said he believes that's how he became infected with hepatitis C.

Poor said he has been coming to the center for about five years and stocks up so he can give clean needles to others. Staff members know him by name.

During his recent visit, he dumped about 35 used syringes into the red bin.

Minutes later, he was back out on the street, holding a small brown lunch bag filled with supplies.

11. Trump Pledges to End HIV Transmission by 2030

*Doable, But Daunting**

CARMEN HEREDIA RODRIGUEZ

Noting that science has "brought a once-distant dream within reach," President Donald Trump pledged to eliminate HIV transmission within 10 years.

"We have made incredible strides, incredible," Trump said in the 2019 State of the Union address. "Together, we will defeat AIDS in America and beyond."

It's a goal long sought by public health advocates. But even given the vital gains made in drug therapies and understanding of the disease over nearly 40 years, it is not an easy undertaking.

"The reason we have an AIDS epidemic is not just for a lack of the medication," said Dr. Kenneth Mayer, medical research director at the Boston LGBT health center Fenway Institute. "There are a lot of social, structural, individual behavioral factors that may impact why people become infected, may impact if people who are infected engage in care and may impact or affect people who are at high risk of HIV."

Health and Human Services Secretary Alex Azar, who provided details of the initiative after Trump's announcement, said the administration will target viral hot spots by providing local groups more resources, using data to track the spread of the disease and creating local task forces to bolster prevention and treatment.

Neither Azar nor other federal officials who briefed reporters offered cost estimates for the program.

Azar said the plan seeks to reduce new infections by 75 percent in the next five years and 90 percent in the next decade.

"That goal is predicated on growing use of current medications that suppress the virus to such low levels that it is not transmitted during sexual intercourse. PrEP, a drug combination available to individuals with a negative HIV status but may become infected, can reduce their risk of getting the virus by 97 percent," Azar said.

"This is not the HIV epidemic of the 1990s," said Terrance Moore, acting executive

---

*Originally published as Carmen Heredia Rodriguez, "Trump Pledges to End HIV Transmission by 2030. Doable, but Daunting," *Kaiser Health News*, https://khn.org/news/trump-pledges-to-end-hiv-transmission-by-2030-doable-but-daunting/ (February 6, 2019). Reprinted with permission of the publisher. Kaiser Health News is a nonprofit news service covering health issues. It is an editorially independent program of the Kaiser Family Foundation that is not affiliated with Kaiser Permanente.

director of NASTAD, a nonprofit organization that represents officials who administer HIV and hepatitis programs. "We have the tools to end this epidemic."

Gay and bisexual men made up two-thirds of the nearly 40,000 new HIV cases in 2017, but one clear signal of that difference in the epidemic today is the geography. The nation's HIV hotbeds are no longer located just in coastal metropolitan areas. In 2017, more than half of the new cases were diagnosed in Southern states.

HHS said it will focus its efforts on the heart of the epidemic: 48 counties across 19 states; the District of Columbia; San Juan, Puerto Rico; and rural areas in seven states, many of which are in the South.

The new federal initiative would expand PrEP access in community health clinics for low-income patients and quickly refer any new clinic patients with HIV to specialized care.

Medications alone are not the answer. Lawmakers must have the political will to move forward with policies based in science, said Moore. Existing programs do not provide enough infrastructure to achieve this goal, he added.

"You can't be simultaneously attacking and undermining the needs of these communities, while claiming that you want to support them and end the AIDS epidemic," said Scott Schoettes, HIV project director for the LGBT advocacy group Lambda Legal.

The Trump administration has pursued policies that may hinder the president's goal. And efforts in the South face additional challenges, like higher levels of poverty, difficulty providing health care in rural areas and historical racial tension.

"I don't think that these things are things that we cannot overcome," said Greg Millett, vice president and director of public policy at the HIV research foundation amfAR. "But I also think that we need to be very clear about what the obstacles are and to start thinking now innovatively about how we're going to be able to obviate them."

Here are some of the challenges that experts said the president's plan could face:

Health Insurance

Insurance coverage plays a crucial role in keeping HIV patients healthy.

Comprehensive insurance helps patients access the expensive medications needed to keep the virus under control and vital tests to check on virus levels and white blood cell counts—key health indicators. HIV patients are also often susceptible to infections because the virus compromises the immune system. And they tend to have higher rates of mental health conditions, which could affect their ability to adhere to HIV medication if left untreated.

The Affordable Care Act opened up coverage for thousands of HIV patients with its guarantee of insurance for people with preexisting conditions, but many Republican officials are still calling for the law's repeal.

In addition, the ACA's Medicaid expansion led to a substantial jump in the number of people with AIDS who got that coverage, according to the Kaiser Family Foundation. But many states, especially in the South, have not expanded Medicaid. (Kaiser Health News is an editorially independent program of the foundation.)

A federal judge in Texas in December ruled the ACA unconstitutional in a lawsuit waged by a faction of conservative states and supported by the president.

"If you're not going to provide it through the Affordable Care Act," Schoettes said, "then there needs to be something that's as comprehensive in terms of getting people care."

Housing

Although the federal government provides some housing assistance for people with HIV, it does not fill the need.

Those who are homeless or have unstable housing have lower access to HIV medications and poorer treatment outcomes.

A study from the Centers for Disease Control and Prevention found that among individuals living with HIV in certain impoverished urban areas across the country, the lower the household income, the higher the rate of HIV in the area.

The federal government provides assistance through a program called Housing Opportunities for Persons With AIDS, known as HOPWA. In 2016, HOPWA changed its funding formula to better allocate its resources to Southern areas hardest hit by HIV.

However, some of these HOPWA programs have waiting lists that can extend years. The nation is also experiencing an affordable housing shortage, which further limits options for low-income individuals living with HIV and their families.

Stigma and Mistrust

Experts continue to cite stigma as a key obstacle for treatment. Twenty-six states have laws that penalize an HIV patient for exposing someone to the virus, including 19 that require people who are aware they are infected to notify sexual partners and 12 that mandate disclosure to needle-sharing partners, according to the CDC.

The problems extend to doctors and medical staff. One study, published in 2016, found widespread stigma against HIV patients among health care staff in Alabama and Mississippi, especially among whites and men.

Gina Brown, a community engagement manager for the Southern AIDS Coalition, in part blames the culture of the South, where religious beliefs often clash with gay culture, for perpetuating these problems. "We are still in Bible Belt country, where religion plays a huge part in how we talk about sex or not talk about sex," she said.

But federal policies, such as the Trump administration's ban on transgender men and women serving in the military, also play a role.

Federal officials acknowledged these difficulties and affirmed the program would not discriminate against transgender patients.

In addition, minority communities hard hit by the HIV epidemic harbor lingering distrust toward the medical system due to historical abuses such as the Tuskegee syphilis trials, said Mayer.

Injection Drug Use

The scourge of addiction has killed tens of thousands across the nation, spread hepatitis C and is now leading to spikes in HIV transmission, as drug users share needles. In

2015, Scott County, Ind., sought to combat an HIV outbreak fueled by injected opioid use that infected 215 people. Drug use has also been connected to multiple HIV clusters in Massachusetts and Kentucky.

HHS reported that injection drug users accounted for 1 in 10 new HIV cases in 2016.

Expanding syringe exchange programs across the country could minimize this problem, experts said.

"Unfortunately, in the United States we haven't done as good a job as other Western countries in making sure that those programs are widely available for those Americans who need them," said Millett.

The CDC and HHS consider syringe exchange programs effective interventions, but some cities, such as Charleston, W.Va., that implemented the programs have now shut them down because of neighborhood complaints, funding concerns and opposition from citizens who object to providing injection equipment.

Federal funds can be used to support this intervention, but these dollars cannot go directly toward purchasing needles.

12. The Unexpected Public Health Emergency*

Jenna Tyler

Emergency managers and public health administrators are charged with identifying and predicting the threats and hazards that have the greatest probability of affecting their local jurisdiction. However, despite their education and experience, very few might have predicted that a localized drug abuse problem would escalate to a declared public health emergency that called for executive orders, the suspension of existing laws and a complex multiagency response. Yet a growing HIV outbreak turned this unexpected threat into a reality as a rural county in southeastern Indiana experienced more than 180 confirmed HIV cases in less than nine months.

The Event

According to the Centers for Disease Control and Prevention (CDC), the Indiana State Department of Health (ISDH) opened an ongoing investigation January 23, 2015, after disease intervention specialists linked 11 confirmed HIV cases to Scott County, Indiana. With a population of less than 25,000 and a historical average of five HIV cases per year, the initial response by ISDH focused on interviewing the newly diagnosed individuals about their sexual behaviors and past drug abuse. These interviews led ISDH to conclude that a majority of the cases were caused by syringe-sharing partners injecting a prescription opioid called Opana.

By mid–March, the outbreak showed no end in sight. The ISDH reported 55 confirmed HIV cases. This prompted the Governor of Indiana to declare a public health emergency and sign Executive Order 15–05, which suspended current Indiana Code and legalized a short-term needle exchange program. This needle exchange program allowed injecting drug users to register with the local health department to obtain enough needles to last for one week and then required the injecting drug user to return their used needles in order to acquire new needles for the following week. Despite the controversial debate of the effectiveness of needle exchange programs, empirical studies have found needle exchange programs to be quite effective in limiting the spread of blood-borne illnesses such as HIV.

---

*Originally published as Jenna Tyler, "The Unexpected Public Health Emergency," *PA Times*, https://patimes.org/unexpected-public-health-emergency/ (September 18, 2015). Reprinted with permission of the publisher.

The needle exchange program was housed within the Community Outreach Center which provided community members free HIV testing and vaccinations, as well as guidance on HIV prevention and treatment. Personnel from local health departments and ISDH staffed the Community Outreach Center while personnel from the CDC focused on patient tracing. Together, these entities strived to contain the outbreak and provide treatment for the individuals who tested positive for HIV.

Best Practices

The Scott County HIV outbreak is not simply a warning to the State of Indiana, but a warning to the entire nation. In fact, state health officials argue there is no distinct reason why the HIV outbreak occurred in Scott County, Indiana, and claim it is only a matter of time before similar incidents develop across the country.

In the interest of this prediction, the following three actions should be considered best practices for similar public health emergencies.

1. Establishing a Community Outreach Center

The Community Outreach Center offered a centralized location for managing the incident and provided critical public services to community members all free of cost. In an effort to attract more community members, supporting state agencies were also stationed in the Community Outreach Center to help people obtain state-issued ID cards, birth certificates and enroll in a health insurance plan. This approach enabled a more coordinated and collaborative multiagency response.

2. Engaging the Public

In order to stop the spread of HIV, response agencies had to ensure the public was aware of the incident and the consequences of not getting tested. As such, ISDH launched the You Are Not Alone campaign focusing on substance abuse, safe sex, needle disposal and HIV testing treatment. Additionally, the local health department identified many members did not have a means of transportation to participate in the needle-exchange program. As such, the local health department began operating a mobile needle-exchange program.

3. Creating a Culture of Acceptance

From the start of this public health emergency, it was clear that in order to stop the spread of HIV, response organizations would have to create a culture of acceptance and attend to the needs of the public. Moreover, it was absolutely critical to establish a cooperative relationship built upon trust with community members. This meant proving that community members could openly admit to abusing prescription drugs without fear of arrest.

Conclusion

Indiana state health officials believe the Scott County HIV outbreak has reached its peak with the response efforts slowly dwindling. Now, it is up to the locals to recover to a community that fosters social resiliency. Keck and Sakdapolrak describe social resilience as the ability of communities to cope with and overcome adversities by learning from experiences to make adjustments that minimize the chances of reoccurrence. In the case of Scott County, building a socially resilient community rests in the hands of community members—not response agencies—who will have to decide if they will let this incident define them or transform them.

13. An Addiction Researcher Shares 6 Strategies to Address the Opioid Epidemic*

Nabila El-Bassel

The devastating opioid epidemic is one of the largest public health problems facing the U.S. Over 2.5 million people in the U.S. suffer from opioid use disorder.

Four in five new heroin users started out misusing prescription painkillers. A 2015 analysis by the Centers for Disease Control and Prevention found people who are addicted to painkillers are 40 times more likely to be addicted to heroin.

The epidemic actually began more than three decades ago. In 1980, crack and cocaine addiction contributed to the thousands of overdose deaths, whereas now people die from pain relievers and synthetic opioids such as fentanyl.

In 1990, I began studying its relationship to HIV and the experiences of people with multiple addictions. My research team and I have recruited research participants from emergency rooms, methadone programs, jails, prisons, alternative to incarceration projects, and HIV and primary care clinics. We have examined barriers to accessing care for drug addiction and HIV, and some of the lessons we have learned apply to the broader population.

Two Faces of the Opioid Addiction

Years ago, I interviewed Jennifer, a former nurse, who was prescribed antidepressants to cope with childhood sexual abuse trauma. When this didn't help, she stole narcotics from her clinic and was fired. With no access to pain pills, Jennifer began using heroin and cocaine. She reported facing stigma from health care providers due to her addiction, and she lacked access to counseling for depression. Jennifer's case is not unique; many women face a lack of access to services addressing trauma and gender-based violence.

More recently, our research team interviewed John, who started using narcotics prescribed for back pain. His need for increasingly higher dosages exceeded the number of pills his physician would prescribe, so he turned to friends and then began heroin and injection drug use.

---

*Originally published as Nabila El-Bassel, "An Addiction Researcher Shares 6 Strategies to Address the Opioid Epidemic," *The Conversation*, https://theconversation.com/an-addiction-researcher-shares-6-strategies-to-address-the-opioid-epidemic-94154 (April 26, 2018). Reprinted with permission of the publisher.

Although incarcerated numerous times for accidents while driving impaired, he said he was never asked about addiction or referred to drug treatment by his primary care office. Since John detoxed "cold turkey" in prison, he often overdosed after his release, reuniting with his "running buddies." Recently, one of John's buddies saved his life by using a free naloxone kit from a health department stall at a street fair. John was lucky: Thousands of opioid users cannot access naloxone.

Not Addressing the Core Causes

Though overprescribing opioids may have contributed to the current epidemic, many addiction experts believe that the root causes remain poverty, incarceration, drug and health policies, stigma toward people who use drugs, and a lack of access to drug treatment.

Yet much of what has been done to end the opioid epidemic has focused mainly on [reducing the amount of prescription painkillers] and improving drug monitoring programs to identify newly filled prescriptions, which are not the real solutions to the growing opioid epidemic. In my view, there has been no clear policy action or plan to address the major root causes of the problem and improve access to drug treatment. President Donald Trump's plan to address the opioid epidemic emphasizes punishment, reduction of supply, and law enforcement strategies with no potential to produce important change in the crisis.

Here are my six recommendations to address the opioid epidemic.

Increase Medicaid Coverage for Drug Treatment in All States

The number of states providing benefits for addiction treatment grew with the creation of Affordable Care Act in 2010 and the expansion of Medicaid benefits—but only for states that opted to expand. Now, 32 states and the District of Columbia have adopted Medicaid expansion, which provides medical coverage including addiction treatment for most low-income adults.

However, an estimated 2.5 million Americans fall into a coverage gap, where they are not eligible for Medicaid because their state did not expand and they make too little to qualify for marketplace subsidies.

Integrate Drug Treatment into Primary Care

Medication assisted treatment—the practice of treating addiction with medicines—must be made available in primary care settings and integrated with health care services. The majority of the 2.5 million individuals with an opioid use disorder do not receive evidence-based MAT. Few states have integrated this treatment.

The Affordable Care Act is designed to promote improved integration of substance use in health care services in a more efficient and cost-effective way. There is extensive scientific evidence supporting integration into primary care.

Some of the major barriers include state and federal regulations on credentialing and provision of medication-assisted treatment, such as strict rules on how and who can prescribe buprenorphine in primary care settings; shortage of physicians with training to treat substance use disorders; and clinic costs to meet the demands of staff training.

Reduce Stigma of Health Care Providers Toward Drug Users

While health care providers understand addiction is a disease, research shows they commonly view addiction as a moral failure. In fact, studies show that negative attitudes by health professionals toward patients with substance use disorders are common. They are a major reason individuals do not seek, receive or complete addiction treatment or access harm reduction services such as syringe access programs.

Increase and Customize Programs That Reduce Harm

I believe harm reduction—access to services aiming to reduce harm from the addiction rather than just treating it—is critical. Syringe exchange programs allow people with addiction trade in used syringes for new ones, reducing exposure to HIV, hepatitis C or other diseases that occur frequently in those with addiction. Supervised injection facilities would provide a safe place for drug users to inject illicit substances with medical staff nearby.

Address Neglected Populations Within the Criminal Justice System

Those addicted to opioids in prison and jails are often left untreated. Medication assisted treatment, such as the use of methadone, buprenorphine and naltrexone should be provided to all inmates. Upon release, individuals should receive naloxone to use on themselves or others. To avoid relapse, access to addiction treatment and other care is imperative.

Make Naloxone Available to All

I have seen countless research participant lives saved by relatives, friends and partners who received naloxone. Recent evidence shows states that actively promoted naloxone experienced 9 to 11 percent reductions in opioid-related deaths. States need strategies to make naloxone available and affordable to everyone, not just first responders. Medicaid should also reimburse naloxone prescriptions for home settings.

Even after 30 years, drug use remains stigmatized and individuals are left untreated. Understanding stories like Jennifer's and John's help destigmatize drug use and convey the need to address addiction in primary health care settings and link individuals to treatment in their communities.

14. Why Are HIV Survival Rates Lower in the Deep South Than the Rest of the U.S.?*

Susan Reif *and* Carolyn McAllaster

The Deep South region has become the epicenter of the US HIV epidemic. Despite having only 28% of the total U.S. population, nine states in the Deep South account for nearly 40% of national HIV diagnoses. This region has the highest HIV diagnosis rates and the highest number of people living with HIV of any U.S. region based on data for 2008–2011. And new research has found that the five-year survival rate for people diagnosed with HIV or AIDS is lower in the Deep South than in the rest of the country.

So why are we seeing higher death rates and lower survival rates among those living with HIV in the Deep South? The reasons are complicated, but poverty, social stigma, lack of health-care infrastructure and more rural geography likely all play a role.

Five-Year Survival Rates Are Poor

Recent research by the Centers for Disease Control and Prevention (CDC) and the Southern HIV/AIDS Strategy Initiative (SASI) at Duke University Law School in nine states of the Deep South—Alabama, Florida, Georgia, Louisiana, Mississippi and North and South Carolina, Tennessee and Texas—found that people diagnosed with HIV or AIDS in these states are dying at higher rates than those diagnosed in the rest of the country. This is the case even after controlling for regional differences in age, sex, race, and area population size.

CDC/SASI research found that 27% of people diagnosed with AIDS in the Deep South region in 2003–2004 had died within five years of diagnosis. Although five-year survival varied among states in the Deep South, no state had a survival percentage at or above the US average, 77%. In Louisiana, one-third of people diagnosed with AIDS and 19% of those diagnosed with HIV had died within five years of diagnosis.

Researchers also compared the characteristics of those diagnosed with HIV/AIDS in the Deep South region to national averages and found higher percentages of young

---

*Originally published as Susan Reif and Carolyn McAllaster, "Why Are HIV Survival Rates Lower in the Deep South Than the Rest of the U.S.?," *The Conversation*, https://theconversation.com/why-are-hiv-survival-rates-lower-in-the-deep-south-than-the-rest-of-the-us-37872 (April 22, 2015). Reprinted with permission of the publisher.

people (aged 13–24), blacks, females and transmission attributed to heterosexual contact among the region's individuals diagnosed with HIV. More than one-quarter of people diagnosed with HIV lived outside a large urban area, which is the highest percentage of any U.S. region.

What Makes the Deep South Different from the Rest of the U.S.?

The Deep South has lower levels of income, education and insurance coverage than the rest of the U.S. Poverty is consistently associated with poorer health so it is not surprising that the Deep South is experiencing high death rates among those diagnosed with HIV. And none of the Deep South states have accepted federal dollars to expand their Medicaid programs under the Affordable Care Act, leaving thousands of people in the region without health insurance.

Geography also plays a role in the Southern HIV epidemic. Much of the Deep South HIV epidemic is concentrated outside of large urban areas. The CDC/SASI research found that living outside a large urban area at the time of HIV diagnosis significantly predicted greater death rates among people living with HIV in the region.

HIV-related stigma has been found to be higher outside the large urban areas and transportation is a significant barrier to medical care for HIV-positive individuals living outside urban areas since most HIV specialty care is located in urban areas. Without reliable transportation, people miss appointments and may lack access to supportive services such as case management, support groups and legal services.

Thanks to advances in HIV treatment, people who are diagnosed with HIV can have normal life expectancies. But that's only if they get linked to HIV medical care and remain on treatment, which is a challenge in a region where so many people live outside of urban areas, live in poverty or lack access to health care.

Stigma Kills

HIV-related stigma has consistently been cited as a driver of the HIV epidemic—especially in the South. In the words of a Deep South focus group participant living with HIV, "HIV doesn't kill. Stigma kills."

HIV care providers in the Deep South region tell stories of patients who don't come to their medical appointments, who won't participate in support groups, who won't disclose their HIV status to their closest family members (and the list goes on) because of stigma and a deep fear of how they will be perceived if others discover their status. Stigma also prevents people from getting tested for HIV, which is a critical step in getting the right treatment and in preventing further transmission of the disease.

Southern laws and policies also contribute to stigma. Most Deep South states have abstinence-based sex education in public schools, which has not been shown to be effective in preventing sexually transmitted infections

Many Southern states also criminalize HIV-related sexual behaviors and prohibit syringe exchange programs, thus further marginalizing people at high risk for becoming HIV positive, such as sex workers and injection drug users. These laws also discourage HIV testing and make interventions that have proven effective, like syringe exchange, illegal.

Overcoming Stigma and Promoting Prevention

The drivers of the Southern HIV epidemic are complicated and to a great extent mirror the causes of poor health outcomes overall in southern states. Creative programs, such as the expansion of telemedicine programs and the co-location of HIV care with other services, such as case management and mental health and substance abuse care, are important to overcome stigma and the lack of transportation and medical care in non-urban areas.

Funding to support anti-stigma interventions, including empowerment initiatives for those living with HIV and educational efforts for churches and community, is critical. Finally, increased prevention funding that is directed at urban and rural areas alike is crucial if we are to stem the new HIV diagnosis rates and lower the death rates in the Deep South.

15. Should You Be Tested for HIV?

Why June 27 Is a Good Day to Do It*

Jodi Sutherland

June 27 is National HIV Testing Day. Have you been tested?

The Centers for Disease Control and Prevention report that of the estimated 1.1 million people in the United States who have the HIV infection, 1 in 7 don't know their status.

That is especially true for youth ages 13 to 24 that make up 21% of the nearly 40,000 new HIV diagnoses made in 2017. More than 50% of youth who have HIV don't know about their infection.

Only 9% of high school students report having been tested for HIV. Many people do not get tested because of lack of access to health care, fear and misperceptions about HIV risk and the testing process, and health care settings that lack HIV testing as a routine part of care.

As a nurse at a clinic that treats sexually transmitted infectious diseases, I frequently saw patients visit the clinic requesting HIV testing because their provider did not want to test them for HIV, or their provider said they did not offer HIV testing. We would also see young people at the clinic because they could not always be assured of confidentiality at their doctors' offices.

Nurse practitioners play a valuable role in testing of HIV in youth. A colleague and I recently published an article on HIV testing that showed nurse practitioners are less likely to perform HIV testing on people younger than 18 years of age. That may be in part because of issues related to patient confidentiality, consent, and linkage to care when a person tests positive.

Nurse practitioners are in a unique position to educate youth about HIV, refer youth to health services including HIV testing and perform HIV testing. But currently, nurse practitioners do not have full practice authority in all states. One way to increase HIV testing for all persons might be to include giving nurse practitioners the full authority under state regulations and practice acts to test for HIV.

Testing a Major Breakthrough

The development of testing technologies has been one of the two leading breakthroughs

---

*Originally published as Jodi Sutherland, "Should You Be Tested for HIV? Why June 27 Is a Good Day to Do It," *The Conversation*, https://theconversation.com/should-you-be-tested-for-hiv-why-june-27-is-a-good-day-to-do-it-119075 (June 27, 2019). Reprinted with permission of the publisher.

to the possibility of ending the HIV epidemic; the other is pharmacological interventions that effectively manage the disease and prevent transmission. Our nurse practitioner study concluded that nurse practitioners have an important role to increase HIV testing rates and could help put an end to HIV.

Nevertheless, many people don't know if they should be tested, and so they are not.

Although it has been nearly 40 years since the beginning of the HIV crisis, the CDC reports that the infection continues to affect gay, bisexual and other men who have sex with men of all races and ethnicities; black and Latino men and women; people who inject drugs; people aged 25–34; and people in the Southern U.S. disproportionately.

There are national recommendations and practice guidelines for nurse practitioners to test for HIV. However, the rate at which they screen for HIV is low, as my colleague Gale Spencer and I reported in our recent study.

We found that the strongest predictor of nurse practitioner HIV testing behavior was the practice setting's social pressures that influence HIV testing. In other words, when office staff supported routine HIV screening, then nurse practitioners were more likely to test for HIV, even when it took more time.

Also, nurse practitioners believed that when "consent from a parent/guardian should be obtained before screening for HIV in a person younger than 18 years," they were less likely to screen for HIV. This means that better policy and procedures are needed to help guide providers for testing those younger than 18. We believe this is pivotal, given that among young people between the ages 13 and 24 with HIV, nearly half are not aware of their status.

Testing Guidelines for All

According to the CDC recommendations, everyone should be tested at least once between the ages of 13 and 64 as part of routine health care.

Also, if you are pregnant or planning to get pregnant, the CDC recommends that you should get tested as early as possible.

You should also get tested at least once a year if:

- You are a sexually active gay or bisexual man
- You have had sex with an HIV-positive partner
- You have had more than one partner since your last HIV test
- You have shared needles or "works" to inject drugs
- You have exchanged sex for drugs or money
- You have another sexually transmitted disease, hepatitis or tuberculosis
- You have had sex with anyone who has done anything in this list, or with someone whose sexual history you do not know.

Also, the CDC recommends testing before having sex for the first time with a new partner. The agency also recommends that you talk about sexual and drug-use history.

In January 2019, the World Health Organization made the proposal to declare 2020 the "Year of the Nurse and Midwife." Nurses provide the essential link between the people of the community and the complex health care system. With their help, more youth—and others—can get tested.

16. Violence Against Women Is Overlooked in Its Role in Opioid Epidemic*

Nabila El-Bassel

One night, a woman I'll call Tonya got a compliment from a guy when she was out with her boyfriend. Tonya's boyfriend cursed her because another man had complimented her. He said: "You give it to everybody, I want it too." In anticipation of his physical abuse, she reasoned, "I could go off to Wonder World." She then injected heroin, to be "in her own world," she later told me.

Tonya is only one of the hundreds of women I've interviewed for my research with similar stories in the span of my nearly 30-year career studying the links between intimate partner violence, sexual coercion, substance use disorders and HIV.

In the early '90s, I was among a few social scientists who identified intimate partner violence as a major risk factor for HIV risk behaviors and transmission and a barrier to treatment access, and engagement among women.

Over the years, I have designed, tested and promoted the use of gender-specific HIV and prevention interventions to address these issues simultaneously for women, men and couples who use drugs.

More recently, I have expanded my substance abuse research to include greater involvement in opioid overdose prevention among women and men. I have begun a cross-university collaboration to tackle the opioid crisis and issues such as partner violence, reproductive health and gender equity are included in the interventions that we will develop, in order improve access to services and treatment for individuals who use opiates.

While progress has been made to address intimate partner violence among women who use drugs, those with opioid use disorders who experience partner violence are still in dire need of help in navigating and engaging in substance use treatment programs and other services.

Our research found that many men with substance use disorders often undermined their female partners' recovery. They can control their ability to engage in treatment, deny them potential sources of protection, and jeopardize the custody of their children to maintain control over them and, for some men, have women take care of them.

---

*Originally published as Nabila El-Bassel, "Violence Against Women Is Overlooked in Its Role in Opioid Epidemic," *The Conversation*, https://theconversation.com/violence-against-women-is-overlooked-in-its-role-in-opioid-epidemic-113604 (March 20, 2019). Reprinted with permission of the publisher.

Medicating to Mitigate Trauma

Stigma often keeps people from caring about women who are victims of violence and have substance use disorders.

Many women in controlling and violent relationships like Tonya's "self-medicate"— or use drugs that are not prescribed to them to help with their medical condition—to mitigate the trauma of physical and sexual assault. As a result, their bodies crave an ever-increasing steady supply of substances to get high in order to feel "better." Today, the drugs of choice are usually opioids.

Research has repeatedly indicated that drug use is associated with partner violence, specifically against women, who may be particularly susceptible to such violence when under the influence of opioids. Living with substance use disorders puts these women into a number of contexts that expose them to HIV and other sexually transmitted diseases that jeopardize their survival in many ways.

In my research with men on partner violence and drug use and HIV, a man reported pushing his partner to the floor and forcing her to have sex. He did not consider this violent, since she reportedly gave him a "signal."

In another study with women who use drugs, a woman said that her husband hit her and forced her to have sex: "I didn't know I was raped because he was my husband."

Treatment must address the need for escape that these women seek. As another woman said, "When I was sober I didn't dare have sex with him. I had to be high to be able … to make love to him."

A Power Imbalance

Many women who use drugs lack the power to negotiate safer sex and reduce drug risk behaviors, such as not sharing syringes with a partner or others, due to imbalanced power dynamics with their partners, and male controlling behaviors. Yet, most available HIV and substance use prevention strategies and treatment put the onus on women to insist on safe sex and drug risk reduction, increasing their risk of physical and sexual abuse.

This can be dangerous. Studies have shown that women are often physically or sexually abused when negotiating safe sex or refusing to engage in drug risk. Thus, a key person is missing from the conversation: her male partner.

My research has shown that counseling the couple may help. In a systematic review, colleagues and I found that couple-based interventions for women and male sex partners who use drugs help reduce sexual- and drug-risk behaviors and promote healthy relationship. Counseling couples allows partners to address gender differences in a safe environment, power imbalances and gender inequalities when sharing needles.

No Easy Fixes

The opioid epidemic is complex and requires many approaches. In April 2018, the U.S. Surgeon General issued a public health advisory emphasizing the necessity of safe prescribing of opioids, accessing evidence-based medication-assisted treatment (MAT) and distributing naloxone to reverse overdose. However, the advisory makes no mention of the need for gender-specific approaches and interventions.

A recent study found that women were nearly three times less likely to receive naloxone during emergency resuscitation efforts than men, which is likely due to their being devalued.

Emergency responders and police officers as well as family members and peers must be trained to overcome this gendered barrier and recognize signs and symptoms of overdose.

Women who use drugs face multilayers of stigma and disbelief, preventing them from disclosing problems such as partner violence. Staying in treatment is difficult for women when services are designed and delivered by men who may not know how to create an environment of trust for women. These issues must be changed if we are serious on addressing the opioid epidemic among women.

Women who use drugs have told our research teams that they feel unsafe in the locations where they are forced to inject. In fact, they face greater risks than men in these locations where men—who may have abused them—share. A movement toward safe injection locations, similar to the site in Vancouver specifically for women, would ensure women can avoid violence and gain access to harm reduction services.

Women with active opioid use disorders and those in recovery need to be at the forefront of discussions of how to move forward effective policies and programs to curb gender disparities and partner violence. Only then can we observe better outcomes for women like Tonya.

17. Fighting HIV in Miami, One Dirty Needle at a Time*

Amy Driscoll

MIAMI—The doctor on a mission met the homeless heroin addict who lived under a tree last year at Jackson Health System's special immunology clinic when both men were struggling to overcome the odds.

Jose De Lemos, infected with HIV and hepatitis C from a shared needle, had gone without treatment for almost a year. He'd dropped 80 pounds, suffered from night sweats and a rash on his leg and chest. Even walking hurt.

He was in no mood for conversation with a well-meaning doc.

But Hansel Tookes, a University of Miami doctor with a degree in public health and a calling to public service, isn't the kind of doctor who is easily put off. He talked to De Lemos anyway. Sent him to dermatology, started him on meds for HIV and hepatitis C, worked to find him a bed in rehab, and talked—about his own uphill battle to create a syringe exchange program in South Florida, the kind of program that might have prevented De Lemos' infection.

A public health advocate in Miami, where new HIV infection rates consistently top the state and national charts, Tookes had been struggling for years to get a bill passed in the Florida legislature to create a program in Miami-Dade County to help end that terrible distinction.

In that time, he had gone from medical student to doctor. Testified before legislative committees over and over. And learned just how hard he would have to fight to get what he considered a very modest proposal to save lives and improve public health through a conservative, Republican-dominated legislature.

For De Lemos, his doctor's commitment to the cause—an unpopular one, at that—was a revelation: "I'm hard-headed. And he's persistent. He's like, 'If you get clean, you can talk about this. You'll be great.... You can help me.' I admire him because he went through a lot but he kept going."

Tookes recalled a different moment with his patient: "He started crying because he said he didn't know people cared."

For the next eight months, as De Lemos kicked heroin, endured a skin condition

---

*Originally published as Amy Driscoll, "Fighting HIV In Miami, One Dirty Needle at a Time," *Kaiser Health News*, https://khn.org/news/fighting-hiv-in-miami-one-dirty-needle-at-a-time/ (August 10, 2016). Reprinted with permission of the publisher. Kaiser Health News is a nonprofit news service covering health issues. It is an editorially independent program of the Kaiser Family Foundation that is not affiliated with Kaiser Permanente.

that caused blisters across his entire torso and finally saw his sky-high viral count drop, Tookes started seeing hope, too. His proposal, which had been stalled for years, started gaining traction. The nationwide heroin epidemic had changed the dialogue about blood-borne diseases. De Lemos' appointments with Tookes now usually included an update on the needle exchange bill in Tallahassee. Sometimes, when there was a big vote, Tookes played video recordings of the committee meetings on his phone for De Lemos to see.

"The reception in the ER isn't great. I had to prop the door open," Tookes said, with a laugh. "But we watched."

In March, a full five years after Tookes published a study in a medical journal when he was still a student that documented the harsh reality of illicit needle use in Miami, Gov. Rick Scott signed the Miami-Dade Infectious Disease Elimination Act (IDEA), making Miami-Dade's program the first legal needle exchange in the American South.

The victory didn't mean his fight was over. Legislators weren't unanimous when they approved the bill, and IDEA reflects that: It creates a five-year test program, only in Miami-Dade and without any public financing. Tookes and UM, which will run the program, must raise all the money for the program privately, through grants and donations. Tookes—doctor, public health advocate and needle exchange crusader—must now also become a fund-raiser.

He's undaunted. His determination has carried him this far, and he is already envisioning the rest.

"When I flew back to Miami after the bill had passed, I looked at the city as we were landing at MIA and I thought, what we just did is going to change the health of tens of thousands of people," Tookes said. "And that was an amazing feeling. And that's an amazing truth. And that's where we are."

Advanced HIV Cases

Tookes, a 35-year-old internist, took on the against-the-odds fight for a needle exchange because he felt he had to. Too many people were coming through the doors of Miami-Dade's public health system with advanced cases of HIV in an era when the virus that causes AIDS is generally treated as a disease you live with, not one that kills you. Injection drug overdoses were rising, too.

The doctor knew getting people into treatment earlier could make a huge difference in their lives and reduce infections of others. ("I'm trained to look for public health solutions," he said.) A needle exchange was a step toward that goal. Florida had never allowed a needle exchange program before. But why couldn't that change?

His grandmother, Gracie Wyche, had set the bar high in his family. She was a pioneering black nurse in Miami who started out in the then-segregated wards of Jackson Memorial and eventually became a head nurse, concentrating on a mysterious illness in the 1980s that later became known as AIDS. Tookes became even more interested in public service during his undergraduate work at Yale University and a stint as an investigator for Project Aware, an HIV testing/counseling clinical trial at UM. He got a public health degree at UM, and then his medical degree.

Now a third-year resident who does his research through UM's division of infectious diseases at the Miller School of Medicine, Tookes said his grandmother's work set him on this path. "She inspired me," he said. "There's just a long history of service on both sides of the family."

The HIV numbers drove him, too. In 2014, the Miami-Fort Lauderdale region ranked No. 1 in the nation by the U.S. Centers for Disease Control and Prevention for the rate of new HIV infections in areas with more than 1 million people. That year, Miami-Dade County had 1,324 new HIV cases, the CDC said, while Broward had 836 cases. Statewide, in 2014, the Florida Department of Health said 110,000 people were diagnosed and living with HIV. People are still dying of the virus: In the United States, 6,955 people died from HIV and AIDS in 2013, according to the CDC.

Tookes saw the toll up close, in the examining room. A man in his 40s who had sex with men, no body fat and pneumocystis pneumonia, a disease often associated with AIDS—who didn't know he'd probably had HIV for years. An impoverished woman from Liberty City with a debilitating bacterial infection from a severely compromised immune system, who had never before been tested for HIV. Or a young man diagnosed with HIV a few months ago who revealed to Tookes during a clinic visit that he uses intravenous methamphetamine.

"Everything with this issue—all of the advocacy that we did for this policy—was to fix an issue that we were seeing in everyday clinical practice.... I think as physicians, we had a duty to intervene," Tookes said. "We knew there was something we could do for these people to help them from getting so sick, and so we decided to fight for it."

He faced deep suspicion about the idea going back to the just-say-no 1980s. Although needle exchange programs have become increasingly common even in GOP-controlled states—Indiana's governor and then Republican vice presidential candidate Mike Pence changed his position after an outbreak of HIV and hepatitis C—Florida remained a holdout. Some lawmakers continued to believe that giving addicts clean needles amounted to government-endorsed drug use.

Starting in 2012, Tookes—backed by a coalition including the Florida Medical Association, the Florida Hospital Association and the Miami-Dade State Attorney's Office—tried to make headway with lawmakers. When he hit the wall of opposition, he didn't give up. He didn't get disillusioned or cynical. He tried again. And again. In the legislative sessions of 2013, '14, '15.

Then 2016 came along. The heroin epidemic created a whole new conversation around the issue of injection-drug use.

State Sen. Oscar Braynon, a Miami Gardens Democrat, sponsored the syringe exchange bill—over and over—because of the high rates of HIV and hepatitis C in his district. He said he saw opposition flag after Florida shut down its "pill mills" starting in 2011, sending opioid users to the needle.

"The first thing people hear is that you're trying to empower drug users to use drugs," Braynon said. "But the narrative changed over time.... What started to happen is that drug use picked up. First it was people in the 'hood. But now it's some of the wealthier people."

And so the legislature's attitude changed. Injection drug use—and the blood-borne diseases that can go with it—were no longer just "a Miami problem," Tookes said.

"In the context of a nationwide heroin epidemic and in the context of what I believe were many more constituents across the state going to see their senators and representatives and telling them that this was something that was ravaging their communities, we had a lot more of a sympathetic ear from the legislature this year," he said.

A needle exchange program won't fix Miami-Dade's problem with HIV and hepatitis C. But Tookes says it will help. And though a small percentage of HIV infections can be traced directly to needle use and the biggest risk factor is still sex, reducing the number of shared needles reduces the community's risk overall. People who share needles don't always tell their sexual partners that they are at risk.

A needle exchange also brings the hard-core, drug-injecting population into the public health system to be tested and treated. That reduces the risk to everyone else and cuts costs of treating their illnesses.

This is not just theory. In Washington, D.C., the number of new HIV infections dropped from an average of 19 a month to six a month after a needle exchange program was introduced in 2008, according to a study released last year by George Washington University's public health school. The reduction in cases saved taxpayers an estimated $45.6 million, using CDC estimates that the average lifetime of care for AIDS patients costs about $380,000.

Miami-Dade stands to save money, too, if addicts stop reusing needles. A study co-authored last year by Tookes showed that the cost of treating patients who had bacterial infections as a result of dirty needles ran about $11.4 million a year at taxpayer-funded Jackson Memorial Hospital.

For Tookes, all of these public health arguments start with what he learned on the streets of Miami interviewing intravenous drug users when he was still a medical student at UM. The study he published in 2011 showed that drug users in Miami were 34 times more likely to dispose of their needles in public than drug users in San Francisco, which has had a needle exchange program since 1988.

Tookes still sees the bits and pieces of drug equipment in bushes and along streets, even in upscale places like Brickell Avenue, lined with high rise condos and financial companies from all over the world.

"I still have syringe radar," he said. "I spot them everywhere."

Street Needles

A few miles away from the Jackson clinics where Tookes works, in the shadow of the Metrorail station in Miami's Overtown neighborhood, Carlos Franco is handing out his precious stash of clean needles to addicts once again.

Franco, 67, says he began his underground one-man operation more than two decades ago after he was horrified to see his girlfriend share needles with other drug users. He buys the sterile syringes, 100 to a box, at his own expense when he has the money, from the North American Syringe Exchange Network.

Franco is instantly recognizable to many in the neighborhood, where orange caps from syringes are sprinkled in vacant, overgrown lots and along sidewalks and under bushes.

"¡Oye!" yells one man, hailing Franco from a block away.

The operation is quick, Franco reaching into his backpack and handing over several packs of needles. The man, identified only as Flaco—"Skinny," in Spanish—nods his thanks, looks both ways and disappears behind a metal gate next to a house across the street.

Around the corner, near the Interstate 95 overpass, Franco points out the improvised "cookers" that litter the shrubbery, bottoms of soda cans fashioned to heat up drugs. As he's talking, a blond, thin guy in a T-shirt and jeans walks up poking a toe into the shrubbery.

Franco pulls the box from his backpack. "You need this?"

The man nods, his face now eager. Franco hands him a packet of syringes. Sean says he is 41, from New Jersey, a construction worker when he can find work. He is a heroin addict.

Sean has hepatitis C, something he shrugs off. "If you're on the streets, it's sort of required," he says, with a short laugh that reveals a few missing teeth.

He walks away. A moment later, only half-hidden by a metal fence, he hunches over his arm.

"What really bothers me," Franco says, "is when the numbers on the side of the syringe are worn off because it's been used so much. That, and when they use a needle so dull it looks like a nail going into the skin—it can't get through."

Franco knows his needle distribution is both illegal and dangerous, but he's not sure if he'll give it up when the official needle exchange program is running. He supports the idea of a legal program but worries about the people who might be too afraid to try it.

"I'll wait and see," he says. "A lot of people on the streets know me. I'm not sure if they will go to an official program. The cops might harass the program."

"People Are Still Dying"

No one knows exactly why Miami-Dade's HIV infection rate remains higher than other metropolitan areas, even as medicines are better than ever, statewide rates have declined and mother-to-child transmissions—AIDS babies—are rare.

Public health officials rattle off a variety of contributing factors: Thirty-five years into this epidemic, younger people think of HIV as a treatable, chronic disease. Drugs like Truvada, which can prevent HIV infection if taken as a precaution, have added to that perception. HIV is largely an urban disease. Immigration brings people to Florida from places without much access to healthcare or health education. Miami is an international party town, and the highest risk for HIV is unprotected sex, especially for men having sex with men. Testing and medication in South Florida can be difficult to find.

Also, HIV has fallen out of the headlines for the most part, added AIDS Healthcare Foundation's advocacy and legislative affairs manager Jason King.

"People are still dying. But you don't get the press coverage.... So it's not at the forefront of people's minds."

Stigma is part of the problem, too. If you can't admit you have HIV, your sexual partners are probably at higher risk.

"It's not a death sentence like before but the stigma still exists," said King, who is HIV positive. "And then they have to be conscientious about disclosing it to their next partner and they fear rejection."

That's definitely true in Miami-Dade, said Dr. Cheryl Holder, a general internist who works at Jessie Trice Community Health Center and is an associate professor at Florida International University.

Holder says stigma, especially in the African American community, is one of the toughest issues she combats when she sees patients with HIV.

"We're seeing changes in communities, but it's still labeled as wrong and there's something wrong with you.... I still have patients who hide their medicine."

Walking out of the health center at the end of a day not long ago, she saw one of her patients, a young man in a hoodie, waiting for a ride from a family member. "If it weren't for his diagnosis, I would have waited with him for his family. But as I walked by, he didn't look at me and I didn't look at him. And that's when I know it's stigma. He couldn't just pull me over and say, this is my doctor. We need to normalize health care so I don't have to walk past my patient and not meet his mom."

Raising Money

In some ways, Tookes' work starts again now. Though Congress lifted a ban on federal funding for needle exchanges late last year, no federal money can be used on needles themselves. And Florida's bill specifies that no public money can be used for the program.

That leaves Tookes, working with UM, raising it all—about $500,000 a year. And the pressure is on: Other counties in Florida are watching to see how well the program works.

"This pilot program is going to make a big dent in the infection rate in Miami. All eyes are on us. We have to make this a success."

He has raised $100,000 from private donors locally—including Joy Fishman, the widow of the inventor of Narcan, the "save shot" for people who are overdosing—and another $100,000 from the MAC AIDS Fund.

Nancy Mahon, global executive director of the fund, said that syringe exchanges are key to fighting HIV/AIDS. "Needle exchange programs like this halt new infections, period. There is still work to do, but providing sterile syringes and supportive services to IV drug users is a solid step in order to begin saving lives."

Miami-Dade's health department is joining the effort.

"Definitely, we will be helping in any way we can," administrator Lillian Rivera said. "We can't buy the syringes, but we definitely will be providing wrap-around services. As the patients come in, we will be ensuring that they will be tested for HIV and hepatitis.... All of the services that we have will be available to the patients that come through the door."

The IDEA Exchange, which will be run through UM, comes too late to prevent De Lemos' infections. But it'll help others as the 35-year war on the epidemic continues—as many as 2,000 in the first year, Tookes said. A project manager will start work in August, and other staff members are next. The AIDS Healthcare Foundation is donating the HIV and hepatitis C test kits with the agreement that those identified with one of the diseases will be linked with medical care. Tookes is hoping that other groups will follow.

And De Lemos—at 53, homeless no longer—will do his part, inspired by the fight of his doctor to pass the law. His viral load is so low it's considered undetectable, and he is looking at life with new eyes. Service is part of his personal plan now. "I really want to be a part of this needle exchange program. If he can do that, I can do anything."

Tookes says he will measure success with each HIV test, each syringe handed out.

"This has been a long journey.... It's a very exciting time for Miami. We're going to save a lot of lives. We're going to save a lot of money. We're going to give people a lot of clean needles. We're going to provide HIV tests. We're going to get people into treatment.... We're going to change the world."

• *B. Hepatitis C* •

18. Addressing Increases in Hepatitis C Infections Linked to the Opioid Epidemic*

Don C. Des Jarlais

The great majority of people living with antibodies to hepatitis C or living with chronic hepatitis C in the U.S. represent infections that happened many years ago. These are primarily baby boomers (individuals born between 1945 and 1965) who became infected through injection drug use in the 1960s and 1970s or through blood transfusions prior to the discovery of the hepatitis C virus, development of antibody testing, and blood supply screening. Baby boomers represent approximately three-quarters of all hepatitis C infections in the U.S., so it is critically important that they are screened for hepatitis C, diagnosed, and treated, as many of them may be approaching end-stage liver disease.

The other important component of the U.S. hepatitis C epidemic is smaller in absolute numbers but is the major source of new hepatitis C infections: infections associated with the opioid epidemic, injection drug use, and the sharing of needles and other drug injection equipment. This problem is a growing one as new hepatitis C infections in the United States nearly doubled between 2011 and 2014. In many parts of the country, persons who became addicted to opioid analgesics are transitioning to heroin injection as heroin is usually much less expensive. In the United States, those newly infected with hepatitis C are more likely to be younger, more likely to be white, more likely to live in rural areas, and more likely to be infected because of injection drug use.

There are effective interventions to reduce the transmission of hepatitis C among persons who inject drugs (PWID). Needle/syringe service programs that provide sterile injection equipment and medication-assisted treatment (methadone and buprenorphine) for opioid use disorders have effectively reduced hepatitis C transmission where utilized. Additionally, we have a cure for hepatitis C infection. The new direct-acting antiviral (DAA) drugs for treating hepatitis C infection cure 90% or more of those treated. DAAs have a much higher cure rate than the previous treatments for hepatitis C infection, require shorter lengths of treatment, and have much less severe side effects.

The combination of evidence-based interventions such as syringe service programs

---

*Originally published as Don C. Des Jarlais, "Addressing Increases in Hepatitis C Infections Linked to the Opioid Epidemic," https://hepvu.org/addressing-increases-hepatitis-c-infections-linked-opioid-epidemic/ (2019). Reprinted with permission of the author.

for prevention and medication-assisted drug treatment with the new DAAs has created the possibility of eliminating hepatitis C infection for PWID populations. There are, however, many structural problems that we need to overcome: the coverage of syringe service programs and medication-assisted treatment is low in many parts of the world, including many parts of the U.S., and the cost of the new DAAs is very high in many countries.

Scaling effective combined prevention and treatment programs for hepatitis C infection is essential to ending the hepatitis C epidemic among PWID. Being cured of hepatitis C infection does not prevent an individual from becoming re-infected with hepatitis C. Many PWID who need treatment for hepatitis C infection are likely to continue injecting drugs, particularly if they do not have access to effective substance use treatment. Additionally, the likelihood of re-infection is also determined by the prevalence of hepatitis C infected persons in the local PWID population. Small-scale prevention efforts will undoubtedly prevent some new infections, and small-scale treatment programs will undoubtedly cure some cases of HCV infection (and save lives), but small-scale efforts will not halt the current epidemic of hepatitis C infections.

Ending the Hepatitis C Epidemic

What should we do about this complex hepatitis C epidemic in the United States? The steps are different for the two main components of the epidemic. For the large number of baby boomer hepatitis C infections, the key is screening tests to identify people living with hepatitis C, about half of whom are not aware of their infection, and linking those living with chronic hepatitis C infection to care and treatment. In fact, the U.S. Centers for Disease Control and Prevention (CDC) recommend that all adults born during 1945–1965 receive one-time testing for hepatitis C.

For the newer PWID population, prevention is of the highest priority, and policies and programs that support safe injection practices, provide effective substance use treatment, and reduce initiation into injecting are important components of an overall plan to reduce hepatitis C transmission. For these efforts to be truly effective, however, they will need to be conducted on a public health scale. Pilot-scale programs will not stop the hepatitis C epidemic.

19. Hepatitis C and Injection Drug Use*
U.S. Department of Health and Human Services

What Is Hepatitis C?

Hepatitis C is a serious liver disease caused by the hepatitis C virus. Some people get only a short term, or acute, infection and are able to clear the virus without treatment. If someone clears the virus, this usually happens within 6 months after infection. However, about 80% of people who get infected develop a chronic, or lifelong, infection. Over time, chronic hepatitis C can cause serious health problems including liver damage, liver failure, and even liver cancer.

What Are the Symptoms?

Symptoms of hepatitis C can include fever, feeling tired, not wanting to eat, upset stomach, throwing up, dark urine, grey-colored stool, joint pain, and yellow skin and eyes. However, many people who get hepatitis C do not have symptoms and do not know they are infected. If symptoms occur with acute infection, they can appear anytime from two weeks to six months after infection. Symptoms of chronic hepatitis C can take decades to develop, and when symptoms do appear, they often are a sign of advanced liver disease.

Should I Get Tested?

Yes. If you have ever injected drugs, you should get tested for hepatitis C. If you are currently injecting, talk to your doctor about how often you should be tested. The hepatitis C Antibody Test is a blood test that looks for antibodies to the hepatitis C virus. A reactive or positive hepatitis C Antibody Test means that a person has been infected at some point in time. Unlike HIV, a reactive antibody test does not necessarily mean a person still has hepatitis C. An additional blood test called an RNA test is needed to determine if a person is currently infected with hepatitis C.

---

*Public document originally published as U.S. Department of Health and Human Services, "Hepatitis C and Injection Drug Use," www.cdc.gov/hepatitis.

How Is Hepatitis C Spread Among People Who Inject Drugs?

The hepatitis C virus is very infectious and can easily spread when a person comes into contact with surfaces, equipment, or objects that are contaminated with infected blood, even in amounts too small to see. The virus can survive on dry surfaces and equipment for up to 6 weeks. People who inject drugs can get hepatitis C from:

- Needles and syringes. Sharing or reusing needles and syringes increases the chance of spreading the hepatitis C virus. Syringes with detachable needles increase this risk even more because they can retain more blood after they are used than syringes with fixed-needles.
- Preparation Equipment. Any equipment, such as cookers, cottons, water, ties, and alcohol swabs, can easily become contaminated during the drug preparation process.
- Fingers. Fingers that come into contact with infected blood can spread Hepatitis C. Blood on fingers and hands can contaminate the injection site, cottons, cookers, ties, and swabs.
- Surfaces. Hepatitis C can spread when blood from an infected person contaminates a surface and then that surface is reused by another person to prepare injection equipment.

Are There Other Ways Hepatitis C Can Spread?

Hepatitis C can also spread when tattoo, piercing, or cutting equipment is contaminated with the hepatitis C virus and used on another person. Although rare, hepatitis C can be spread through sex. Hepatitis C seems to be more easily spread through sex when a person has HIV or a STD. People who have rough sex or numerous sex partners are at higher risk of getting hepatitis C. Hepatitis C can also be spread from a pregnant woman to her baby.

Can Hepatitis C Be Prevented?

Yes. The best way to prevent hepatitis C is to stop injecting. Drug treatment, including methadone or buprenorphine, can lower your risk for hepatitis C since there will no longer be a need to inject. However, if you are unable or unwilling to stop injecting drugs, there are steps you can take to reduce the risk of becoming infected.

- Do not share any equipment used to inject drugs with another person.
- Always use new, sterile needles, syringes and preparation equipment—cookers, cottons, water, ties, and alcohol swabs—for each injection.
- Set up a clean surface before placing down your injection equipment.
- Do not divide and share drug solution with equipment that has already been used.
- Avoid using syringes with detachable needles to reduce the amount of blood remaining in the syringe after injecting.
- Thoroughly wash hands with soap and water before and after injecting to remove blood or germs.

- Clean injection site with alcohol or soap and water prior to injecting.
- Apply pressure to injection site with a sterile pad to stop any bleeding after injecting.
- Only handle your own injection equipment. If you do inject with other people, separate your equipment from others to avoid accidental sharing.

Use New Syringes and Equipment with Every Injection

The hepatitis C virus is difficult to kill. The best way to prevent hepatitis C is to use new, sterile syringes and equipment with every injection. If using a new syringe is not possible, bleach has been found to kill the hepatitis C virus in syringes when used as a solution of 1 part bleach to 10 parts water for two minutes. Bleach, however, may not be effective when used to clean other types of equipment used to prepare or inject drugs. Although boiling, burning, or using common cleaning fluids, alcohol, or peroxide can reduce the amount of virus, this may not prevent you from getting infected. Cleaning previously used equipment and syringes should only be done if new, sterile equipment is not available.

Can Hepatitis C Be Treated?

Yes. New and improved treatments are available that can cure most people with hepatitis C. Most of the new treatments are taken as pills and do not require interferon injections. However, treatment for hepatitis C depends on many different factors, so it is important to talk to a doctor about options.

Can Someone Get Re-Infected with Hepatitis C?

Yes. Someone who clears the virus, either on their own or from successful treatment, can become infected again.

Does Injecting Put You at Risk for Other Types of Hepatitis?

Yes. People who inject are more likely to get hepatitis A and hepatitis B. Getting vaccinated for hepatitis A and B will prevent these types of hepatitis. There is currently no vaccine for hepatitis C.

20. A "Safe" Space to Shoot Up

Worth a Try?*

Stephanie O'Neill

Tawny Biggs' seemingly happy childhood in the northern Los Angeles County suburb of Santa Clarita, Calif., showed no outward sign that she would one day struggle with drug addiction.

As Biggs tells it, she was raised with two siblings "in a very good family" by an assistant fire-chief dad and a stay-at-home mom. Her after-school hours were filled with hockey and soccer.

But paradise was lost sometime during her late teens, when emotional problems, drugs and alcohol turned Biggs into a self-described "nightmare." One night, when she was amped up on cocaine, her boyfriend gave her a hit of something different to help her sleep: heroin.

Before she even knew what had happened, she was addicted. Six months later, she learned she had contracted hepatitis C from a dirty needle.

Biggs, now 37, finally got sober 14 years ago. Now, she helps others get clean as an admissions coordinator at Action Family Counseling drug and alcohol treatment centers, in her hometown. Based in part on her own arduous experience, she strongly supports a controversial proposal to establish venues where adult intravenous drug users can shoot up with clean needles under medical supervision and get referrals to addiction treatment.

The only injection facility currently operating in North America is in Vancouver, Canada. Australia and several countries in Europe also have such centers.

"I think it's a great idea," said Biggs. "Right now, in this climate, we have to think out of the box because we're fighting an uphill battle."

A bill pending in the state legislature, AB 186, would authorize eight California counties—Alameda, Fresno, Humboldt, Los Angeles, Mendocino, San Francisco, San Joaquin and Santa Cruz—to test so-called "safe injection sites."

The legislation faces tough opposition. Critics say it essentially endorses the use of illicit drugs. And it is not likely to sit well with the federal government, particularly under Attorney General Jeff Sessions, whose hard line on drugs is well-known.

---

*Originally published as Stephanie O'Neill, "A 'Safe' Space to Shoot Up: Worth a Try?," *Kaiser Health News*, https://khn.org/news/a-safe-space-to-shoot-up-worth-a-try-in-california/ (June 19, 2017). Reprinted with permission of the publisher. Kaiser Health News is a nonprofit news service covering health issues. It is an editorially independent program of the Kaiser Family Foundation that is not affiliated with Kaiser Permanente. This story was produced by Kaiser Health News, which publishes California Healthline, an editorially independent service of the California Health Care Foundation.

Advocates argue, however, that a different approach is needed to stem the rising tide of addiction and related deaths.

Earlier this spring, San Francisco's Board of Supervisors instructed the Department of Public Health to form a task force to make recommendations on the establishment of safe injection venues.

Nationwide, several major cities—including Seattle, Baltimore and Philadelphia—are considering such publicly sanctioned locations as a means to curb escalating heroin drug overdoses and deaths; slow the spread of infectious diseases such as hepatitis C; and help people kick their lethal habits.

Across the United States, an exploding opioid epidemic has sent overdose deaths skyrocketing and policymakers scrambling for solutions. In 2015, opioid overdoses—both from prescription drugs and from more potent and easier-to-obtain street heroin—took the lives of 2,018 Californians and 33,091 Americans, according to data from the Kaiser Family Foundation. (California Healthline is produced by Kaiser Health News, an editorially independent service of the foundation.)

"This is a medical issue, it is a brain disease, and we have to get out of our shell of thinking that these are bad people and … they have to hit bottom and then decide to pull themselves up by their own bootstraps," said Barbara A. Garcia, director of health at the public health department in San Francisco, where 22,000 residents are known IV drug users. "That's the pathway to death."

Safe injection sites would go beyond existing needle exchanges by allowing drug use on the premises. Under the proposed California measure, introduced by Assemblywoman Susan Talamantes Eggman (D–Stockton), health care providers stationed at the sites would be armed with the emergency medication naloxone, which is used to help revive people from opioid overdoses.

"What we're talking about here is essentially a medical facility," said Christian Burkin, a spokesman for Eggman. "This is an opportunity to take drug abuse off the streets and put it into a safe and sterile environment."

Opponents of the measure, including many law enforcement organizations, fear such sites would only serve to normalize illicit drug use and harm local neighborhoods.

"It creates a danger for the communities that these safe consumption program sites would be located in," said Cory Salzillo, legislative director for the California State Sheriffs' Association. "It doesn't require anybody to undergo treatment. … It's just effectively: 'Here's a safe place for you where you can come; here's your needle, your paraphernalia and here you go, shoot up.'"

Even if the state measure were to pass, it might face significant resistance from the federal government, since the drugs that would be injected are illegal under U.S. law, said Stanley Goldman, a criminal law professor at Loyola Law School in Los Angeles.

"So you'd have to be fairly assured that the federal government was not going to proceed against such operations before people could feel completely comfortable with participating," Goldman said.

Cary Quashen, president and founder of the Santa Clarita rehabilitation center where Biggs works, said that while he also has some reservations, he'd be likely to support the concept as long as drug users are offered access to recovery services at the centers.

"We got to do something different. People are dying everywhere," Quashen said. "We lose more people in this country to accidental overdoses than to car crashes and gun violence."

Burkin noted that the proposed safe injection clinics would be restricted to areas "where they are experiencing a high rate of opioid abuse, including death."

A 2011 study published in *The Lancet* found that overdose deaths on the streets surrounding Vancouver's safe injection site dropped 35 percent in the two years after it opened, compared with the two prior years. In the rest of the city, overdose deaths dropped 9.3 percent during the same period.

Another study showed a 30 percent increase in the use of addiction treatment services associated with the opening of the Vancouver site. Studies also suggest that supervised injection facilities in Australia and Europe have reduced overdoses without an increase of drug injecting or trafficking in their communities.

"We are not supporting what people call 'shooting galleries,'" said Garcia, the San Francisco public health director. "I don't believe in allowing people to just sit in a room and shoot drugs with each other—that is not something I'm going to support. What I will support is how do we engage those who are using drugs to help them reduce their harm and get better and go into recovery eventually."

Another argument in favor of supervised injection sites is financial: Two recent studies showed that a single supervised injection site would save $3.5 million a year on health care costs in San Francisco and $6 million in Baltimore.

Burkin believes that, given a chance, the safe injection pilot programs will prove their worth.

"Someone addicted to opioids who is going to come to a facility like this is someone starting on the first step toward recovery," he said. "This is not someone who is going to ignore appeals or attempts to get them connected to services."

Tawny Biggs agrees. If it were not for a work colleague in recovery who introduced her to a 12-step program years ago, she said, she would not have survived.

When her boyfriend gave her that first hit of heroin, she said, it didn't seem like a big deal.

"I was thinking, 'I can handle this,'" Biggs recalled. "Then something snapped in my brain and there became no control over needing it. I knew at that point it was either I gave up my son to my mom and shot up dope until I died, or I got some sort of help."

21. Treating the New Hep C Generation on Their Turf*

Pauline Bartolone

UKIAH, Calif.—Once a week, Dr. Diana Sylvestre puts her medical expertise to use in a rickety old house frequented by drug users in this small Northern California city.

She sets up in a stuffy office no bigger than a walk-in closet, just feet from a room where people who shoot heroin or methamphetamine drop off used needles and pick up clean ones. The needle exchange and Sylvestre's makeshift clinic are under the same roof, part of a program run by the Mendocino County AIDS/Viral Hepatitis Network.

Sylvestre comes here in part to treat young drug users, people who are often homeless or suffering from mental illness, many of them newly infected with hepatitis C. She doesn't see many of them at a hepatitis C clinic she runs in Oakland.

"They are the ones who are spreading hepatitis C," she said. "They're the ones who have the high-risk behaviors."

The opioid addiction crisis has engendered an unfortunate side effect—an epidemic of new hepatitis C infections, mainly among young people who share infected needles. Although people over age 52 still account for the largest share of chronic hepatitis C cases, the highest number of new infections occurs among people in their 20s.

From 2009 to 2015, the rate of acute hepatitis C cases in the United States roughly tripled among people in their 20s, and it more than doubled among people ages 30 to 39, according to the Centers for Disease Control and Prevention.

In California, newly reported cases shot up 55 percent among men in their 20s and 37 percent for women in that age range from 2007 to 2015, the California Department of Public Health (CDPH) said.

The wave of hepatitis C infections among young people is "cause for alarm," said John Ward, the CDC's viral hepatitis director. The agency is studying the best ways to treat this population, he said, adding that a new "front of attack" is needed. Health experts and doctors like Sylvestre say that battle may be best waged outside traditional health care settings, in places frequented by young drug users.

At the needle exchange in Ukiah, caseworkers give $7 Subway gift cards to people who agree to be tested for hepatitis C. Those who test positive can visit Sylvestre and try

---

*Originally published as Pauline Bartolone, "Treating the New Hep C Generation on Their Turf," *Kaiser Health News*, https://khn.org/news/treating-the-new-hep-c-generation-on-their-turf/ (December 7, 2017). Reprinted with permission of the publisher. Kaiser Health News is a nonprofit news service covering health issues. It is an editorially independent program of the Kaiser Family Foundation that is not affiliated with Kaiser Permanente. This KHN story first published on California Healthline, a service of the California Health Care Foundation.

to qualify for expensive new medications that wipe out the virus. Drug users can also get help for their substance abuse.

Patient advocates say this kind of on-site treatment is an anomaly in California, where only a few needle exchanges offer such services.

Treating young drug users is not easy, Sylvestre said. Their lives are chaotic, which makes it difficult to start or continue their medication. "They're frequently homeless; they have untreated mental illness," she said. "They aren't the most reliable people in the world."

The surge in hepatitis C cases among young people doesn't surprise 28-year-old Stephanie Clarizio of San Francisco. She injected heroin for about six years, starting in her home town of Atlanta. Clarizio said many of her friends who used intravenous drugs there knew about the risk of hepatitis C, and many of them contracted the virus.

"Everyone kind of knows about it," Clarizio said. "You just don't care."

Clarizio had hepatitis C for a couple of years before she was cured in San Francisco while in rehab for heroin addiction.

Experts and government officials say they're concerned about the surge among young people, who are more challenging to treat because many of them do not regularly see a doctor.

Many people who have been recently infected don't experience symptoms of the viral disease. Left untreated, hepatitis C can cause severe liver damage or cancer later in life.

While the baby boomer generation, defined by the CDC as those people born between 1945 and 1965, still accounts for three-quarters of chronic cases, University of California–Berkeley epidemiologist Art Reingold suggests the public health response should target the newly infected population.

"The prevention opportunity is much greater" when treating the younger generation, Reingold explained. "If you're working on a group that's already got [75 percent] of the people infected, your opportunity to prevent new infections is much smaller."

Dr. Heidi Bauer, chief of the sexually transmitted diseases control branch at the state Department of Public Health, said she encourages local health departments and community-based organizations to be creative about treating the younger population.

"We ask for people to think beyond that baby boomer box," Bauer said. Public health organizations "can take their services on the road, so to speak, and they can make an extra effort to reach populations that may be more at risk."

Dr. Sylvestre has been doing just that for more than a year. "If they're not going to show up in our medical facilities, we need to go out where they are there," she said.

Ashley Greene, a 29-year-old resident of Eureka, Calif., said treating young drug users for hepatitis C at needle exchanges is a good strategy. Greene recently recovered from the disease, which she said she contracted injecting cocaine as a teenager. She also used heroin on and off until 2011.

Greene feels much more energetic, clear-minded and optimistic about life since she was cured of hepatitis C, and she supports anything that educates young drug users about treatment, she said.

Not all will be ready for treatment, but at least "you can lead them to water," she said.

Part III

Practices, Programs, and Policies of Governments and Nonprofits

• *A. Federal* •

22. New Rules for Safe and Secure Prescription Drug Disposal Options*

U.S. Drug Enforcement Administration

(WASHINGTON)—The U.S. Drug Enforcement Administration's Final Rule for the Disposal of Controlled Substances, which implements the Secure and Responsible Drug Disposal Act of 2010, was made available online for preview by the Federal Register at https://s3.amazonaws.com/public-inspection.federalregister.gov/2014-20926.pdf. The Act, in an effort to curtail the prescription drug abuse epidemic, authorized DEA to develop and implement regulations that outline methods to transfer unused or unwanted pharmaceutical controlled substances to authorized collectors for the purpose of disposal. The Act also permits long-term-care facilities to do the same on behalf of residents or former residents of their facilities.

"These new regulations will expand the public's options to safely and responsibly dispose of unused or unwanted medications," said DEA Administrator Leonhart. "The new rules will allow for around-the-clock, simple solutions to this ongoing problem. Now everyone can easily play a part in reducing the availability of these potentially dangerous drugs."

Prior to the passage of the Act, the Controlled Substances Act made no legal provisions for patients to rid themselves of unwanted pharmaceutical controlled substances except to give them to law enforcement, and banned pharmacies, doctors' offices, and hospitals from accepting them. Most people flushed their unused drugs down the toilet, threw them in the trash, or kept them in the household medicine cabinet.

Unused medications in homes create a public health and safety concern, because they are highly susceptible to accidental ingestion, theft, misuse, and abuse. Almost twice as many (6.8 million) currently abuse pharmaceutical controlled substances than the number of those using cocaine, hallucinogens, heroin, and inhalants *combined*, according to the 2012 National Survey on Drug Use and Health. Nearly 110 Americans die every day from drug-related overdoses, and about half of those overdoses are related to opioids, a class of drug that includes prescription painkillers and heroin. About 70 percent of people who misuse prescription painkillers for the first time report obtaining the drugs from friends or relatives, including from the home medicine cabinet.

---

*Public document originally published as Drug Enforcement Administration, "New Rules for Safe and Secure Prescription Drug Disposal Options," https://www.dea.gov/press-releases/2014/09/08/dea-releases-new-rules-create-convenient-safe-and-secure-prescription (September 8, 2014).

As a temporary measure, DEA began hosting National Prescription Drug Take-Back events in September 2010. Since then, the DEA has sponsored eight take-back days. Enormous public participation in those events resulted in the collection of more than 4.1 million (over 2,100 tons) of medication at over 6,000 sites manned by law enforcement partners throughout all 50 states, the District of Columbia, and several U.S. territories.

"Every day, I hear from another parent who has tragically lost a son or daughter to an opioid overdose. No words can lessen their pain," said Michael Botticelli, Acting Director of National Drug Control Policy. "But we can take decisive action, like the one we're announcing today, to prevent more lives from being cut short far too soon. We know that if we remove unused painkillers from the home, we can prevent misuse and dependence from ever taking hold. These regulations will create critical new avenues for addictive prescription drugs to leave the home and be disposed of in a safe, environmentally friendly way."

The public may visit www.dea.gov or call 1–800–882–9539 to find a nearby collection site.

DEA's goal in implementing the Act is to expand the options available to safely and securely dispose of potentially dangerous prescription medications on a routine basis.

- The Final Rule authorizes certain DEA (manufacturers, distributors, reverse distributors, narcotic treatment programs, retail pharmacies, and hospitals/clinics with an on-site pharmacy) to modify their registration with the DEA to become authorized collectors.
- All collectors may operate a collection receptacle at their registered location, and collectors with an on-site means of destruction may operate a mail-back program.
- Retail pharmacies and hospitals/clinics with an on-site pharmacy may operate collection receptacles at long-term care facilities.
- The public may find authorized collectors in their communities by calling the DEA Office of Diversion Control's Registration Call Center at 1–800–882–9539.
- Law enforcement continues to have autonomy with respect to how they collect pharmaceutical controlled substances from ultimate users, including holding take-back events. Any person or entity-DEA registrant or non-registrant-may partner with law enforcement to conduct take-back events.
- Patients also may continue to utilize the guidelines for the disposal of pharmaceutical controlled substances listed by the Food and Drug Administration on their website at http://www.fda.gov/downloads/Drugs/ResourcesForYou/Consumers/
- BuyingUsingMedicineSafely/UnderstandingOver-the-CounterMedicines/ucm107163.pdf
- Any method of disposal that was valid prior to these new regulations being implemented continues to be valid.

23. Safely Using Sharps (Needles and Syringes) at Home, at Work and on Travel*

U.S. Food and Drug Administration

Sharps is a medical term for devices with sharp points or edges that can puncture or cut skin. They may be used at home, at work, and while traveling to manage the medical conditions of people or their pets, including allergies, arthritis, cancer, diabetes, hepatitis, HIV/AIDS, infertility, migraines, multiple sclerosis, osteoporosis, blood clotting disorders, and psoriasis.

Examples of sharps include:

- Needles—hollow needles used to inject drugs (medication) under the skin.
- Syringes—devices used to inject medication into or withdraw fluid from the body.
- Lancets, also called "fingerstick" devices—instruments with a short, two-edged blade used to get drops of blood for testing. Lancets are commonly used in the treatment of diabetes.
- Auto Injectors, including epinephrine and insulin pens—syringes pre-filled with fluid medication designed to be self-injected into the body.
- Infusion sets—tubing systems with a needle used to deliver drugs to the body.
- Connection needles/sets—needles that connect to a tube used to transfer fluids in and out of the body. This is generally used for patients on home hemodialysis.

How to Dispose of Sharps

Used sharps should be immediately placed in a sharps disposal container. FDA-cleared sharps containers are generally available through pharmacies, medical supply companies, health care providers and online. These containers are made of puncture-resistant plastic with leak-resistant sides and bottom. They also have a tight fitting, puncture-resistant lid.

If an FDA-cleared container is not available a heavy-duty plastic household container, such as a laundry detergent container can be used as an alternative.

---

*Public document originally published as Food and Drug Administration, "Safely Using Sharps (Needles and Syringes) at Home, at Work and on Travel," https://www.fda.gov/medical-devices/consumer-products/safely-using-sharps-needles-and-syringes-home-work-and-travel (August 30, 2018).

Used needles and other sharps are dangerous to people and pets if not disposed of safely because they can injure people and spread infections that cause serious health conditions. The most common infections are:

- Hepatitis B (HBV),
- Hepatitis C (HCV), and
- Human Immunodeficiency Virus (HIV).
- Safe sharps disposal is important whether you are at home, at work, at school, traveling, or in other public places such as hotels, parks, and restaurants.

Never place loose needles and other sharps (those that are not placed in a sharps disposal container) in the household or public trash cans or recycling bins, and never flush them down the toilet. This puts trash and sewage workers, janitors, housekeepers, household members, and children at risk of being harmed.

Pet owners who use needles to give medicine to their pets should follow the same sharps disposal guidelines used for humans.

What to Do If You Are Accidentally Stuck by a Used Needle or Other Sharp

If you are accidently stuck by another person's used needle or other sharp:

- Wash the exposed area right away with water and soap or use a skin disinfectant (antiseptic) such as rubbing alcohol or hand sanitizer.
- Seek immediate medical attention by calling your physician or local hospital.
- Follow these same instructions if you get blood or other bodily fluids in your eyes, nose, mouth, or on your skin.

FDA-Cleared Sharps Containers

The FDA recommends that used needles and other sharps be immediately placed in FDA-cleared sharps disposal containers. FDA-cleared sharps disposal containers are generally available through pharmacies, medical supply companies, health care providers, and online.

The FDA has evaluated the safety and effectiveness of these containers and has cleared them for use by health care professionals and the public to help reduce the risk of injury and infections from sharps.

FDA-cleared sharps disposal containers are made from rigid plastic and come marked with a line that indicates when the container should be considered full, which means it's time to dispose of the container.

FDA-cleared sharps disposal containers are available in a variety of sizes, including smaller travel sizes to use while away from home.

A list of products and companies with FDA-cleared sharps disposal containers can be found here. Although the products on this list have received FDA clearance, all products may not be currently available on the market.

Alternative Sharps Disposal Containers

If an FDA-cleared container is not available, some organizations and community guidelines recommend using a heavy-duty plastic household container as an alternative. The container should be leak-resistant, remain upright during use and have a tight fitting, puncture-resistant lid, such as a plastic laundry detergent container.

Household containers should also have the basic features of a good sharps disposal container described below.

All sharps disposal containers should be:

- made of a heavy-duty plastic;
- able to close with a tight-fitting, puncture-resistant lid, without sharps being able to come out;
- upright and stable during use;
- leak-resistant; and
- properly labeled to warn of hazardous waste inside the container.

When your sharps disposal container is about three-quarters (3/4) full, follow your community guidelines for proper disposal methods.

Best Way to Get Rid of Used Needles and Other Sharps

The FDA recommends a two-step process for properly disposing of used needles and other sharps.

Step 1: Place all needles and other sharps in a sharps disposal container immediately after they have been used.

This will reduce the risk of needle sticks, cuts, and punctures from loose sharps. Sharps disposal containers should be kept out of reach of children and pets.

Note: Overfilling a sharps disposal container increases the risk of accidental needle-stick injury. When your sharps disposal container is about three-quarters (3/4) full, follow your community guidelines for getting rid of the container (Step 2, below).

DO NOT reuse sharps disposal containers.

Be prepared when leaving home. Always carry a small, travel-size sharps disposal container in case other options are not available.

If traveling by plane, check the Transportation Security Administration (TSA) website for up-to-date rules on what to do with your sharps. To make your trip through airport security easier, make sure your medicines are labeled with the type of medicine and the manufacturer's name or a drug store label, and bring a letter from your doctor.

Step 2: Dispose of used sharps disposal containers according to your community guidelines.

Sharps disposal guidelines and programs vary depending on where you live. Check with your local trash removal services or health department (listed in the city or county government [blue] pages in your phone book) to see which of the following disposal methods are available in your area:

Other Methods

Drop Box or Supervised Collection Sites: You may be able to drop off your sharps disposal containers at appropriate chosen collection sites, such as doctors' offices, hospitals, pharmacies, health departments, medical waste facilities, and police or fire stations. Services may be free or have a nominal fee.

Household Hazardous Waste Collection Sites: You may be able to drop off your sharps disposal containers at local public household hazardous waste collection sites. These are sites that also commonly accept hazardous materials such as household cleaners, paints and motor oil.

Mail-Back Programs: You may be able to mail certain FDA-cleared sharps disposal containers to a collection site for proper disposal, usually for a fee. Fees vary, depending on the size of the container. Follow the container manufacturer's instructions because mail-back programs may have specific requirements on how to label sharps disposal containers.

Residential Special Waste Pick-Up Services: Your community may provide special waste pick-up services that send trained special waste handlers to collect sharps disposal containers from your home. These services are typically fee-based and many have special requirements for the types of containers they will collect. Some programs require customers to call and request pick-ups, while other offer regular pick-up schedules.

For more information specific to your state, call Safe Needle Disposal at 1–800–643–1643 or e-mail info@safeneedledisposal.org. Information they can provide for your state includes:

- types of sharps containers that can be used,
- disposal programs in your area,
- how to label your sharps disposal containers,
- how to secure the lid of your sharps disposal container, and
- whether sharps disposal containers can be thrown away in the common trash.

What to Do if You Can't Find a Sharps Disposal Container: The safest way to dispose of a used needle is to immediately place it in a sharps disposal container to reduce the risk of needle sticks, cuts and punctures from loose sharps. If you cannot find a sharps disposal container right away, you may need to recap the needle or use a needle clipper until you have an opportunity to dispose of sharps in an appropriate sharps disposal container. Never throw away loose needles and other sharps in trash cans or recycling bins, and never flush them down the toilet.

Recapping

If you need to put the cap back on the needle (recap), do not bend or break the needle and **never** remove a hypodermic needle from the syringe by hand. This may result in accidental needle sticks, cuts or punctures. Recapping should be performed using a mechanical device or the one-handed technique (see below for step-by-step instructions). Recapped needles should be placed in a disposal container at the next available opportunity.

The One-Handed Needle Recapping Method

> Step 1: Place the cap on a flat surface like the table or counter with something firm to "push" the needle cap against
> Step 2: Holding the syringe with the needle attached in one hand, slip the needle into the cap without using the other hand
> Step 3: Push the capped needle against a firm object to "seat" the cap onto the needle firmly using only one hand.

Needle Clippers

Needle clippers make syringes unusable by clipping off the needle. Clippers may be used for needle disposal of small syringes (such as insulin syringes), but not for clipping lancets.

After the needle clipper clips off the needle from the syringe, the needle is automatically and safely retained within the clipper.

Do not attempt to clip a needle with any tool except a needle clipper designed to safely clip a needle.

Before using any of the above procedures, check your community guidelines for acceptable sharps disposal methods.

Tips for Health Care Providers

Health care providers should advise their patients on the safe disposal of needles and other sharps. The following information should help health care providers counsel their patients about safe sharps disposal:

- Find out about the sharps disposal programs available in your area and share this information with your patients. If pamphlets are available, consider placing them in your office waiting area.
- To learn about sharps disposal guidelines and programs in your community, visit the Safe Needle Disposal Website for more information specific to your state.
- Print out the DOs and DON'Ts of proper sharps disposal for your patients.

Tips for Employers and Businesses

The risk of needle sticks, cuts and punctures from needles and other sharps is high in facilities such as airports, hotels, restaurants, and office buildings. In these places, people are more likely to throw their used needles and sharps into the trash.

Employers and businesses should consider providing sharps disposal containers in restrooms or other designated areas and make employees and guests aware of the location of the containers. Businesses with sharps disposal containers in their restrooms may need to register with their state and/or local authorities as a "sharps collection station" because they may be considered "waste generators." Contact your state and/or local authorities for legal requirements that apply to the waste generated on their premises.

Dos and Don'ts of Proper Sharps Disposal

- DO immediately place used needles and other sharps in a sharps disposal container to reduce the risk of needle sticks, cuts or punctures from loose sharps.
- DO use an FDA-cleared sharps disposal container, if possible. If an FDA-cleared container is not available, some organizations and community guidelines recommend using a heavy-duty plastic household container as an alternative.
- DO make sure that if a household container is used, it has the basic features of a good disposal container.
- DO carry a portable sharps disposal container for travel.
- DO follow your community guidelines for getting rid of your sharps disposal container.
- DO call your local trash or public health department (listed in the county and city government section of your phone book) to find out about sharps disposal programs in your area.
- DO ask your health care provider, veterinarian, local hospital or pharmacist where and how to get an FDA-cleared sharps disposal container, if they can dispose of your used needles and other sharps, or if they know of sharps disposal programs near you.
- DO keep all sharps and sharps disposal containers out of reach of children and pets.
- DO seal sharps disposal containers when disposing of them, label them properly and check your community guidelines on how to properly dispose of them.
- DO ask your medical or prescription insurer whether they cover sharps disposal containers.
- DO ask the manufacturer of your drug products that are used with a needle or other sharps if they provide a sharps disposal container to patients at no charge.
- DO report a problem associated with sharps and disposal containers.
- DON'T throw loose needles and other sharps into the trash.
- DON'T flush needles and other sharps down the toilet.
- DON'T put needles and other sharps in your recycling bin—they are not recyclable.
- DON'T try to remove, bend, break, or recap needles used by another person. This can lead to accidental needle sticks, which may cause serious infections.
- DON'T attempt to remove the needle without a needle clipper because the needle could fall, fly off, or get lost and injure someone.

24. HRSA Implementation Guidance of Syringe Services Programs*

U.S. DEPARTMENT OF HEALTH AND HUMAN SERVICES

This guidance was developed in accordance with the Department of Health and Human Services Implementation Guidance to Support Certain Components of Syringe Services Programs, 2016.

Background

The Consolidated Appropriations Act, 2016 (Pub. L. 114–113), signed by President Barack Obama in December 2015, modifies the ban on the use of federal funds to support programs distributing sterile needles or syringes (referred to as "SSP") for Department of Health and Human Services (HHS) programs, including Health Resources and Services Administration (HRSA) programs. Federal funds may not be used to purchase sterile needles or syringes for the purpose of injecting illegal drugs. However, federal funds may be used to support various components of SSPs as outlined in the Department of Health and Human Services Implementation Guidance to Support Certain Components of Syringe Services Programs, 2016.

The following conditions must be met when federal funds are used for SSP.

1. The applicable state, local, territorial, or tribal health department must determine, in consultation with the Centers for Disease Control and Prevention (CDC), that the jurisdiction in which federal funds will be used for SSP is experiencing or is at risk of experiencing a significant increase in hepatitis or HIV infections due to injection drug use.

2. SSPs must adhere to federal, state and local laws, regulations, and other requirements related to such programs or services.

Process for HRSA Recipients to Use HRSA Funding to Support SSPs

HRSA recipients must obtain prior approval for use of HRSA funding to support SSPs.

---

*Public document originally published as U.S. Department of Health and Human Services, "HRSA Implementation Guidance of Syringe Services Programs," https://www.aids.gov/pdf/hhs-ssp-guidance.pdf (April 7, 2016).

Required Documentation

In accordance with Department of Health and Human Services Implementation Guidance to Support Certain Components of Syringe Services Programs, 2016, HRSA recipients that wish to use new or existing HRSA funds for SSPs are required to obtain the following documents:

- the CDC notification to the applicable state, local, territorial, or tribal health department that the evidence submitted by the health department is sufficient to demonstrate that the jurisdiction is experiencing, or is at risk for, a significant increase in hepatitis infections or an HIV outbreak due to injection drug use; and
- a certification in the form of a letter signed by the Health Officer from the state, local, territorial, or tribal health department that such program is operating in accordance with applicable law.

Approval Process

HRSA recipients must contact the corresponding HRSA project officer or contract officer, as applicable for the grant, cooperative agreement, or contract, to discuss their interest in using HRSA funds for SSPs. Requests to use HRSA funds for SSPs will require electronic submission of the required documentation described above. Recipients that wish to reallocate existing HRSA funding to support SSPs must follow standard procedures established for the awarded grant, cooperative agreement, or contract. Following submission of required documentation and HRSA approval, as applicable, funds may be reallocated starting in Fiscal Year (FY) 2016, and may continue in future FYs unless otherwise indicated. The HRSA project officer or contract officer will instruct the HRSA recipient of any additional requirements to implement use of HRSA funds for SSPs under the grant, cooperative agreement, or contract.

Future Plans

Beginning in FY 2017 and thereafter, HRSA FOAs will identify whether the programs funded under the FOA or contract will permit support of SSPs, including criteria for eligibility and any budgetary or programmatic requirements.

25. Implementation Guidance for Syringe Services Programs*

U.S. Department of Health and Human Services

SAMHSA-specific Guidance for Minority HIV/AIDS Initiative (MAI) Programs Implementing SSPs. This guidance was developed in accordance with HHS's Implementation Guidance for Syringe Services Programs (SSPs).

On December 18, 2015, President Barack Obama signed the Consolidated Appropriations Act, 2016 (Pub. L. 114–113),[1] which modifies the restriction on use of federal funds for programs distributing sterile needles or syringes (referred to as SSPs, or as syringe exchange programs) for HHS programs. The Consolidated Appropriations Act, 2016, Division H states:

SEC. 520. Notwithstanding any other provision of this Act, no funds appropriated in this Act shall be used to purchase sterile needles or syringes for the hypodermic injection of any illegal drug: Provided, That such limitation does not apply to the use of funds for elements of a program other than making such purchases if the relevant State or local health department, in consultation with the Centers for Disease Control and Prevention, determines that the State or local jurisdiction, as applicable, is experiencing, or is at risk for, a significant increase in hepatitis infections or an HIV outbreak due to injection drug use, and such program is operating in accordance with State and local law.

Pertinent language of the Consolidated Appropriations Act of 2016 (the Act) is found here: http://docs.house.gov/billsthisweek/20151214/CPRT-114-HPRT-RU00-SAHR2029-AMNT1final.pdf.

While the provision still prohibits the use of federal funds to purchase sterile needles or syringes for the purposes of hypodermic injection of any illicit drug, it allows for federal funds to be used for other aspects of SSPs based on evidence of a demonstrated need (i.e., experiencing, or at risk for, increases in hepatitis infections or an HIV outbreak due to injection drug use) by the state or local health department and in consultation with the Centers for Disease Control and Prevention (CDC). State and local health departments interested in redirecting federal funds to support SSPs should consult with CDC by providing evidence that their jurisdiction is (1) experiencing or, (2) at risk for increases in viral hepatitis infections or an HIV outbreak due to injection drug use. The scope of the presented evidence should address the geographic

---

*Public document originally published as U.S. Department of Health and Human Services, "Implementation Guidance for Syringe Services Programs," https://www.hiv.gov/sites/default/files/hhs-ssp-guidance.pdf (July 28, 2016).

area that will be served by the SSPs and include county, city and state level data, as appropriate.

Applicable Cooperative Agreements and Grants

Grants funded under the following six (6) FY 2016 Funding Opportunity Announcements (FOAs), the Targeted Capacity Expansion-HIV program FOAs (TI-12-007, TI-13-011, TI-15-006, TI-15-013, and TI-16-011) and the Minority AIDS Initiative Continuum of Care program (TI-14-013) may support SSP services with fiscal year 2016 and 2017[2] funds, with certain approvals, as an optional activity. Requests for funding for SSPs can be considered only if "the State or local health department, in consultation with the Centers for Disease Control and Prevention, determines that the State or local jurisdiction, as applicable, is experiencing, or is at risk for, a significant increase in hepatitis infections or an HIV outbreak due to injection drug use," as stated in the Act. Beginning in FY 2017, newly issued FOAs will include guidance on the use of funding to support SSP activities. SAMHSA funds cannot be used to supplant or replace state or other non-federal funds currently supporting SSP activities within a state or jurisdiction. In other words, SAMHSA funds cannot be used to fund an existing SSP so that state or other non-federal funding can be used for other activities or program services.

The grantee, in collaboration with the local public health department, may propose to use their SAMHSA funds to implement or support an SSP in accordance with State and local law and the following requirements:

1. Provide documentation that the state or local jurisdiction has submitted data and supporting documentation to CDC for review and determination of applicability and approval for an SSP has been granted.
2. Demonstrate how an SSP fits with the objectives of the FOA and assess the effectiveness of SSP activities in referring individuals to substance use disorder prevention and treatment, and co-occurring mental health services and in reducing HIV risk behaviors.
3. Receive approval from your Government Project Officer (GPO) and SAMHSA to proceed with submission of the request.
4. Once approved continue with the reporting requirements specified in your FOA and include reporting of the number of participants receiving SSP services, the number and types of services directly provided or provided by referrals and the amount of federal funds expended on SSP activities.

Allowed Use of Federal Funding to Support SSPs

1. Personnel to support SSP implementation and management (e.g., program staff, as well as staff for planning, monitoring, evaluation, and quality assurance).
2. Supplies to promote sterile injection and reduce infectious disease transmission through injection drug use, exclusive of sterile needles, syringes and other drug preparation equipment.
3. Testing kits for viral hepatitis (i.e., HBV and HCV) and HIV.

4. Syringe disposal services (e.g., contract or other arrangement for disposal of biohazardous material).

5. Navigation services to ensure linkage to: HIV and viral hepatitis prevention, testing, treatment and care services, including antiretroviral therapy for HCV and HIV, pre-exposure prophylaxis (PrEP), post-exposure prophylaxis (PEP), prevention of mother to child transmission and partner services; substance use disorder treatment, and medical and mental health care.

6. Educational materials, including information about: safer injection practices; reversing a drug overdose; HIV and viral hepatitis prevention, testing, treatment and care services; and mental health and substance use disorder treatment, including medication assisted treatment.

7. Male and female condoms to reduce sexual risk of HIV and other STD infections.

8. Referral to hepatitis A and hepatitis B vaccinations to reduce risk of viral hepatitis infection.

9. Communication, including use of social media technologies, and outreach activities designed to raise awareness about, and increase utilization, of SSPs.

10. SSP planning and non-research evaluation activities.

SAMHSA funds can only be used to establish new or expand existing SSPs with prior approval from the project officer and grants management officer. SSPs are subject to the terms and conditions incorporated or referenced in the recipient's federal funding. SAMHSA funds cannot be used to supplant or replace state or other non-federal funds currently supporting SSP activities within a jurisdiction. In other words, SAMHSA funds cannot be used to fund an existing SSP so that state or other non-federal funding can then be used for another program.

Grantee Process for Consideration of SSPs

Approval must be secured from the State Health Department, CDC, and the SAMHSA GPO. SAMHSA GPOs may require additional information such as:

- Description of proposed model(s) and plans, including MOUs with SSP providers who can supply needles;
- Timeline for implementation;
- Copy of existing SSP protocols or guidelines, if available;
- Description of current training and technical assistance needs;
- Location of SSP related activities to be supported with federal funds; and
- Signed statement (i.e., Annual Certification) that the grantee will comply with the language in the Consolidated Appropriations Act of 2016.

Additionally, any changes impacting your current program budget must be submitted to and approved by the Division of Grants Management. Budget revisions must include a revised budget form SF424a, detailed budget and budget narrative. The budget narrative must include a justification for budget changes, including any disposal equipment. The narrative must also clearly identify how these costs are related to activities in the budget.

Awardees implementing new or expanding existing SSPs will need to collect basic

SSP metrics information (e.g., number of syringes distributed, estimated number of syringes returned for safe disposal, number of persons tested for HIV or viral hepatitis, referrals to HIV, viral hepatitis and substance use disorder treatment) and amount of federal funds used for this program.

If you have any questions, contact your SAMHSA Project Officer.

Notes

1. https://www.congress.gov/114/bills/hr2029/BILLS-114hr2029enr.pdf. Accessed on December 22, 2015.

2. Use of 2017 funds for elements of syringe services programs is subject to an authorized appropriation for the fiscal year involved.

26. Injection Drug Use*

CENTERS FOR DISEASE CONTROL AND PREVENTION

Sharing needles, syringes, or other equipment (works) to inject drugs puts people at high risk for getting or transmitting HIV and other infections. People who inject drugs account for about 1 in 10 HIV diagnoses in the United States. Syringe services programs (SSPs) can play a role in preventing HIV and other health problems among PWID, by providing access to sterile syringes. These programs can also provide comprehensive services such as help with stopping substance misuse; testing and linkage to treatment for HIV, hepatitis B, and hepatitis C; education on what to do for an overdose; and other prevention services.

HIV and People Who Inject Drugs

People who inject drugs (PWID) are at high risk for getting HIV if they use needles, syringes, or other drug injection equipment—for example, cookers—that someone with HIV has used. New HIV diagnoses among PWID have declined in recent years in the 50 states and District of Columbia. However, injection drug use in nonurban areas has created prevention challenges and placed new populations at risk for HIV.

PWID accounted for 9% (3,641) of the 38,739 diagnoses of HIV in the US and dependent areas in 2017 (2,389 cases were attributed to injection drug use and 1,252 to male-to-male sexual contact and injection drug use).

Injection Drug Use and HIV Risk

Sharing needles, syringes, or other drug injection equipment—for example, cookers—puts people at risk for getting or transmitting HIV and other infections.

Risk of HIV

The risk for getting or transmitting HIV is very high if an HIV-negative person uses injection equipment that someone with HIV has used. This is because the needles,

---

*Public document originally published as Centers for Disease Control and Prevention, "Injection Drug Use," https://www.cdc.gov/hiv/risk/drugs/index.html.

syringes, or other injection equipment may have blood in them, and blood can carry HIV. HIV can survive in a used syringe for up to 42 days, depending on temperature and other factors.

Substance use disorder can also increase the risk of getting HIV through sex. When people are under the influence of substances, they are more likely to engage in risky sexual behaviors, such as having anal or vaginal sex without protection (like a condom or medicine to prevent or treat HIV), having sex with multiple partners, or trading sex for money or drugs.

Risk of Other Infections and Overdose

Sharing needles, syringes, or other injection equipment also puts people at risk for getting viral hepatitis. People who inject drugs should talk to a health care provider about getting a blood test for hepatitis B and C and getting vaccinated for hepatitis A and B.

In addition to being at risk for HIV and viral hepatitis, people who inject drugs can have other serious health problems, like skin infections and heart infections. People can also overdose and get very sick or even die from having too many drugs or too much of one drug in their body or from products that may be mixed with the drugs without their knowledge (for example, fentanyl).

Reducing the Risk

The best way to reduce the risk of getting or transmitting HIV through injection drug use is to stop injecting drugs.

The best way to reduce the risk of getting or transmitting HIV through injection drug use is to stop injecting drugs. People who inject drugs can talk with a counselor, doctor, or other health care provider about treatment for substance use disorder, including medication-assisted treatment. People can find treatment centers in their area by using the locator tools on Substance Abuse and Mental Health Services Administration (SAMHSA) or www.hiv.govexternal, or call 1–800–662-HELP (4357).

People who continue injecting drugs should never share needles, syringes, or other injection equipment such as cookers.

People who continue injecting drugs should never share needles, syringes, or other injection equipment such as cookers. Many communities have syringe services programs (SSPs) where people can get free sterile needles and syringes and safely dispose of used ones. SSPs can also refer people to treatment for substance use disorder and help them get tested for HIV and hepatitis. People can contact their local health department or the North American Syringe Exchange Network (NASEN) to find an SSP. Also, some pharmacies may sell needles and syringes without a prescription.

Other things people can do to lower their risk of getting or transmitting HIV, if they continue to inject drugs, include:

- Using bleach to clean needles, syringes, cookers, and surfaces where drugs are prepared. This may reduce the risk of HIV and hepatitis C but doesn't eliminate it. Bleach can't be used to clean water or cotton. New, sterile water or cotton should be used each time.

- Being careful not to get someone else's blood on their hands, needles, syringes, or other injection equipment.
- Disposing of syringes and needles safely after one use. People can put them in a sharps container or another container like an empty bleach or laundry detergent bottle. Keep all used syringes and needles away from other people.
- Asking their health care provider about taking daily medicine to prevent HIV (called pre-exposure prophylaxis or PrEP). People who take PrEP must take an HIV test before beginning PrEP and every 3 months while they're taking it.
- Taking HIV medicine if they have HIV. People with HIV who take HIV medicine as prescribed and get and keep an undetectable viral load have effectively no risk of transmitting HIV through sex. We don't know whether keeping an undetectable viral load prevents HIV transmission through sharing needles, syringes, or other injection equipment. It very likely reduces the risk, but we don't know by how much.
- Using a condom the right way every time they have anal or vaginal sex. Condom Dos and Don'ts:
- DO use a condom every time you have sex.
- DO put on a condom before having sex.
- DO read the package and check the expiration date.
- DO make sure there are no tears or defects.
- DO store condoms in a cool, dry place.
- DO use latex or polyurethane condoms.
- DO use water-based or silicone-based lubricant to prevent breakage.
- DON'T store condoms in your wallet as heat and friction can damage them.
- DON'T use nonoxynol-9 (a spermicide), as this can cause irritation.
- DON'T use oil-based products like baby oil, lotion, petroleum jelly, or cooking oil because they will cause the condom to break.
- DON'T use more than one condom at a time.
- DON'T reuse a condom.

27. Syringe Services Programs (SSPs) FAQs*

CENTERS FOR DISEASE CONTROL AND PREVENTION

Syringe services programs (SSPs) are also referred to as syringe exchange programs (SEPs) and needle exchange programs (NEPs). Although the services they provide may vary, SSPs are community-based programs that provide access to sterile needles and syringes, facilitate safe disposal of used syringes, and provide and link to other important services and programs such as:

- Referral to substance use disorder treatment programs.
- Referral to substance use disorder treatment programs.
- Screening, care, and treatment for viral hepatitis and HIV.
- Education about overdose prevention and safer injection practices.
- Vaccinations, including those for hepatitis A and hepatitis B.
- Screening for sexually transmitted diseases.
- Abscess and wound care.
- Naloxone distribution and education.
- Referral to social, mental health, and other medical services.

Are SSPs Legal?

Some states have passed laws specifically legalizing SSPs because of their life-saving potential. SSPs may also be legal in states where possession and distribution of syringes without a prescription are legal.

Decisions about use of SSPs as part of prevention programs are made at the state and local levels. The Federal Consolidated Appropriations Act of 2016 includes language that gives states and local communities meeting certain criteria the opportunity to use federal funds provided through the Department of Health and Human Services to support certain components of SSPs, with the exception of provision of needles, syringes, or other equipment used solely for the purposes of illicit drug use.

---

*Public document originally published as Centers for Disease Control and Prevention, "Syringe Services Programs (SSPs) FAQs," https://www.cdc.gov/ssp/syringe-services-programs-faq.html (May 23, 2019).

Do SSPs Help People to Stop Using Drugs?

Yes. When people who inject drugs use an SSP, they are more likely to enter treatment for substance use disorder and stop injecting than those who don't use an SSP.[1,2,3,4] New users of SSPs are five times as likely to enter drug treatment as those who don't use the programs. People who inject drugs and who have used an SSP regularly are nearly three times as likely to report a reduction in injection frequency as those who have never used an SSP.

Do SSPs Reduce Infections?

Yes. Nonsterile injections can lead to transmission of HIV, viral hepatitis, bacterial, and fungal infections and other complications. By providing access to sterile syringes and other injection equipment, SSPs help people prevent transmitting bloodborne and other infections when they inject drugs. In addition to being at risk for HIV, viral hepatitis, and other blood-borne and sexually transmitted diseases, people who inject drugs can get other serious, life-threatening, and costly health problems, such as infections of the heart valves (endocarditis), serious skin infections, and deep tissue abscesses. Access to sterile injection equipment can help prevent these infections, and health care provided at SSPs can catch these problems early and provide easy-to-access treatment to a population that may be reluctant to go to a hospital or seek other medical care.[5,6,7]

Do SSSPs Cause More Needles in Public Places?

No. Studies show that SSPs protect the public and first responders by providing safe needle disposal and reducing the presence of needles in the community.[8,9,10,11,12,13]

Do SSPs Lead to More Crime and/or Drug Use?

No. SSPs do not cause or increase illegal drug use. They do not cause or increase crime.[14,15]

Are SSPs Cost Effective?

Yes. SSPs reduce health care costs by preventing HIV, viral hepatitis, and other infections, including endocarditis, a life-threatening heart valve infection. The estimated lifetime cost of treating one person living with HIV is more than $450,000.[16] Hospitalizations in the U.S. for substance-use-related infections cost over $700 million each year.[17] SSPs reduce these costs and help link people to treatment to stop using drugs.

Do SSPs Reduce Drug Use and Drug Overdoses?

SSPs help people overcome substance use disorders. If people who inject drugs use an SSP, they are more likely to enter treatment for substance use disorder and reduce or stop injecting. A Seattle study found that new users of SSPs were five times as likely to enter drug treatment as those who didn't use the programs. People who inject drugs and who have used an SSP regularly are nearly three times as likely to report reducing or stopping illicit drug injection as those who have never used an SSP. SSPs play a key role in preventing overdose deaths by training people who inject drugs how to prevent, rapidly recognize, and reverse opioid overdoses. Specifically, many SSPs give clients and community members "overdose rescue kits" and teach them how to identify an overdose, give rescue breathing, and administer naloxone, a medication used to reverse overdose.[18,19,20,21,22,23]

Notes

1. Wodak, A., Cooney, A. Do needle syringe programs reduce HIV infection among injecting drug users: a comprehensive review of the international evidence. *Subst Use Misuse.* 2006;41(6–7):777–813.
2. Hagan, H., McGough, J.P., Thiede, H., Hopkins, S., Duchin, J., Alexander, E.R. Reduced injection frequency and increased entry and retention in drug treatment associated with needle-exchange participation in Seattle drug injectors. *J Subst Abuse Treat.* 2000;19(3):247–252.
3. Strathdee, S.A., Celentano, D.D., Shah, N., et al. Needle-exchange attendance and health care utilization promote entry into detoxification. *J Urban Health.* 1999;76(4):448–460.
4. Bluthenthal, R.N., Gogineni, A., Longshore, D., Stein, M. (2001). Factors associated with readiness to change drug use among needle-exchange users. *Drug Alcohol Depend.* 2001;62(3):225–230.
5. Robinowitz, N., Smith, M.E., Serio-Chapman, C., Chaulk, P., Johnson, K.E. Wounds on wheels: implementing a specialized wound clinic within an established syringe exchange program in Baltimore, Maryland. *Am J Public Health.* 2014;104(11):2057–2059. doi:10.2105/ AJPH.2014.302111.
6. Grau, L.E., Arevalo, S., Catchpool, C., Heimer, R. Expanding harm reduction services through a wound and abscess clinic. *Am J Public Health.* 2002;92(12):1915–1917.
7. Pollack, H.A., Khoshnood, K., Blankenship, K.M., Altice, F.L. The impact of needle exchange-based health services on emergency department use. *J Gen Intern Med.* 2002;17(5):341–348.
8. Tookes, H.E., Kral, A.H., Wenger, L.D., et al. A comparison of syringe disposal practices among injection drug users in a city with versus a city without needle and syringe programs. *Drug Alcohol Depend.* 2012;123(1–3):255–259. doi:10.1016/j.drugalcdep.2011.12.001.
9. Riley, E.D., Kral, A.H., Stopka, T.J., Garfein, R.S., Reuckhaus, P., Bluthenthal, R.N. Access to sterile syringes through San Francisco pharmacies and the association with HIV risk behavior among injection drug users. *J Urban Health.* 2010;87(4):534–542. doi:10.1007/s11524–010–9468-y.
10. Klein, S.J., Candelas, A.R., Cooper, J.G., et al. Increasing safe syringe collection sites in New York State. *Public Health Rep.* 2008;123(4):433–440. doi:10.1177/003335490812300404.
11. De Montigny, L., Vernez, Moudon A., Leigh, B., Kim, S.Y. Assessing a drop box program: a spatial analysis of discarded needles. *Int J Drug Policy.* 2010; 21(3):208–214. doi:10.1016/j.drugpo.2009.07.003.
12. Doherty, M.C., Junge, B., Rathouz, P., Garfein, R.S., Riley, E., Vlahov, D. The effect of a needle exchange program on numbers of discarded needles: a 2-year follow-up. *Am J Public Health.* 2000;90(6):936–939.
13. Bluthenthal, R.N., Anderson, R., Flynn, N.M., Kral, A.H. Higher syringe coverage is associated with lower odds of HIV risk and does not increase unsafe syringe disposal among syringe exchange program clients. *Drug Alcohol Depend.* 2007;89(2–3):214–222.
14. Marx, M.A., Crape, B., Brookmeyer, R.S., et al. Trends in crime and the introduction of a needle exchange program. *Am J Public Health.* 2000;90(12),1933–1936.
15. Galea, S., Ahern, J., Fuller, C., Freudenberg, N., Vlahov, D. Needle exchange programs and experience of violence in an inner city neighborhood. *J Acquir Immune Defic Syndr.* 2001;28(3),282–288.
16. Farnham, P.G., Gopalappa, C., Sansom, S.L., et al. Updates of lifetime costs of care and quality of life estimates for HIV-infected persons in the United States: Late versus early diagnosis and entry into care. *J Acquir Immune Defic Syndr.* 2013;64(2):183–189. doi:10.1097/ QAI.0b013e3182973966.
17. Ronan, M., & Herzig, S. (2016). Hospitalizations related to opioid abuse/dependence and associated serious infections increased sharply, 2002–12. *Health Affairs* (Millwood). 2016;35(5):832–837. doi: 10.1377/hlthaff.2015.1424.
18. Seal, K.H., Thawley, R., Gee, L. Naloxone distribution and cardiopulmonary resuscitation training for injection drug users to prevent heroin overdose death: A pilot intervention study. *J Urban Health.* 2005;82(2):303–311. doi:10.1093/jurban/jti053.
19. Galea, S., Worthington, N., Piper, T.M., Nandi, V.V., Curtis, M., Rosenthal, D.M. Provision of naloxone to injection drug users as an overdose prevention strategy: Early evidence from a pilot study in New York City. *Addict Behav.* 2006;31(5):907–912. doi:10.1016/j. addbeh.2005.07.020.

20. Tobin, K.E., Sherman, S.G., Beilenson, P., Welsh, C., Latkin, C.A. Evaluation of the Staying Alive program: Training injection drug users to properly administer naloxone and save lives. *Int J Drug Policy.* 2009;20(2):131–136. doi:10.1016/j.drugpo.2008.03.002.

21. Doe-Simkins, M., Walley, A.Y., Epstein, A., Moyer, P. Saved by the nose: Bystander-administered intranasal naloxone hydrochloride for opioid overdose. *Am J Public Health.* 2009;99(5):788–791. doi:10.2105/ajph.2008.146647.

22. Bennett, A.S., Bell, A., Tomedi, L., Hulsey, E.G., Kral, A.H. Characteristics of an overdose prevention, response, and naloxone distribution program in Pittsburgh and Allegheny County, Pennsylvania. *J Urban Health.* 2011;88(6):1020–1030. doi:10.1007/s11524-011-9600-7.

23. Leece, P.N., Hopkins, S., Marshall, C., Orkin, A., Gassanov, M.A., Shahin, R.M. Development and implementation of an opioid overdose prevention and response program in Toronto, Ontario. *Can J Public Health.* 2013;104(3):e200–204.

28. The Safety and Effectiveness of Syringe Services Programs*

CENTERS FOR DISEASE CONTROL AND PREVENTION

The nation is currently experiencing an opioid crisis involving the misuse of prescription opioid pain relievers as well as heroin and fentanyl.[1,2] The increase in substance use has resulted in concomitant increases in injection drug use across the country.[3] This has caused not only large increases in overdose deaths,[4] but also tens of thousands of viral hepatitis infections annually[5] and is threatening recent progress made in HIV prevention.[6] The most effective way for individuals who inject drugs to avoid the negative consequences of injection drug use is to stop injecting.[7,8] However, many people are unable or unwilling to do so, or they have little or no access to effective treatment. Approximately 775,000 Americans report having injected a drug in the past year.[9] In 2017, 14% of high school students reported using opioids without a prescription and 1.5% reported having ever injected drugs.[10]

Syringe services programs (SSPs) are proven and effective community-based prevention programs that can provide a range of services, including access to and disposal of sterile syringes and injection equipment, vaccination, testing, and linkage to infectious disease care and substance use treatment. SSPs reach people who inject drugs, an often hidden and marginalized population. Nearly 30 years of research has shown that comprehensive SSPs are safe, effective, and cost-saving, do not increase illegal drug use or crime, and play an important role in reducing the transmission of viral hepatitis, HIV and other infections.[11,12] Research shows that new users of SSPs are five times more likely to enter drug treatment and about three times more likely to stop using drugs than those who don't use the programs.[13] SSPs that provide naloxone also help decrease opioid overdose deaths. SSPs protect the public and first responders by facilitating the safe disposal of used needles and syringes.

Appropriations language from Congress in fiscal years 2016–2018 permits use of funds from the Department of Health and Human Services (HHS), under certain circumstances, to support SSPs with the exception that funds may not be used to purchase needles or syringes.[14] State, local, tribal, or territorial health departments must first consult with CDC and provide evidence that their jurisdiction is experiencing or at risk for significant increases in hepatitis infections or an HIV outbreak due to injection drug

---

*Public document originally published as Centers for Disease Control and Prevention, "The Safety and Effectiveness of Syringe Services Programs," https://www.cdc.gov/ssp/syringe-services-programs-summary.html (May 23, 2019).

use.[15] CDC has developed guidance and consults with state, local, or tribal and territorial health departments on determining if they have adequately demonstrated need according to federal law. Decisions about use of SSPs to prevent disease transmission and support the health and engagement of people who inject drugs are made at the state and local level.

Prevention of Infectious Diseases

Viral hepatitis, HIV, and other blood-borne pathogens can spread through injection drug use if people use needles, syringes, or other injection materials that were previously used by someone who had one of these infections. Injecting drugs can also lead to other serious health problems, such as skin infections, abscesses and endocarditis. The best way to reduce the risk of acquiring and transmitting disease through injection drug use is to stop injecting drugs. For people who do not stop injecting drugs, using sterile injection equipment for each injection can reduce the risk of infection and prevent outbreaks.

During the last decade, the United States has seen an increase in injection drug use—primarily the injection of opioids. Outbreaks of hepatitis C, hepatitis B and HIV infections have been correlated with these injection patterns and trends.[16,17] The majority of new hepatitis C virus (HCV) infections are due to injection drug use, and the nation has seen a 3.5-fold increase in reported cases of HCV from 2010 to 2016, reaching a 15-year high. New HCV virus infections are increasing most rapidly among young people, with the greatest incidence among individuals under 30.

Until recently, CDC had observed a steady decline since the mid–1990s in HIV diagnoses attributable to injection drug use. However, recent data show progress has stalled. Notably, new HIV infections among white people who inject drugs, the group most affected by the expanding opioid epidemic, increased 10% from 2014 to 2015.[18] The estimated lifetime cost of treating one person living with HIV is near $450,000.[19] Hospitalization in the US due to substance-use related infections alone costs over $700 million annually.[20] In the United States, the estimated cost of providing health care services for people living with chronic HCV infection is $15 billion annually.[21] SSPs can help reduce these healthcare costs by preventing viral hepatitis, HIV, endocarditis and other infections.

SSPs are a tool that can help reduce transmission of viral hepatitis, HIV, and other blood-borne infections. SSPs are associated with an approximately 50% reduction in HIV and HCV incidence. When combined with medications that treat opioid dependence (also known as medication-assisted treatment) HIV and HCV transmission is reduced by more than two-thirds.[22,23]

Linkage to Substance Use Treatment, Naloxone, and Other Healthcare Services

Syringe services programs serve as a bridge to other health services including, HCV and HIV diagnosis and treatment and MAT for substance use.[24] The majority of SSPs offer referrals to MAT,[25] and people who inject drugs who regularly use an SSP are more than five times as likely to enter treatment for a substance use disorder and nearly three times as likely to report reducing or discontinuing injection as those who have never used an SSP. SSPs facilitate entry into treatment for substance use disorders by people who inject drugs.[26,27,28] People who use SSPs show high readiness to reduce or stop their drug use.[29] There is also evidence that people who inject drugs who work with a nurse at an SSP or other community-based venue are more likely to access primary care than those who don't, also increasing access to MAT.[30] Many comprehensive community-based SSPs offer a range of preventative services including vaccination, infectious disease testing, and linkage to healthcare services.

Syringe services programs can reduce overdose deaths by teaching people who inject drugs how to prevent and respond to a drug overdose, providing them training on how to use naloxone, a medication used to reverse overdose, and providing naloxone to them. Many SSPs provide "overdose prevention kits" containing naloxone to people who inject drugs.[31,32] SSPs have partnered with law enforcement, providing naloxone to local police departments to help them keep their communities safer.[33]

Public Safety

Syringe services programs can benefit communities and public safety by reducing needlestick injuries and overdose deaths, without increasing illegal injection of drugs or criminal activity. Studies show that SSPs protect first responders and the public by providing safe needle disposal and reducing community presence of needles.[34,35,36,37,38] As many as one in every three officers may be stuck by a used needle during his or her career.[39] Needle stick injuries are among the most concerning and stressful events experienced by law officers.[40,41] A study compared the prevalence of improperly disposed of syringes and self-reported disposal practices in a city with SSPs (San Francisco) to a city without SSPs (Miami) and found eight times as many improperly disposed of syringes in Miami, the city without SSPs.[34] People who inject drugs in San Francisco also reported higher rates of safe disposal practices than those in Miami. Data from CDC's National HIV Behavioral Surveillance system in 2015 showed that the more syringes distributed at SSPs per people who inject drugs in a geographic region, the more likely people who inject drugs in that region were to report safe disposal of used syringes.[42]

Evidence demonstrates that SSPs do not increase illegal drug use or crime.[43,44] Studies in Baltimore[44] and New York City[43] have found no difference in crime rates between areas with and areas without SSPs. In Baltimore, trends in arrests were examined before and after a SSP was opened and found that there was not a significant increase in crime rates. The study in New York City assessed whether proximity to an SSP was associated with experiencing violence in an inner city neighborhood and found no association.

SSP Implementation

Not all SSPs are alike. Programs differ in size, scope, geographic location, and delivery venue (e.g., mobile vs. fixed sites). Community acceptance and legality also impact program success. Prior to establishing an SSP, it is important for public health agencies (or others) to assess the needs of potential clients, their families, key stakeholders, law enforcement, and the community at large.

The decision to incorporate SSPs as part of a comprehensive prevention program is made at the state and local level. Laws vary by state and can either increase or reduce access to SSPs. CDC created a guidance document to aid state and local health departments in managing HIV and hepatitis C outbreaks among people who inject drugs, which provides best practices to consider when establishing an SSP.[45] Conducting a needs assessment prior to the establishment of an SSP, developing evaluation tools, and careful planning of the operational tasks can increase the chances the SSP will be successful in a community.

HHS guidance states that SSPs should be part of a comprehensive service program that includes, as appropriate,[46]

- Provision of sterile needles, syringes, and other drug preparation equipment (purchased with non-federal funds) and disposal services.
- Education and counseling to reduce sexual, injection and overdose risks.
- Provision of condoms to reduce risk of sexual transmission of viral hepatitis, HIV or other sexually transmitted diseases.
- Provision of HIV, viral hepatitis, STD and tuberculosis screening.
- Provision of naloxone to reverse opioid overdoses.
- Referral and linkage to HIV, viral hepatitis, STD, and TB prevention, treatment, and care services, including antiretroviral therapy for HCV and HIV, pre-exposure prophylaxis (PrEP), post-exposure prophylaxis (PEP), prevention of mother-to-child transmission, and partner services.
- Referral and linkage to hepatitis A virus (HAV) and hepatitis B virus vaccination.
- Referral and linkage to and provision of substance use disorder treatment, including MAT for opioid use disorder, which combines drug therapy (e.g., methadone, buprenorphine, or naltrexone) with counseling and behavioral therapy.
- Referral to medical care, mental health services, and other support services.

Emerging Issues

In addition to the concerning increases in hepatitis and HIV rates, CDC has also identified additional emerging infectious disease risks related to injection drug use, including increases in methicillin-resistant *Staphylococcus aureus* (MRSA) infection rates, which increased 124% between 2011 and 2016 among people who inject drugs.[47] In addition, people who inject drugs are 16 times as likely as other people to develop invasive MRSA infections.

Rates of endocarditis, a life-threatening infection of the heart valves that can occur in people who inject drugs, has also increased. For example, in North Carolina alone, the rate of hospital discharge diagnoses for endocarditis related to drug dependence increased more than 12-fold from 2010 to 2015, with unadjusted hospital costs increasing from $1.1 million in 2010 to over $22 million in 2015.[48] Identifying and responding to these emerging infectious disease threats is critical to alleviate the subsequent harms of opioid misuse and abuse. These infections have been linked to frequency of injecting and to syringe sharing.[49] SSPs may help reduce bacterial infections by providing sterile injection equipment and linkage to substance use treatment.

Notes

1. What is the U.S. Opioid Epidemic? https://www.hhs.gov/opioids/about-the-epidemic/index.html.
2. Office of National Drug Control Policy. (n.d.) Prescription opioid misuse, heroin and fentanyl.
3. Zibbell, J. E., Asher, A. K., Patel, R. C., Kupronis, B., Iqbal, K., Ward, J. W., & Holtzman, D. (2018). Increases in Acute Hepatitis C Virus Infection Related to a Growing Opioid Epidemic and Associated Injection Drug Use, United States, 2004 to 2014. *Am J Public Health*, 108(2), 175–181. doi:10.2105/ ajph.2017.304132.
4. Centers for Disease Control and Prevention. (2018). Drug overdose death data.
5. Centers for Disease Control. (2018). Surveillance for Viral Hepatitis—United States, 2016.
6. Centers for Disease Control and Prevention. (2016). Vital signs: HIV and injection drug use [PDF—2.4 MB, 4 pages].
7. MacArthur, G. J., Minozzi, S., Martin, N., Vickerman, P., Deren, S., Bruneau, J., Hickman, M. (2012). Opiate substitution treatment and HIV transmission in people who inject drugs: systematic review and meta-analysis. Bmj, 345, e5945. doi:10.1136/bmj.e5945.
8. Martin, N. K., Hickman, M., Hutchinson, S. J., Goldberg, D. J., & Vickerman, P. (2013). Combination interventions to prevent HCV transmission among people who inject drugs: modeling the impact of antiviral treatment, needle and syringe programs, and opiate substitution therapy. *Clin Infect Dis*, 57 Suppl 2, S39–45. doi:10.1093/cid/cit329.
9. Lansky, A., Finlayson, T., Johnson, C., Holtzman, D., Wejnert, C., Mitsch, A., … Crepaz, N. (2014). Estimating the number of persons who inject drugs in the United States by meta-analysis to calculate national rates of HIV and hepatitis C virus infections. *PLoS ONE*, 9(5), e97596.
10. National Center for HIV/AIDS, Viral Hepatitis, STD, and TB Prevention: Division of Adolescent and School Health Centers for Disease Control and Prevention. *Youth Risk Behavior Survey Data Summary & Trends Report 2007–2017*.
11. Aspinall, E. J., Nambiar, D., Goldberg, D. J., Hickman, M., Weir, A., Van Velzen, E., … Hutchinson, S.J. (2014). Are needle and syringe programs associated with a reduction in HIV transmission among people who inject drugs: a systematic review and meta-analysis. *Int J Epidemiol*, 43(1), 235–248. doi:10.1093/ije/dyt243.
12. Bernard, C. L., Owens, D. K., Goldhaber-Fiebert, J. D., & Brandeau, M.L. (2017). Estimation of the cost-effectiveness of HIV prevention portfolios for people who inject drugs in the United States: A model-based analysis. *PLoS Med*, 14(5). doi:10.1371/journal.pmed.1002312.
13. Hagan, H., McGough, J.P., Thiede, H., Hopkins, S., Duchin, J., Alexander, E.R., "Reduced injection frequency and increased entry and retention in drug treatment associated with needle-exchange participation in Seattle drug injectors," *Journal of Substance Abuse Treatment*, 2000; 19:247–252.
14. Department of Defense and Labor, Health and Human Services, and Education Appropriations Act, 2019 (P.L. 115–245).
15. Centers for Disease Control and Prevention. (2018). Syringe service program determination of need.
16. Comer, M., Matthias, J., Nicholson, G., Asher, A., Holmberg, S., Wilson, C. Notes from the field: Increase in acute hepatitis B infections—Pasco County, Florida, 2011–2016. *MMWR Morb Mortal Wkly Rep 2018*;67:230–231.
17. Harris, A.M., Iqbal, K., Schillie, S., et al. Increases in acute hepatitis B virus infections—Kentucky, Tennessee, and West Virginia, 2006–2013. *MMWR Morb Mortal Wkly Rep 2016*;65:47–50.
18. Centers for Disease Control and Prevention. *HIV Surveillance Report*, 2016; vol. 28. Published November 2017. Accessed 7/30/2018.
19. Farnham, P.G. et al. Updates of lifetime costs of care and quality of life estimates for HIV-infected persons in the United States: Late versus early diagnosis and entry into care. *JAIDS 2013*; 64: 183–189. Estimates updated to 2017
20. Ronan, M., & Herzig, S. (2016). Hospitalizations related to opioid abuse/ dependence and associated serious infections increased sharply, 2002–12. *Health Affairs*, 35(5), 832–837.
21. Chahal, H. S., Marseille, E. A., Tice, J. A., Pearson, S. D., Ollendorf, D. A., Fox, R. K., et al. (2016, January). Cost-effectiveness of early treatment of hepatitis C virus genotype 1 by stage of liver fibrosis in a U.S. treatment-naive population. *The Journal of the American Medical Association*, 176(1), 65–73. Retrieved October 25, 2017.
22. Platt, L., Minozzi, S., Reed, J., Vickerman, P., Hagan, H., French, C., Jordan, A., Degenhardt, L., Hope, V., Hutchinson, S., Maher, L., Palmateer, N., Taylor, A., Bruneau, J., Hickman, M. Needle syringe programs and opioid substitution therapy for preventing hepatitis C transmission in people who inject drugs. *Cochrane Database of Systematic Reviews 2017*, Issue 9. Art. No.: CD012021. DOI: 10.1002/14651858.CD012021.pub2
23. Fernandes, R. M., Cary, M., Duarte, G., Jesus, G., Alarcao, J., Torre, C., … Carneiro, A.V. (2017). Effectiveness of needle and syringe programs in people who inject drugs—An overview of systematic reviews. *BMC Public Health*, 17(1), 309. doi:10.1186/s12889-017-4210-2
24. HIV and Injection Drug Use: Syringe Services Programs for HIV Prevention. (2016). CDC Vital Signs.
25. Des Jarlais, D., Nugent, A., Solberg, A. Syringe service programs for persons who inject drugs in urban, suburban, and rural areas—United States, 2013 *MMWR Morb Mortal Wkly Rep 2015*;64: 1337–1341
26. Strathdee, S.A., Celentano, D.D., Shah, N., Lyles, C., Stambolis, V.A., Macal, G., Nelson, K., Vlahov, D.,

"Needle-exchange attendance and health care utilization promote entry into detoxification," *J Urban Health* 1999; 76(4):448–60.

27. Heimer, R. (1998). Can syringe exchange serve as a conduit to substance abuse treatment? *Journal of Substance Abuse Treatment* 15:183–191.

28. Bluthenthal, R.N., Gogineni, A. Longshore, D., Stein, M. (2001). Factors associated with readiness to change drug use among needle-exchange users. *Drug & Alcohol Dependence* 62:225–230.

29. Artenie, Andreea, Jutras-Aswad, D., Roy, É., Zang, G., Bamvita, J.-M., Lévesque, Annie, and Bruneau, J. (2015). Visits to primary care physicians among persons who inject drugs at high risk of hepatitis C virus infection: Room for improvement. *Journal of Viral Hepatitis*. 22. 10.1111/jvh.12393.

30. Chou, R., Korthuis, P.T., Weimer, M., et al. Medication-Assisted Treatment Models of Care for Opioid Use Disorder in Primary Care Settings. Rockville (MD): Agency for Healthcare Research and Quality (U.S.); 2016 Dec. (Technical Briefs, No. 28).

31. Seal, K.H., Thawley, R., Gee, L., Bamberger, J., Kral, A.H., Ciccarone, D., Edlin B.R. (2005). "Naloxone distribution and cardiopulmonary resuscitation training for injection drug users to prevent heroin overdose death: A pilot intervention study," *Journal of Urban Health: Bulletin of the New York Academy of Medicine*, 2005; 82(2): 303–311.

32. Leece, P.N., Hopkins, S., Marshall, C., Orkin, A., Gassanov, M.A., Shahin, R.M., "Development and implementation of an opioid overdose prevention and response program in Toronto, Ontario," *Canadian Journal of Public Health*, 2013;104(3):e200–4.

33. Childs, R. Law Enforcement and Naloxone Utilization in the United States.

34. Tookes, H.E., Kral, A.H., Wenger, L.D., Cardenas, G.A., Martinez, A.N., Sherman, R.L., Pereyra, M., Forrest, D.W., Laota, M., Metsch, L.R., "A comparison of syringe disposal practices among injection drug users in a city with versus a city without needle and syringe programs," *Drug and Alcohol Dependence*, 2012 ;123(1–3):255–9

35. Riley, E.D., Kral, A.H., Stopka, T.J., Garfein, R.S., Reuckhaus, P., Bluthenthal, R.N., "Access to sterile syringes through San Francisco pharmacies and the association with HIV risk behavior among injection drug users," *Journal of Urban Health*, 2010; 87(4):534–42

36. Klein, S.J., Candelas, A.R., Cooper, J.G., Badillo, W.E., Tesoriero, J.M., Battles, H.B., Plavin, H.A., "Increasing safe syringe collection sites in New York State," *Public Health Reports*, 2008; 123(4):433–40.

37. De Montigny, L., Vernez Moudon, A., Leigh, B., Kim, S.Y., "Assessing a drop box programme: a spatial analysis of discarded needles," *International Journal of Drug Policy*, 2010; 21(3):208–14. Doherty, M.C., Junge, B., Rathouz, P., Garfein, R.S., Riley, E., Vlahov, D., "The effect of a needle exchange program on numbers of discarded needles: a 2-year follow-up," *American Journal of Public Health*. 2000 Jun; 90(6):936–9.

38. Bluthenthal, R.N., Anderson, R., Flynn, N.M., Kral, A.H., "Higher syringe coverage is associated with lower odds of HIV risk and does not increase unsafe syringe disposal among syringe exchange program clients," *Drug and Alcohol Dependence*, 2007; 89(2–3):214–22

39. Lorentz, J., Hill, L., & Samimi, B. (2000). Occupational Needlestick Injuries. *American Journal of Preventive Medicine*, 18(2), 146–150.

40. Cepeda, J. A., Beletsky, L., Sawyer, A., Serio-Chapman, C., Smelyanskaya, M., Han, J., Sherman, S.G. (2017). Occupational Safety in the Age of the Opioid Crisis: Needle. *Journal of Urban Health*, 94(1), 100–103.

41. Davis, C., Johnston, J., de Saxe Zerden, L., Clark, K., Castillo, T., & Childs, R. (2014). Attitudes of North Carolina law enforcement officers toward syringe. *Drug and Alcohol Dependence* (144), 265–269.

42. Centers for Disease Control and Prevention. HIV Infection, Risk, Prevention, and Testing Behaviors among Persons Who Inject Drugs—National HIV Behavioral Surveillance: Injection Drug Use, 20 U.S. Cities, 2015. HIV Surveillance Special Report 18. Revised edition. Published May 2018. Accessed 7/30/2018.

43. Galea, S., Ahern, J., Fuller, C., Freudenberg, N., & Vlahov, D. (2001). Needle exchange programs and experience of violence in an inner city neighborhood. *Journal of Acquired Immune Deficiency Syndromes* (28), 282–288.

44. Marx, M. A., Crape, B., Brookmeyer, R. S., Junge, B., Latkin, C., Vlahov, D., & Strathdee, S.A. (2000). Trends in crime and the introduction of a needle exchange program. *American Journal of Public Health*, 90(12), 1933–1936.

45. Centers for Disease Control and Prevention. Managing HIV and hepatitis C outbreaks among people who inject drugs—A guide for state and local health departments. March 2018.

46. Department of Health and Human Services Implementation Guidance to Support Certain Components of Syringe Services Programs, 2016. (2016, March). Department of Health and Human Services.

47. Jackson, K.A., Bohm, M.K., Brooks, J.T., et al. Invasive Methicillin-Resistant Staphylococcus aureus Infections Among Persons Who Inject Drugs—Six Sites, 2005–2016. *MMWR Morb Mortal Wkly Rep 2018*; 67:625–628.

48. Fleischauer, A.T., Ruhl, L., Rhea, S., & Barnes, E. (2017). Hospitalizations for Endocarditis and Associated Health Care Costs Among Persons with Diagnosed Drug Dependence—North Carolina, 2010–2015. *MMWR Morb Mortal Wkly Rep*, 66(22), 569–573. doi:10.15585/mmwr.mm6622a1

49. Dahlman, D., Hakansson, A., Kral, A., Wenger, L., Ball, E., & Novak, S. (2017). Behavioral characteristics and injection practices associated with skin and soft tissue infections among people who inject drugs: A community-based observational study. *Substance Abuse*, 38(1), 105–112.

29. CDC's Role in Safe Injection Practices*

Centers for Disease Control and Prevention

CDC works with numerous partners to conduct a range of activities to improve injection safety and prevent transmission of bloodborne pathogens and other infectious diseases. Below are some of CDC's current injection safety activities.

Promotion of Safe Injection Practices

CDC is collaborating with the Safe Injection Practices Coalition (SIPC) to develop and implement an educational campaign to promote safe injection practices by raising awareness among patients and healthcare providers about safe injection practices.

Development of Infection Control Guidelines

CDC and the Healthcare Infection Control Practices Advisory Committee (HICPAC), a federal advisory committee, developed recommendations on Safe Injection Practices which are applicable in all healthcare settings. These recommendations are part of Standard Precautions and can be found in the 2007 Guideline for Isolation Precautions. CDC and HICPAC are in the process of further developing documents specifically targeting infection control practices in outpatient healthcare settings.

Improved Basic Infection Control through Collaborations with CMS

CDC is improving basic infection control practices and safe injection practices through collaborations with the Centers for Medicaid and Medicare Services (CMS) to enhance survey and oversight capacity of non-acute healthcare settings.

---

*Public document originally published as Centers for Disease Control and Prevention, "CDC's Role in Safe Injection Practices," https://www.cdc.gov/injectionsafety/cdcsrole.html.

Improved Safety through Collaborations with FDA

CDC is collaborating with the Food and Drug Administration (FDA) to address issues associated with medication packaging, labeling and instructions for safe use as well as to promote safe injection practices and prevent the misuse of injectable medications, injection equipment, and related devices.

Improved Healthcare Personnel Protections from Sharps Injuries

CDC has developed guidance, toolkits and surveillance packages aimed at protecting healthcare personnel from blood and body fluid exposures and sharps injuries.

Responding to Outbreaks in Healthcare Settings

There has been a steady increase in the number of requests to CDC from state health departments and healthcare facilities for assistance in investigating infections and outbreaks potentially stemming from unsafe injection practices or related breakdowns in safe care. Support from CDC includes technical guidance and consulting from epidemiologists, on-site assistance with field investigations, and laboratory assistance.

Identification and Promotion of Best Practices for Patient Notification

CDC hosted a meeting to discuss and obtain input on the ethical and communication issues surrounding patient notification when a serious lapse in infection control (e.g., syringe reuse) has been identified. To supplement the input obtained at the meeting, CDC conducted a series of focus groups to further evaluate patient notification practices. CDC is in the process of further developing and disseminating these investigation, risk assessment and patient notification tools.

Efforts to Improve Injection Safety through Collaborations with Industry

CDC is working to promote innovation in product development and identify education and marketing improvements through industry partner meetings in May 2010 with leaders from injection equipment and medication industries and other partners.

Improved Capacity in State Health Departments

CDC is building infrastructure and capacity in state health departments to address healthcare-associated infection and patient safety issues through Healthcare-Associated Infection (HAI) Recovery Act Funding.

Expansion of the HHS Action Plan to Prevent HAIs in Outpatient Healthcare Settings

CDC collaborated closely with HHS, AHRQ, CMS, and other federal agencies to expand the HHS Action Plan to Prevent HAIs to include ambulatory surgical centers and hemodialysis centers. CDC continues to play a lead role as these modules are developed, helping focus attention on the need to assure that safe injection and other basic infection control standards are met in all settings where healthcare is delivered.

Identification of Drug Diversion as an Infection Risk

CDC and health departments continue to investigate and identify outbreaks stemming from drug diversion activities involving healthcare providers.

30. CDC Program Guidance for Syringe Services Programs*

Centers for Disease Control and Prevention

The purpose of this document is to provide implementation guidance for programs directly funded by CDC interested in implementing new or expanding existing syringe services programs (SSPs) for persons who inject drugs (PWID). This program guidance was developed in accordance with the Department of Health and Human Services (HHS) Implementation Guidance to Support Certain Components of Syringe Service Programs, 2016.

As described in the 2012 summary guidance for prevention of HIV, viral hepatitis, STDs and TB for persons who inject drugs from CDC and HHS,[1] the term SSPs includes provision of sterile needles, syringes and other drug preparation equipment and disposal services, as well as some or all of the following services: comprehensive sexual and injection risk reduction counseling; HIV, viral hepatitis, other sexually transmitted diseases (STD) and tuberculosis (TB) screening; provision of naloxone to reverse opioid overdoses; referral and linkage to HIV, viral hepatitis, other STDs and TB prevention, care and treatment services; referral and linkage to hepatitis A virus (HAV) and hepatitis B virus (HBV) vaccination; and referral to integrated and coordinated substance use disorder services, mental health services, physical health care, social services, and recovery support services. A directory of current SSPs is maintained by the North American Syringe Exchange Network.

On December 18, 2015, President Barack Obama signed the Consolidated Appropriations Act, 2016, (Pub. L. 114–113),[2] which modified the restriction on use of federal funds for programs distributing sterile needles or syringes (referred to as SSPs, or as syringe exchange programs) for HHS programs. The Consolidated Appropriations Act, 2016, Division H states:

> SEC. 520. Notwithstanding any other provision of this Act, no funds appropriated in this Act shall be used to purchase sterile needles or syringes for the hypodermic injection of any illegal drug: Provided, That such limitation does not apply to the use of funds for elements of a program other than making such purchases if the relevant State or local health department, in consultation with the Centers for Disease Control and Prevention, determines that the State or local jurisdiction, as applicable, is experiencing, or is at risk for, a significant increase in

---

*Public document originally published as Centers for Disease Control and Prevention, "CDC Program Guidance for Syringe Services Programs," https://www.cdc.gov/hiv/pdf/risk/cdc-hiv-syringe-exchange-services.pdf (2016).

hepatitis infections or an HIV outbreak due to injection drug use, and such program is operating in accordance with State and local law.

While the provision still prohibits the use of federal funds to purchase sterile needles or syringes for the purposes of hypodermic injection of any illegal drug, it allows for federal funds to be used for other aspects of SSPs based on evidence of a demonstrated need (i.e., experiencing, or at risk for, significant increases in hepatitis infections or an HIV outbreak due to injection drug use) by the state or local health department and in consultation with the CDC.

The HHS SSP guidance outlines the process for health departments to request a determination of need. For areas in which a determination of need has been made, this guidance details which SSP activities can be supported with CDC funds, which relevant CDC cooperative agreements can be used to support SSPs, and the process for how CDC funded programs can direct resources to implement new or expand existing SSPs. As always, requests to direct program funding to a different emergent activity are subject to approval from the CDC project officer and grants management officer.

Principles Guiding the Use of HHS Funding for SSPs

As noted in the HHS SSP Guidance, the following principles should be considered when planning, implementing, and evaluating an SSP:

- Programs that use federal funding for SSPs must adhere to federal, state and local laws, regulations, and other requirements related to such programs or services. State and local laws may vary and will impact the ability of federally funded recipients to implement these programs.
- Recipients should coordinate with and work toward obtaining cooperation from local law enforcement officials when implementing SSPs.
- SSPs, as they are implemented, should be a part of a comprehensive service program[3] that includes, as appropriate:
- Provision of sterile needles, syringes and other drug preparation equipment (purchased with non-federal funds) and disposal services;
- Education and counseling to reduce sexual, injection and overdose risks;
- Provision of condoms to reduce risk of sexual transmission of viral hepatitis, HIV or other STDs;
- HIV, viral hepatitis, STD and TB screening;
- Provision of naloxone to reverse opioid overdoses;
- Referral and linkage to HIV, viral hepatitis, STD and TB prevention, treatment and care services, including medication for hepatitis C virus (HCV)and HIV, pre-exposure prophylaxis (PrEP), post-exposure prophylaxis (PEP), prevention of mother-to-child transmission and partner services;
- Referral and linkage to [sic] hepatitis A virus (HAV) and hepatitis B virus (HBV) vaccination;
- Referral and linkage to and provision of substance use disorder treatment (including medication-assisted treatment for opioid use disorder which combines drug therapy [e.g., methadone, buprenorphine, or naltrexone] with counseling and behavioral therapy);
- Referral to medical care, mental health services, and other support services.

- Recipients should ensure that SSPs supported with federal funds provide referral and linkage to HIV, viral hepatitis, and substance use disorder prevention, care and treatment services, as appropriate.
- HHS funding recipients should coordinate and collaborate with other local agencies, organizations, and providers involved in comprehensive prevention programs for PWID to minimize duplication of effort.
- SSPs are subject to the terms and conditions incorporated or referenced in the recipient's federal funding.
- Federal funds can only be used to establish a new or expand an existing SSP with prior approval from the respective federal agency.

Use of CDC Funds

The Consolidated Appropriations Act, 2016 (P.L. 114–113) has modified the prohibition on federal funding for SSPs, and this change can be applied by CDC funded programs starting in Fiscal Year (FY) 2016 and can continue in future FYs, unless otherwise notified. CDC funded SSPs should be in accord with this guidance and remain subject to the terms and conditions as described in the recipient's Notice of Award. CDC funds can only be used to establish new or expand existing SSPs, with prior approval from the project officer and grants management officer. CDC funds cannot be used to supplant or replace state or other non-federal funds currently supporting SSP activities within a jurisdiction. In other words, CDC funds cannot be used to fund an existing SSP so that state or other non-federal funding can then be used for another program.

Applicable CDC Funding Opportunity Announcements

CDC has reviewed the scope of its various funding opportunity announcements (FOAs) to identify those whose awardees are best positioned to effectively support the implementation of SSPs in communities and to directly monitor local SSP activities to ensure compliance with national, as well as state and local laws, which vary by jurisdiction. As a result, two FOAs have been selected. Organizations receiving funds through these FOAs may request to direct funds to support SSPs. These applicable FOAs and their respective allowable SSP activities are outlined below.

PS12–1201, "Comprehensive HIV Prevention Programs for Health Departments"

- Allowed uses for funding include:
- Personnel to support SSP implementation and management (e.g., program staff, as well as staff for planning, monitoring, evaluation, and quality assurance);
- Supplies to promote sterile injection and reduce infectious disease transmission through injection drug use, exclusive of sterile needles, syringes and other drug preparation equipment;
- Testing kits for viral hepatitis (i.e., HBV and HCV) and HIV;

- Syringe disposal services (e.g., contract or other arrangement for disposal of biohazardous material);
- Navigation services to ensure linkage to: HIV and viral hepatitis prevention, testing, treatment and care services, including antiretroviral therapy for HCV and HIV, pre-exposure prophylaxis (PrEP), post-exposure prophylaxis (PEP), prevention of mother to child transmission and partner services; substance use disorder treatment, and medical and mental health care;
- Educational materials, including information about: safer injection practices; reversing a drug overdose; HIV and viral hepatitis prevention, testing, treatment and care services; and mental health and substance use disorder treatment, including medication assisted treatment;
- Male and female condoms to reduce sexual risk of infection with HIV and other STDs;
- Referral to hepatitis A and hepatitis B vaccinations to reduce risk of viral hepatitis infection;
- Communication, including use of social media technologies, and outreach activities designed to raise awareness about and increase utilization of SSPs; and
- SSP planning and non-research evaluation activities.

PS14-004, "Reduce Hepatitis Infections by Treatment and Integrated Prevention Services (Hepatitis-TIPS) among Non-urban Young Persons Who Inject Drugs"

- Allowed uses for funding include:
- Personnel to support SSP implementation and management (e.g., program staff, as well as staff for planning, monitoring, evaluation, and quality assurance);
- Supplies to promote sterile injection and reduce infectious disease transmission through injection drug use, exclusive of sterile needles, syringes and other drug preparation equipment;
- Testing kits for viral hepatitis (i.e., HBV and HCV) and HIV;
- Syringe disposal services (e.g., contract or other arrangement for disposal of biohazardous material);
- Navigation services to ensure linkage to viral hepatitis prevention, treatment and care services, prevention of mother to child transmission and partner services; substance use disorder treatment, and medical and mental health care;
- Educational materials, including information about: safer injection practices; reversing a drug overdose; viral hepatitis prevention, testing, treatment and care services; and mental health and substance use disorder treatment, including medication assisted treatment;
- Male and female condoms to reduce sexual risk of infection with HIV and other STDs;
- Referral to hepatitis A and hepatitis B vaccinations to reduce risk of viral hepatitis infection;
- Communication, including use of social media technologies, and outreach activities designed to raise awareness about and increase utilization of SSPs; and
- SSP planning and non-research evaluation activities.

During FY 2016, CDC resources to support allowable SSP activities must come from current CDC HIV and/or viral hepatitis program funding. Beginning in FY 2017, newly issued FOAs for HIV and viral hepatitis prevention programs will include guidance on the use of funding to support SSP activities. Below are the eligibility criteria and budgetary and programmatic requirements and restrictions.

Process for Requesting Use of CDC Funds for SSPs

Step 1: As described in the HHS SSP Guidance, state, local, territorial, and tribal health departments interested in directing federal funds to support SSPs must first demonstrate need in consultation with CDC. Health departments should provide CDC evidence that their jurisdiction is (1) experiencing or, (2) at risk for a significant increase in viral hepatitis infections or an HIV outbreak due to injection drug use. The scope of the presented evidence should address the geographic area that will be served by the SSPs and include state, county, and city level data, as appropriate.

At any time, health departments may submit a request for CDC's determination of need to SSPCOORDINATOR@CDC.GOV, with a courtesy copy to their project officer. Within 30 days of receipt of this consultation request, CDC will notify the requestor whether the evidence is sufficient to demonstrate need for SSPs. If the evidence is sufficient, the requesting health department will receive notice of approval regarding determination of need for the jurisdiction. This notice may be used by state, local, territorial, or tribal health departments or eligible HHS funded recipients to apply to the respective federal agency for directing funds to SSPs. If the evidence is insufficient, no programmatic or budgetary changes will be authorized. However, jurisdictions may choose to revise and resubmit their request with additional evidence based on feedback from CDC.

Upon notification of CDC's concurrence with the jurisdictional need for SSPs, health departments and other eligible HHS funded recipients are strongly encouraged to discuss their plans to direct funds for SSPs with their respective federal funding agency. An HHS funded health department or other eligible recipient may elect to either (1) immediately request to direct FY16 funds to support SSPs or (2) delay its request to direct funds to support SSPs until a subsequent fiscal year.

Note: Only CDC directly funded, eligible awardees may submit a request to CDC to direct CDC funding to SSP activities.

CDC directly funded, eligible awardees seeking to direct FY16 funds for SSPs are strongly encouraged to request a determination of need according to the below deadlines. Adherence to these recommended deadlines will ensure adequate time to have a determination of need request reviewed and process a subsequent request to direct FY16 funds for SSPs. If CDC directly funded, eligible awardees are unable to meet these deadlines, requests to direct funds for SSPs may be delayed until the next fiscal year.

- For PS12–1201, "Comprehensive HIV Prevention Programs for Health Departments": These awardees should submit their requests for jurisdictional determination of need for SSPs by May 27, 2016
- For PS14–004, "Reduce Hepatitis Infections by Treatment and Integrated Prevention Services (Hepatitis-TIPS) among Non-urban Young Persons Who Inject Drugs": These awardees should collaborate with their respective state

health departments to submit requests for jurisdictional determination of need for SSPs by May 27, 2016

Step 2: Upon notification of CDC's concurrence with the need for SSPs within a jurisdiction, eligible CDC awardees may then discuss their plans to direct funds to support SSP activities with their project officer prior to submitting a proposal to the CDC Office of Grant Services (CDC/OGS). In accordance with CDC/OGS guidelines, eligible awardees must prepare a proposal which identifies the SSP activities that will be supported by CDC funds. The proposal should include (1) a proposed program plan and (2) a revised budget.

The proposal, including the proposed program plan and revised budget, must be submitted to CDC/OGS with a courtesy copy to the CDC project officer. This submission should include a copy of the CDC notification that the jurisdiction has sufficiently demonstrated need to use federal funding for SSP activities. Once approved by both the CDC/OGS grants management specialist and the CDC Project Officer, the requestor will receive a revised Notice of Award signed by the CDC/OGS grants management officer. Awardees must obtain this approval before using their awarded funding to implement any SSP activities.

- **For PS12–1201, "Comprehensive HIV Prevention Programs for Health Departments":** Once the jurisdiction has obtained a CDC notification stating that the jurisdiction has sufficiently demonstrated need to use federal funding for SSPs, and following their decision to implement or expand existing SSPs, awardees should:
- Develop a detailed program plan and budget describing the SSP activities that will be implemented in the jurisdiction. **All requests to direct FY16 funds to support SSPs must be submitted no later than 60 days following receipt of CDC approval of determination of need.**
- Submit an addendum to the current Integrated HIV Prevention and Care Plan to include revisions to planned activities and priority populations as indicated by the addition of SSP components.
- Send an additional courtesy copy of all requests to direct funds for SSP activities to PS12–1201@CDC.GOV.
- **For PS14–004, "Reduce Hepatitis Infections by Treatment and Integrated Prevention Services (Hepatitis-TIPS) among Non-urban Young Persons Who Inject Drugs":** Once the jurisdiction has obtained a CDC notification stating that the jurisdiction has sufficiently demonstrated need to use federal funding for SSPs, and following their decision to implement new or expand existing SSPs, awardees should:
- Develop a detailed program plan and budget describing the SSP activities that will be implemented in the jurisdiction. All requests to direct FY16 funds to support SSPs must be submitted no later than 60 days following receipt of CDC approval of determination of need.

Step 3: CDC will approve or disapprove requests to direct funding to support SSPs activities within 30 days of receipt of all requested information. If seeking to implement SSP activities with FY16 funds, CDC strongly encourages eligible awardees to submit all requests according to the recommended submission deadlines.

After approving requests to direct funding for SSPs, CDC will work in partnership with awardees to determine the appropriate process measures related to SSPs. Awardees implementing new or expanding existing SSPs will need to collect basic SSP metrics information (e.g., number of syringes distributed, estimated number of syringes returned for safe disposal, number of persons tested for HIV or viral hepatitis, referrals to HIV, viral hepatitis and substance use disorder treatment).

Outline of SSP Proposal to CDC

All proposals to request the use of CDC funds to support SSPs should include the following elements, unless otherwise noted:

- Description of proposed new or expanded SSP related activities;
- Timeline for implementation:
- Awardees without prior experience with SSPs should include preparatory activities as part of their timeline, including development of protocols and guidelines, and staff training.
- Impact on current activities funded under the respective FOA;
- Copy of existing protocols and guidelines for SSP related activities, if available;
- Budget and budget justification, proposed activities and measures;
- Description of current training and technical assistance needs related to planning, implementing, and evaluating SSPs, as appropriate; and
- Location of SSP related activities to be supported with federal funds.

Technical Assistance and Resources

Awardees should first review the HHS SSP Guidance and this guidance for instruction, tools, and resources. While requesting either (1) determination of need for SSPs or (2) authority to direct CDC fund to support SSPs, awardees should contact their project officer to discuss specific needs for technical assistance. Project officers can provide guidance and facilitate access to capacity building assistance or other resources.

Additional information about using CDC funds for SSPs is available at http://www.cdc.gov/hiv/risk/syringes.html.

Notes

1. CDC. (2012) Integrated Prevention Services for HIV Infection, Viral Hepatitis, Sexually Transmitted Diseases, and Tuberculosis for Persons Who Use Drugs Illicitly: Summary Guidance from CDC and the U.S. Department of Health and Human Services. MMWR;61(RR05):1–40.
2. https://www.congress.gov/114/bills/hr2029/BILLS-114hr2029enr.pdf. Accessed on December 22, 2015.
3. CDC. (2012) Integrated Prevention Services for HIV Infection, Viral Hepatitis, Sexually Transmitted Diseases, and Tuberculosis for Persons Who Use Drugs Illicitly: Summary Guidance from CDC and the U.S. Department of Health and Human Services. MMWR; 61(RR05):1–40.

31. Medical Waste*

U.S. Environmental Protection Agency

Medical waste is a subset of wastes generated at health care facilities, such as hospitals, physicians' offices, dental practices, blood banks, and veterinary hospitals/clinics, as well as medical research facilities and laboratories. Generally, medical waste is healthcare waste that that may be contaminated by blood, body fluids or other potentially infectious materials, including sharps and needles, and is often referred to as regulated medical waste. These

Who Regulates Medical Waste?

Since the 1988 Medical Waste Tracking Act Expired in 1991, Medical waste is primarily regulated by state environmental and health departments. EPA has not had authority, specifically for medical waste, since the Medical Waste Tracking Act (MWTA) of 1988 expired in 1991. It is important to contact your state environmental program first when disposing of medical waste. Contact your state environmental protection agency and your state health agency for more information regarding your state's regulations on medical waste.

Other federal agencies have regulations regarding medical waste. These agencies include Centers for Disease Control (CDC), Occupational Safety and Health Administration (OSHA), U.S. Food and Drug Administration (FDA), and potentially others.

History

For historical information regarding EPA's work under the Medical Waste Tracking Act of 1989 including several draft studies related to medical waste management, please search EPA's archive using the term "medical waste."

Concern for the potential health hazards of medical wastes grew in the 1980s after medical wastes were washing up on several east coast beaches. This prompted Congress to enact The MWTA of 1988. The MWTA was a two-year federal program in which EPA was required to promulgate regulations on management of medical waste. The Agency did so on March 24, 1989. The regulations for this two-year program went into effect on

---

*Public document originally published as U.S. Environmental Protection Agency, "Medical Waste," https://www.epa.gov/rcra/medical-waste (November 7, 2017).

June 24, 1989, in four states—New York, New Jersey, Connecticut, and Rhode Island and Puerto Rico. The regulations expired on June 21, 1991.

EPA concluded from the information gathered during this period that the disease-causing potential of medical waste is greatest at the point of generation and naturally tapers off after that point. Thus, risk to the general public of disease caused by exposure to medical waste is likely to be much lower than risk for the healthcare workers.

After the MWTA expired in 1991, states largely took on the role of regulating medical waste under the guidance developed from the two-year program.

Most states have since further developed their own programs resulting in each state program differing significantly from each other.

Treatment and Disposal of Medical Waste and Sharps Needles

Disposal of Medical Sharps/Needles. Improper management of discarded needles and other sharps can pose a health risk to the public and waste workers. For example, discarded needles may expose waste workers to potential needle stick injuries and potential infection when containers break open inside garbage trucks or needles are mistakenly sent to recycling facilities. Janitors and housekeepers also risk injury if loose sharps poke through plastic garbage bags. Used needles can transmit serious diseases, such as human immunodeficiency virus (HIV) and hepatitis.

Community Options for Safe Needle Disposal. Sharps disposal by self-injectors is not typically regulated, and self-injectors do not always know the safest disposal methods. This situation could lead to haphazard disposal habits and increased community exposure to sharps. People at the greatest risk of being stuck by used sharps include sanitation and sewage treatment workers, janitors and housekeepers, and children.

Protect Yourself, Protect Others: Safe Options for Home Needle Disposal. All needles should be treated as if they carry a disease. That means that if someone gets stuck with a needle, they have to get expensive medical tests and worry about whether they have caught a harmful or deadly disease. You must be sure you get rid of your used needles the safe way to avoid exposing other people to harm.

Centers for Disease Control and Prevention: Sharps Safety for Healthcare Settings. Occupational exposure to bloodborne pathogens from needlesticks and other sharps injuries is a serious problem, resulting in approximately 385,000 needlesticks and other sharps-related injuries to hospital-based healthcare personnel each year. Similar injuries occur in other healthcare settings, such as nursing homes, clinics, emergency care services, and private homes. Sharps injuries are primarily associated with occupational transmission of hepatitis B virus (HBV), hepatitis C virus (HCV), and human immunodeficiency virus (HIV), but they have been implicated in the transmission of more than 20 other pathogens.

Treatment and Disposal of Other Medical Wastes

Medical Waste Incineration

More than 90 percent of potentially infectious medical waste was incinerated before 1997. In August of 1997, EPA promulgated regulations creating stringent emission standards for medical waste incinerators due to significant concerns over detrimental air quality affecting human health. EPA's Office of Air Quality Planning and Standards continues to review and revise the Hospital Medical Infectious Waste Incinerator (HMIWI) standards as required most recently in May of 2013.

Alternative Treatment and Disposal Technologies for Medical Waste

Potential alternatives to incineration of medical waste include the following:

- Thermal treatment, such as microwave technologies;
- Steam sterilization, such as autoclaving;
- Electropyrolysis; and
- Chemical mechanical systems, among others.

With EPA's tighter HMIWI standards, the number of HMIWIs in the United States has declined since 1997. This has led to an increase in the use of alternative technologies for treating medical waste. The alternative treatments are generally used to render the medical waste non-infectious then the waste can be disposed of as solid waste in landfills or incinerators. Many states have regulations requiring medical waste treatment technologies to be certified, licensed or regulated. Check with your state for additional regulation regarding treatment of medical waste.

EPA has jurisdiction over medical waste treatment technologies, which claim to reduce the infectiousness of the waste (i.e., that claim any antimicrobial activity) by using chemicals. This jurisdiction comes from the Federal Insecticide, Fungicide and Rodenticide Act (FIFRA).

Companies wishing to make such claims must register their product under FIFRA through EPA's Office of Prevention, Pesticide, and Toxic Substances (OPPTS), Antimicrobial Division.

32. Opioid Overdose Reversal with Naloxone*

NATIONAL INSTITUTE ON DRUG ABUSE

What Is Naloxone?

Naloxone is a medication designed to rapidly reverse opioid overdose. It is an opioid antagonist—meaning that it binds to opioid receptors and can reverse and block the effects of other opioids. It can very quickly restore normal respiration to a person whose breathing has slowed or stopped as a result of overdosing with heroin or prescription opioid pain medications.

How Is Naloxone Given?

There are three FDA-approved formulations of naloxone:

Injectable: Generic brands of injectable naloxone vials are offered by a variety of companies that are listed in the FDA Orange Book under "naloxone" (look for "injectable"). There has been widespread use of improvised emergency kits that combine an injectable formulation of naloxone with an atomizer that can deliver naloxone intranasally. Use of this product requires the user to be trained on proper assembly and administration. These improvised intranasal devices may not deliver naloxone levels equivalent to FDA-approved products. In fact, the manufacturer of an internasal atomizer device issued a voluntary recall on 10/27/16 noting that some of the devices "may not deliver a fully atomized plume of medication, making the drug potentially less effective." An approved, prefilled nasal spray is now available

Autoinjectable: EVZIO is a prefilled auto-injection device that makes it easy for families or emergency personnel to inject naloxone quickly into the outer thigh. Once activated, the device provides verbal instruction to the user describing how to deliver the medication, similar to automated defibrillators.

Prepackaged Nasal Spray: NARCAN Nasal Spray is a prefilled, needle-free device that requires no assembly and is sprayed into one nostril while patients lay on their back. Both NARCAN Nasal Spray and EVZIO are packaged in a carton containing two doses

---

*Public document originally published as National Institute on Drug Abuse, "Opioid Overdose Reversal with Naloxone," https://www.drugabuse.gov/related-topics/opioid-overdose-reversal-naloxone-narcan-evzio (April 2018).

to allow for repeat dosing if needed. They are relatively easy to use and suitable for home use in emergency situations.

Who Can Give Naloxone to Someone Who Has Overdosed?

The liquid for injection is commonly used by paramedics, emergency room doctors, and other specially trained first responders. To facilitate ease of use, NARCAN Nasal Spray is now available, which allows for naloxone to be sprayed into the nose. While improvised atomizers have been used in the past to convert syringes for use as nasal spray, these may not deliver the appropriate dose. Depending on the state you live in, friends, family members, and others in the community may give the auto-injector and nasal spray formulation of naloxone to someone who has overdosed. Some states require a physician to prescribe naloxone; in other states, pharmacies may distribute naloxone in an outpatient setting without bringing in a prescription from a physician. To learn about the laws regarding naloxone in your state, see the Prescription Drug Abuse Policy System website.

What Dose Can Be Provided?

The dose varies depending on the formulation, and sometimes more than one dose is needed to help the person start breathing again. Anyone who may have to use naloxone should carefully read the package insert that comes with the product. You can find copies of the package insert for EVZIO® and NARCAN® Nasal Spray on the FDA website.

What Precautions Are Needed When Giving Naloxone?

People who are given naloxone should be observed constantly until emergency care arrives and for at least 2 hours by medical personnel after the last dose of naloxone to make sure breathing does not slow or stop.

What Are the Side Effects of Naloxone?

Naloxone is an extremely safe medication that only has a noticeable effect in people with opioids in their systems. Naloxone can (but does not always) cause withdrawal symptoms which may be uncomfortable, but are not life-threatening; on the other hand, opioid overdose is extremely life-threatening. Withdrawal symptoms may include headache, changes in blood pressure, rapid heart rate, sweating, nausea, vomiting, and tremors.

How Much Does Naloxone Cost?

The cost varies depending on where and how you get it. Patients with insurance should check with their insurance company to see what their co-pay is for EVZIO or

NARCAN Nasal Spray. Patients without insurance can check on the retail costs with their local pharmacies. Kaleo, the maker of EVZIO, has a cost assistance program for patients with financial difficulties and no insurance.

Where Can I Get Naloxone?

Naloxone is a prescription drug. You can buy naloxone in many pharmacies, in some cases without bringing in a prescription from a physician. Law enforcement, EMS, and community-based naloxone distribution programs can apply to be a Qualified Purchaser to order naloxone or work with their state or local health departments. Here are some resources to help you find naloxone in your area:
- Naloxone finder at https://www.getnaloxonenow.org/#home —This website also offers access to training for first responders and potential bystanders.

Pennsylvania and Washington have their own websites.

Some pharmacies offer naloxone in an outpatient setting (without bringing in a prescription from a physician). Check with your local pharmacy.

• **B. State** •

33. Syringe Exchange Programs in California

An Overview*

CALIFORNIA DEPARTMENT OF PUBLIC HEALTH

Syringe exchange programs (SEPs) have been operating in California, providing sterile syringes, collecting used ones, and acting as points of access to health education and care for people who inject drugs since the late 1980s. SEPs are a critical part of efforts to protect and improve the health of all Californians, and are one of the cornerstones of Office of AIDS' efforts to improve the health and wellbeing of people who inject drugs.

SEPs were soon established in other cities and counties in the state, and in 1999 Governor Gray Davis signed legislation that sanctioned local authorization of SEPs. The counties and cities in California that provided this authorization were among the first in the country to fund syringe exchange with public dollars.

Scientific research conducted over the more than two decades since those first street-based efforts has conclusively demonstrated that syringe exchange is highly effective in reducing the spread of HIV among people who inject drugs (PWID) and in linking them to other essential services. Research has consistently demonstrated that SEPs do not result in negative consequences such as increased drug use or increased syringe litter in the communities that are host to these programs.

In December 2015, President Barack Obama signed legislation that responded to calls from the scientific, medical and public health communities to allow federal funding of efforts to expand access to sterile syringes. Federal agencies, including the Department of Health and Human Services, the Centers for Disease Control and Prevention (CDC), the Health Resources and Services Administration (HRSA) and the Substance Abuse and Mental Health Administration (SAMHSA), issued guidance to allow grantees to use their funds to support syringe services programs (SSPs).

"SSP" is the term used by CDC and other federal agencies to denote programs that provide syringe exchange, distribution, and/or disposal for PWID. SSPs include SEPs, but may also include other programs or initiatives, such as nonprescription syringe sale in pharmacies, physician prescription for disease prevention purposes, and sharps disposal for PWID.

---

*Public document originally published as California Department of Public Health, "Syringe Exchange Programs in California: An Overview," https://www.cdph.ca.gov/Programs/CID/DOA/Pages/OA_prev_sep.aspx (April 2018).

In a separate but equally impactful action, the California State Legislature passed and Governor Edmund G. Brown signed Senate Bill 75, Committee on Budget, Chapter 18, Statutes of 2015, which authorized funding that allowed the California Department of Public Health (CDPH), Office of AIDS (OA) to establish a Syringe Exchange Supply Clearinghouse. The Supply Clearinghouse provides a baseline level of supplies to authorized SEPs in order to enhance the health and wellness of people who inject drugs and increase the organizational stability of California SEPs.

OA considers access to sterile syringes to be a critical component of HIV prevention and care in California. OA supports an approach to working with PWID that fosters overall health and wellness through such services as wound care, overdose prevention, viral hepatitis testing and medication-assisted treatment, and involving drug users in the development of the programs that are meant to serve them. OA encourages its local partners to include syringe exchange funding among their locally funded initiatives, where such local funds are available, and to include SEPs among the AIDS service organizations with which they consult on matters of policy and practice.

Currently

- There are more than 40 SEPs operating in California.
- California SEPs provide a wide range of services in addition to syringe exchange and disposal. These services may include HIV and hepatitis C testing, overdose prevention training, and referrals to drug treatment, housing, and mental health services. Most SEPs also provide first aid and basic supplies, such as clean socks and bottled water, to meet the needs of homeless clients.
- California SEPs operate in a variety of settings, including in health clinics, mobile vans, storefronts and churches. Some offer street-based services in multiple locations; others offer services daily during standard business hours; still others provide home delivery services.
- Since 1999 the California State Legislature has acted several times to expand access to sterile syringes through SEPs authorized by local government. Most syringe exchange programs currently operating in California have been authorized by their county boards of supervisors or city councils.
- In 2012, Assembly Bill (AB) 604, (Skinner, Chapter 744, Statutes of 2011) also granted authority to the California Department of Public Health, Office of AIDS to permit organizations to apply directly to the Department for authorization to provide syringe exchange services. Existing SEPs are not required to apply for state certification, and local governments may continue to authorize local programs.

Research in California: the CalSEP Study[1]

- The California Syringe Exchange Program (CalSEP) study by the Centers for Disease Control and Prevention examined the impact of syringe exchange legislation over several years in sixteen counties. Researchers found that for most SEP clients, contact with SEPs was the only contact they had with health care or social services of any kind. Of 10 recommended preventive services received by SEP clients, 76 percent were received exclusively from SEPs.

- In addition to syringe exchange, eighty-three percent of SEPs participating in the study offered HIV counseling and testing on site and 63 percent offered screening for hepatitis C virus. All SEPs offered safer sex materials, first aid, and referrals to drug treatment.
- In a survey of 75 clients recruited from 25 California SEPs, more than 90 percent would recommend SEPs to friends with similar needs.

Additional Research Findings

- A study of 81 cities around the world compared HIV infection rates among IDUs in cities that had SEPs to cities that did not. In the 29 cities with SEPs, HIV infection rates decreased by an average of 5.8 percent per year. By contrast, in the 52 cities without SEPs, HIV infection rates increased by 5.9 percent per year.[2]
- Researchers studying a San Francisco SEP found that the program did not encourage drug use, either by recruiting young or new IDUs, or by increasing drug use among current IDUs. In fact, during the five-year study period, injection frequency among IDUs decreased from 1.9 injections per day to 0.7, and the percentage of new IDUs in the community decreased from 3 percent to 1 percent.[3]
- Economic studies have predicted that SEPs could prevent HIV infections among clients, their sex partners, and offspring at a cost of about $13,000 per infection averted.[4] This is significantly less than the lifetime cost of treating an HIV-infected person, which is estimated to be $385,200.
- Hundreds of studies of SEPs have been conducted and have been summarized in a series of federally funded reports beginning in 1991. Each of the eight reports has concluded that SEPs do not appear to lead to increased drug use, increased neighborhood crime, or increased syringe litter in the communities that are home to these programs.[5]
- A comprehensive review of international studies on syringe access programs, including both syringe exchange and nonprescription pharmacy sale concluded, "There is compelling evidence that increasing the availability, accessibility, and both the awareness of the imperative to avoid HIV and utilization of sterile injecting equipment by IDUs reduces HIV infection substantially."[6]
- The National Institutes of Health Consensus Panel on HIV Prevention stated, "An impressive body of evidence suggests powerful effects from needle exchange programs.... Studies show reduction in risk behavior as high as 80 percent, with estimates of a 30 percent or greater reduction of HIV in IDUs."[7]

Related California Legislation

- AB 1743 (Ting, Statutes of 2014) allows licensed pharmacies throughout California to sell syringes to adults without a prescription and removes prior limits on the number of syringes that may be sold. It allows adults 18 years of age and older to purchase and possess an unlimited number of syringes for personal use when acquired from a pharmacy, physician or authorized SEP.
- AB 604 (Skinner, Statutes of 2011) added CDPH/OA to the list of government

entities that may authorize SEPs. As of January 1, 2012, OA has authority to establish a program that allows entities to provide syringe exchange services anywhere in the state where OA determines that the conditions exist for rapid spread of HIV, viral hepatitis, or other blood-borne diseases.

Syringe Exchange Certification Program

In July 2013, CDPH/Office of AIDS established the Syringe Exchange Certification Program, which allows qualified entities to apply directly to CDPH/OA for authorization to provide syringe exchange services. This option allows providers to seek either local authorization from their city council or county board of supervisors, or state authorization through CDPH/OA.

The Syringe Exchange Certification Program does not provide funding to applicants, however all authorized SEPs are eligible to participate in the California Syringe Exchange Supply Clearinghouse, which provides a baseline level of supplies to authorized programs.

Notes

1. Bluthenthal, R. Syringe Exchange Program Diversity and Correlates of HIV Risk: Preliminary results from the California Syringe Exchange Program Study. Presentation to the California Department of Health Services, Office of AIDS, April 22, 2003. Sacramento, CA.
2. Hurley, S.F., Jolley, D.J., Kaldor, J.M. Effectiveness of needle-exchange programs for prevention of HIV infection. *Lancet* 1997; 349:1797–1800.
3. Watters, J.K., Estilo, M.J., Clark, G.L., et al. Syringe and needle exchange as HIV/AIDS prevention for injection drug users. *Journal of the American Medical Association* 1994; 271:115–120.
4. Cohen, D.A., Wu, S-Y., Farley, T.A. Cost-effective allocation of government funds to prevent HIV infection. *Health Affairs* 2005; 24:915–926.
5. Report from the NIH Consensus Development Conference. February 1997.
6. Wodak, A., Cooney, A. Do needle syringe programs reduce HIV infection among injecting drug users: a comprehensive review of the international evidence. *Subst Use Misuse.* 2006;41(6–7):777–813.
7. National Institutes of Health. Consensus development statement. Interventions to prevent HIV risk behaviors, February 11–13,1997;7–8.

34. California Legal Code Related to Access to Sterile Needles and Syringes*

CALIFORNIA DEPARTMENT OF PUBLIC HEALTH

The following sections of California Health and Safety Code and Business and Professions Code regulate the possession of hypodermic needles and syringes and other injection equipment, authorization of syringe services programs (also known as syringe exchange programs, or SEPs), sale or provision of syringes by physicians and pharmacies, and syringe disposal.

Individual Possession of Needles and Syringes and Other Injection Equipment

Health and Safety Code (HSC) Section 11364 governs the possession of drug paraphernalia. Adults age 18 and older may possess syringes for personal use if acquired from a physician, pharmacist, authorized syringe exchange program (SEP) or any other source that is authorized by law to provide sterile syringes or hypodermic needles without a prescription. There are no limits on the number of hypodermic needles and syringes adults may possess for personal use. Additionally, it is lawful to possess hypodermic needles or syringes that are containerized for safe disposal in a container that meets state and federal standards for disposal of sharps waste, such as a standard sharps container distributed by SEPs.

H&S Code Section 121349.1 states that SEP participants shall not be subject to criminal prosecution for possession of needles or syringes or any materials deemed by a local or state health department to be necessary to prevent the spread of communicable diseases, or to prevent drug overdose, injury, or disability acquired from an authorized SEP.

Syringe Services Programs

California Health and Safety (H&S) Code Section 11364.7(a) establishes that no public entity, its agents, or employees shall be subject to criminal prosecution for distribution

---

*Public document originally published as California Department of Public Health, "California Legal Code Related to Access to Sterile Needles and Syringes," https://www.cdph.ca.gov/Programs/CID/DOA/CDPH%20Document%20Library/CA%20Legal%20Code_Final.pdf (June 2019).

of syringes or any materials deemed by a local or state health department to be necessary to prevent the spread of communicable diseases, or to prevent drug overdose, injury, or disability to participants in SEPs authorized by the public entity.

California Business and Professions (B&P) Code Section 4145.5(e) requires SEPs to counsel consumers on safe disposal and provide them with one or more of the following disposal options: (1) onsite disposal, (2) provision or sale of sharps containers that meet applicable state and federal standards, and/or (3) provision or sale of mail-back sharps containers.

Local Authorization of Syringe Exchange Programs and Responsibilities of Local Health Officer

H&S Code Section 121349.1 allows local governments to authorize SEPs in consultation with the California Department of Public Health (CDPH), as part of a network of comprehensive services, including treatment services, to combat the spread of HIV and blood-borne hepatitis infection among people who inject drugs.

H&S Code Section 121349.2 requires that local government and health officials, law enforcement and the public be given an opportunity to comment on SEPs on a biennial basis in order to address and mitigate any potential negative impact of SEPs.

H&S Code Section 121349.3 requires the local health officer to present biennially at an open meeting of the board of supervisors or city council a report detailing the status of SEPs, including, but not limited to, relevant statistics on blood-borne infections associated with needle sharing activity and the use of public funds for these programs. Notice to the public shall be sufficient to ensure adequate participation in the meeting by the public. For SEPs authorized by CDPH, a biennial report shall be provided by the department based on the reports to CDPH from SEPs within the jurisdiction of the local health officer.

State Authorization of Syringe Services Programs

H&S Code Section 121349 allows CDPH to authorize SEPs in locations where the conditions exist for the rapid spread of viral hepatitis, HIV or other potentially deadly diseases.

Sale or Provision of Syringes by Licensed Pharmacists and Physicians

B&P Code Section 4145.5(b) permits pharmacists and physicians to furnish or sell, without a prescription, an unlimited number of hypodermic needles and syringes to adults age 18 and older for disease prevention purposes.

H&S Code Section 11364 permits adults age 18 and older to possess syringes for personal use if acquired from a physician, pharmacist, authorized SEP, or any other source that is authorized by law to provide sterile syringes or hypodermic needles without a prescription.

Nonprescription Sale of Syringes in Pharmacies

B&P Code Section 4145.5 permits the nonprescription sale of hypodermic needles and syringes by California pharmacies. AB 1743 (Ting, Chapter 331, Statutes of 2014) removed the prior limit on the number of hypodermic needles and syringes that California pharmacies and physicians had been permitted to furnish or sell. As of January 1, 2015, pharmacists and physicians may furnish or sell an unlimited number of hypodermic needles and syringes to adults age 18 and older.

A pharmacy that furnishes nonprescription syringes must store them so that they are only available to authorized personnel and are not accessible to other persons. Such pharmacies must also counsel consumers on safe disposal and provide written information or verbal counseling at the time of syringe sale on how to do the following: (1) access drug treatment, (2) access testing and treatment for HIV and hepatitis C, and (3) safely dispose of sharps waste. A Patient Information Sheet that includes this written information can be downloaded from the Office of AIDS website. Pharmacies must also make sharps disposal available to customers by selling or furnishing sharps disposal containers or mail-back sharps containers, or by providing on-site disposal.

Syringe Disposal

B&P Code Section 4146 permits pharmacies to accept the return of needles and syringes from the public if contained in a sharps container, which is defined in H&S Code Section 117750 as "a rigid puncture-resistant container that, when sealed, is leak resistant and cannot be reopened without great difficulty."

H&S Code Section 118286 prohibits individuals from discarding home-generated sharps waste in home or business recycling or waste containers.

H&S Code Section 118286 also requires that home-generated sharps waste be transported only in a sharps container or other container approved by the applicable enforcement agency, which may be either the state (CalRecycle program) or a local government agency. Home-generated sharps waste may be managed at household hazardous waste facilities, at "home-generated sharps consolidation points," at the facilities of medical waste generators, or by the use of medical waste mail-back containers approved by the state.

B&P Code 4145.5 requires SEPs and pharmacies that sell or provide nonprescription syringes to counsel consumers on safe disposal and also provide them with one or more of the following disposal options: (1) onsite disposal, (2) provision of sharps containers that meet applicable state and federal standards, and/or (3) provision of mail-back sharps containers.

35. Florida Is the Latest Republican-Led State to Adopt Clean Needle Exchanges*

Sammy Mack

A green van was parked on the edge of downtown Miami, on a corner shadowed by overpasses. The vehicle serves as a mobile health clinic and syringe exchange, where people who inject drugs like heroin and fentanyl could swap dirty needles for fresh ones.

One of the clinic's regular visitors, a man with heavy black arrows tattooed on his arms, waited on the sidewalk to get clean needles.

"I'm Arrow," he said, introducing himself. "Pleasure."

This mobile unit in Miami-Dade County is part of the IDEA Exchange, the only legal needle exchange program operating in the state. But Florida's Republican governor, Ron DeSantis, signed a new law last week that aims to change that.

Needle exchanges have been legal in many other states for decades, but Southern, Republican-led states like Florida have only recently started to adopt this public health intervention.

The timing of the statewide legalization of needle exchanges comes as Florida grapples with a huge heroin and fentanyl problem. When people share dirty needles to inject drugs, it puts them at high risk for spreading bloodborne infections like HIV and hepatitis C. For years, Florida has had America's highest rates of HIV.

Even so, Arrow said, he and every user he knew always put the drugs first. Clean needles were an afterthought.

"Every once in a while, I did use someone else's and that was a thrill ride—wondering whether or not I was going to catch anything. But I'm blessed; I'm 57 and I don't have anything," Arrow told a reporter at the mobile clinic over a year ago.

Kaiser Health News agreed not to use his full name because of his illegal drug use.

"Now I can shoot with a clean needle every time," he said.

---

*Originally published as Sammy Mack, "Florida Is the Latest Republican-Led State to Adopt Clean Needle Exchanges," *Kaiser Health News*, https://khn.org/news/florida-is-the-latest-republican-led-state-to-adopt-clean-needle-exchanges/ (July 2, 2019). Reprinted with permission of the publisher. Kaiser Health News is a nonprofit news service covering health issues. It is an editorially independent program of the Kaiser Family Foundation that is not affiliated with Kaiser Permanente. This story is part of a partnership that includes WLRN, NPR and Kaiser Health News.

The Miami Experiment

According to the Centers for Disease Control and Prevention, needle exchanges prevent the spread of viruses among users of injection drugs.

But the advocates who want to offer needle exchanges face challenges. For example, carrying around loads of needles to hand out without prescriptions can violate drug paraphernalia laws.

Many states mapped out legal frameworks decades ago to allow needle exchanges as a public health intervention. But in Florida, it was illegal to operate exchanges. Then, in 2016, the state legislature gave Miami-Dade County temporary permission to pilot a needle exchange program for five years.

"This is more than just a needle exchange," said Democratic state Sen. Oscar Braynon. "This has become a roving triage and health center."

In three years of operation, Miami's pilot program has pulled more than a quarter-million used needles out of circulation, according to reports the program filed with the Florida Department of Health. By handing out Narcan—a drug that reverses opioid overdoses—the exchange has prevented more than a thousand overdoses. The program also offers clients testing for HIV and hepatitis C. Finally, the program connects people to medical care and drug rehab.

This year, Braynon introduced Senate Bill 366 to allow the rest of Florida's counties to authorize similar programs.

"We have made it so easy for people to get into HIV care now, and we have so many people who we never would have known were infected—and would have infected countless other people—who are on their medications," said Dr. Hansel Tookes, who heads Miami's needle exchange pilot program.

Tookes was in Tallahassee, the state capital, in May when the expansion bill passed its final vote—a long shot in the conservative-dominated legislature that nonetheless passed by an overwhelming margin. He said he spent the return flight home to Miami staring out the window.

"I looked down at Florida the entire ride," he said, "and I just had this overwhelming feeling like, 'Oh, my God, we just did the impossible and we're going to save so many people in this state.'"

Why Harm Reduction Trumped Politics

Six years ago, Republican state Sen. Rob Bradley cast a "no" vote after considering a proposal for needle exchanges.

"You're trying to make sure the person has a clean needle, which is outweighing the idea of the person breaking the law," he declared in 2013.

This is the primary objection of conservative lawmakers: the concern that these programs promote illegal drug abuse. Responding to this skepticism with data has been central to changing lawmakers' minds.

Decades of research shows that needle exchanges do not encourage drug abuse, and that they lower other health risks for people who are vulnerable and often hard to reach. It's part of a public health approach known as "harm reduction."

In Miami, the needle exchange pilot project has also earned the support of law enforcement.

Officers say it's a relief to know more injection drug users are keeping their syringes in special sharps containers, provided by the exchange, to safely dispose of dirty needles.

"Now, for our officers, when they're doing a pat-down … that sharps container is really protecting you from a loose needle," said Eldys Diaz, executive officer to the Miami police chief. "That's an extraordinary source of comfort for us."

This year, when Bradley heard discussion of the needle exchange bill again, he had a different response.

"I just want to say, when I started my career in the Senate, I voted against the pilot project—and I was wrong," he said as he voted for the bill this time. "And the results speak for themselves. It's very good public policy."

The bill passed unanimously in the Florida Senate and by a 111–3 vote in the Florida House.

Arrow Points to His Future

If it weren't for the tattoos running down his arms, it would be hard today to recognize Arrow as the man who once slept under highway overpasses. His skin is now clear, and he has some meat on his bones. He looks healthier during a visit to a clinic where needle exchange clients get follow-up care, but it's been a rough year.

In May of last year, Arrow's girlfriend died from a heart infection—a serious condition that can happen to people who inject drugs. After that, Arrow said, he overdosed on purpose. Narcan from the needle exchange brought him back.

But he kept using.

Arrow said he doesn't remember a lot from that period but does remember using so much heroin that he ran out of fresh needles between visits to the exchange. So he grabbed other people's used needles.

And then he tested positive for HIV and hepatitis C.

Tookes and his colleagues threw Arrow another life raft: They got him an inpatient drug treatment bed.

Now Arrow sports a string of keychains from Narcotics Anonymous.

"My chain of sobriety," he said of the links. "I got 30-days, 60-days and 90-days chips," he said.

Arrow's HIV is under control. And he connected with health services for people living with HIV, including getting medication that cured his hepatitis C.

Now, he's focused on staying sober, one day at a time. He has been sober for about six months.

Tookes, Braynon and other supporters hope additional needle exchanges across Florida will give more people the chance to recover from addiction—and protect themselves from needle-borne illnesses.

36. Syringe Exchange in Southern Indiana to Respond to an Increase in HIV Cases*

Jeannie D. DiClementi

The recent upsurge in HIV cases linked to injection drug use in southern Indiana has thrust the issue of syringe exchange programs (SEPs) into the headlines. While authorities are linking these cases of HIV infection directly to injecting drugs, it is unknown how many are caused by sexual activity with an infected drug user.

Nearly all states prohibit possession of syringes other than for medical need through their drug paraphernalia laws. Syringe access laws that require ID and proof of medical need to purchase them from pharmacies also exist in the majority of states, including Indiana. Federal funding of syringe exchange programs is banned as well.

To respond to the current outbreak, Indiana Governor Mike Pence signed a 30-day exception to the state's restriction on needle exchange programs. The governor has extended the exception for another 30 days, as the state's legislature considers legalizing needle exchanges in some areas. The Centers for Disease Control and Prevention as well as other federal and state personnel are working to contain the outbreak.

This upsurge in HIV cases in Indiana hasn't exactly come out of nowhere. An increase in Hepatitis C cases (which can also be spread through re-used syringes) began nearly fifteen years ago in Scott County, so officials should not have been surprised that a corresponding rise in HIV cases would eventually follow.

Injection Drug Use and HIV

Injection drug use (IDU) is a well-known risk factor for HIV, as well as Hepatitis B and C infections. The fact is that injection drug use accounts for about one-third of HIV infections in the country since the beginning of the epidemic.

Transmission of HIV occurs through an exchange of bodily fluids. In the case of injection drug use, transmission can occur not only by sharing needles, but by sharing

---

*Originally published as Jeannie D. DiClementi, "Syringe Exchange in Southern Indiana to Respond to an Increase in HIV Cases," *The Conversation*, https://theconversation.com/syringe-exchange-in-southern-indiana-to-respond-to-an-increase-in-hiv-cases-better-late-than-never-40550 (April 28, 2015). Reprinted with permission of the publisher.

any of the materials used to prepare and inject the drug, such as water or cotton used to filter the solution.

Women are particularly vulnerable, either from injecting drugs themselves, or from having unprotected sex with injection drug users, and women account for about twenty percent of new HIV infections yearly.

Why Do People Reuse Syringes?

In most states, access to syringes is severely restricted. This forces injection drug users to reuse or borrow syringes.

These laws intending to prevent illegal injection drug use, while perhaps well-intentioned, do not prevent it. Drug users do not quit because they don't have access to new syringes. Not having access to a clean glass doesn't keep me from being thirsty. Glass or no, I will find a way to get a drink of water.

Being forced to re-use dirty syringes places not only the drug user at risk of greater harm, but the public as well.

In my twenty years of work in the HIV field, I have seen patients who borrowed family members' insulin syringes, migrant workers who shared syringes used to inject liquid vitamins, hospital workers who recovered used syringes from the trash. These syringes are used repeatedly until the needle is too dull to pierce skin. One HIV-positive person places the entire needle-sharing network at risk.

For example, a 73-year-old grandmother was referred to our HIV clinic after her grandson, a 29-year-old addict, had infected her by using and returning her insulin syringes.

We saw groups of migrant workers who had shared needles to inject the liquid vitamins needed to withstand the hard labor, and who were all now HIV positive. We also saw diabetics who shared insulin syringes to save the expense of new ones. The substance being used doesn't matter—only the syringe.

Injection Drugs and Poverty: A Few Hours of Escape

Research also shows an association between poverty and both illegal drug use and HIV infection. The stresses of living in poverty are well known, and often people feel the only ways to relieve the stress include escaping through drug use.

In research conducted in 2011, at Indiana University-Purdue University Fort Wayne (IPFW), located in the center of northeast Indiana counties similar to Scott County, the epicenter of the latest outbreak, we interviewed fifty injection drug users about their drug use. Of the people we interviewed, only one was employed and the rest were living in impoverished situations. Some of the women survived by trading sex for drugs, others in the sample sold drugs—either illegal drugs or legal prescription medications.

They all agreed that getting high was one of the only times they felt good, and while they felt guilty about using drugs, they couldn't give up those few hours of escape that the drugs gave them. Becoming addicted, they then couldn't quit.

None of the people in our sample used drugs alone; they were accompanied by at least one other person, and everyone shared needles at least "several times." Frequent unprotected sex was reported, and only one person reported knowing their HIV status.

Frequently, as the CDC has reported for Scott County, families use drugs together, making it a multigenerational issue. In this case some cases also involve pregnant women who, in a resource-poor area, may or may not have access to treatments that would prevent transmission to their unborn child.

That isn't unusual. Many people with HIV don't know about their positive status. According to the Centers for Disease Control and Prevention, about 14% of 1.2 million HIV positive persons in the US do not know they are HIV positive.

Syringe exchanges can also provide medical services and drug treatment information

Given the incidence of HIV infection in rural, impoverished areas, plus the transmission routes of shared injection syringes and unprotected sex, the situation in southern Indiana is not surprising, and a syringe exchange program (SEP) is a logical response. These programs have been around nearly as long as we have known how HIV is transmitted.

I worked with one such program. A typical SEP trades one sterile syringe for each used syringe. This approach does not put additional syringes on the street. Many programs also include bleach kits and instructions for properly cleaning syringes when clean ones are not available. They also provide condoms and information about safer sexual practices and includes the opportunity for HIV testing.

Research has consistently shown that SEPs do not increase drug use or the number of used syringes discarded in streets and playgrounds. Further, SEPs provide a point of contact for obtaining HIV testing, substance abuse counseling, screening for tuberculosis (TB), hepatitis B, hepatitis C, and other infections as well as referral for medical services.

When I handed out a sterile syringe, bleach kit, and condoms, I also included information about drug rehabilitation, jobs, housing, and my business card. More than once, I received phone calls months later from drug users I had contacted through the SEP who then wanted help with recovery.

Syringe Exchanges Should Be the Rule, Not the exception

The response to the Scott County situation seems reasonable. However, given the predictability of this current outbreak based on the Hepatitis C increase beginning 15 years ago, the Scott County response comes late in the game.

Any HIV statistics are likely underestimates of the true numbers, and given the percentage of persons who are positive and do not know it, the incidence of known HIV cases in Scott and other Indiana counties is quite likely to increase.

Officials would have served the population better with preventative services in place. Governor Pence and the Indiana State Legislature would do well to put establishment of syringe exchange programs on a fast-track to-do list so there is a way to stem the tide of new HIV infections.

37. HIV, STDs, and Hepatitis C*

NEW YORK STATE DEPARTMENT OF HEALTH

The New York State Department of Health (NYSDOH) is the department of the New York state government responsible for public health. It is headed by Health Commissioner Howard A. Zucker, M.D., J.D., who was appointed by Governor Andrew M. Cuomo and confirmed by the State Senate on May 5, 2015. Its regulations are compiled in title 10 of the New York Codes, Rules and Regulations.

Core Services

Promoting the health of all New Yorkers designing and delivering strategies & initiatives to promote population health and prevention ; ensuring access to high-quality, affordable health care; addressing the issues related to and delivering programs to reduce chronic diseases (cancer, heart disease, obesity, diabetes, etc.); promoting maternal, infant and child health; anti-tobacco initiatives; assuring a healthy environment (environmental programs and surveillance, water quality, lead, etc.); eliminating health disparities (ensuring NYs health care delivery system provides accessible, high-quality, affordable services to all New Yorkers across all populations).

AIDS Institute

The New York State Department of Health, AIDS Institute has lead responsibility for coordinating state programs, services and activities relating to HIV/AIDS, sexually transmitted diseases (STDs) and hepatitis C.

NYS Safe Sharps Collection Program

There are many individuals with serious health conditions who manage their care at home and use syringes. For example, people with diabetes use syringes to inject their own insulin and use lancets every day to test their blood glucose. In addition, injection drug users use syringes and needles. Safe disposal of sharps is critically important to optimize

---

*Public document originally published as New York State Department of Health, "HIV, STDs, and Hepatitis C," https://www.health.ny.gov/diseases/aids/consumers/prevention/ (October 2019).

health, safety and protection of the environment. The best way to ensure that people are protected from potential injury or disease transmission of blood borne diseases due to needle sticks is to follow established guidelines for the proper containment of "sharps" syringes, needles and lancets and other safer disposal practices. The Department offers three directories that identify sharps collection sites in communities across New York State.

All hospitals and nursing homes in New York State are mandated by law to accept home-generated sharps as a free community service through their sharps collection programs. In addition, pharmacies, health clinics, community-based organizations, mobile van programs, public transportation facilities, housing projects, police stations, waste transfer stations and other venues have become settings for safe sharps and offer syringe collection drop boxes (or "kiosks") to help facilitate the safe collection of used sharps.

Service providers may share the above directories to educate clients and to refer them to convenient places in the community where they can safely dispose of their household sharps.

Although every attempt has been made to keep the directories updated, service information may have changed since data was collected. Before visiting the location, we suggest calling the phone number alongside the site you are interested in to confirm program information.

Facilities wishing to update information about their community sharps collection sites should e-mail their updated information to New York State Department of Health, AIDS Institute—Sharps Collection Program.

Drug User Health Hubs

The Drug User Health Hubs are expected to improve the availability and accessibility of an array of appropriate health, mental health, and medication assisted treatment services for people who use drugs, especially but not solely injection drug users (IDUs). These services can be provided on-site and/or through facilitated linkage to culturally competent care and treatment services. Drug User Health Hubs operate within a harm reduction framework of prevention with a special emphasis on preventing and responding to opioid overdose. Although the source of contact is self-referral by people who use drugs, funded programs work to foster relationships with law enforcement, emergency departments, emergency medical services and families. Perhaps the most important element of this work is the relationship that is established between the person who is drug involved and the hub organization. It can be a critical turning point in a person's life to have support and guidance that is not predicated on cessation of drug use.

Health Hubs:

- Community Action for Social Justice: Long Island
- Catholic Charities AIDS Services: Albany
- Community Health Action of Staten Island: Staten Island
- Evergreen Health Services: Buffalo
- Southern Tier AIDS Program: Ithaca
- After Hours Project: Brooklyn

- ACR Health: Syracuse
- Alliance for Positive Health: Plattsburgh
- St. Ann's Corner of Harm Reduction: Bronx
- Hudson Valley Community Services: Newburgh
- New York Harm Reduction Educators: Manhattan/Bronx
- Trillium Health: Rochester

Sexually Transmitted Infections (STIs)

Why STI not STD? The New York State Department of Health now uses the term sexually transmitted infection (STI) in place of sexually transmitted disease (STD). The word "disease" suggests noticeable medical problems, while many of the most common sexually transmitted infections have no signs or symptoms, or they are very mild. Even with no signs or symptoms, STIs can cause serious health problems, so it is still necessary to get tested and treated for STIs.

What are STIs? There are more than 30 infections that are spread through vaginal, anal, and oral sex. Some STIs can also be spread through blood, particularly among intravenous (IV) drug users who may be sharing drug equipment (needles, syringes, or "works"). In addition, pregnant people with STIs may pass the infection to infants in the uterus (womb), during birth, or through breast-feeding. Without treatment these infections can cause major health problems such as not being able to get pregnant (infertility), permanent brain damage, heart disease, cancer, and even death. If you think you have been exposed to a sexually transmitted infection, you and your sex partner(s) should visit a health clinic, hospital, or doctor for testing and treatment.

Hepatitis C

Hepatitis C virus (HCV) causes liver disease and it is found in the blood of persons who are infected. HCV is spread by contact with the blood of an infected person.

Hepatitis C infects about 25,000 people each year with most developing chronic infection. However, many of those with chronic hepatitis C do not even know they are infected. Those individuals with chronic infection are at risk for developing chronic liver diseases such as cirrhosis and cancer of the liver. Individuals who injected drugs are at highest risk for infection even if they injected only once many years ago.

Unlike hepatitis A and hepatitis B there is not a vaccine to prevent hepatitis C. Over the years, the treatments for hepatitis C have become more effective. However, treatment is not for everyone and a specialist should be consulted when determining if someone should get treated.

Lesbian, Gay, Bisexual and Transgender Health

One of the goals of the New York State Department of health is to eliminate disparities in health care access by increasing the availability and quality of health care services for New York's underserved populations.

The AIDS Institute has a long and unprecedented history of dedicating resources specifically for LGBT New Yorkers. In 1994, the AIDS Institute developed Lesbian, Gay, Bisexual, and Transgender (LGBT) Health. This initiative supports the provision of effective behavior-based HIV prevention interventions and HIV-related supportive services—including alcohol, substance use and mental health counseling—that address the needs to gay men/men who have sex with men (MSM), lesbians/women who have sex with women (WSW), persons who have sex with multiple genders, and transgender individuals.

In 2008, in a cooperative effort with NYSDOH Center for Community Health, the AIDS Institute developed the LGBT Health and Human Services Unit in an effort to address the non–HIV related health disparities of LGBT persons in NYS. This initiative supports improved access to health care and supportive services, improving health outcomes and quality of life for LGBT individuals, capacity building and increasing community awareness of the health and human service needs of LGBT communities across New York State.

38. Utah Syringe Exchange Program*

UTAH DEPARTMENT OF HEALTH

In 2016, the Utah Legislature passed legislation that legalized syringe exchange programs. The legislation provided limited guidance for the structural elements of a syringe exchange program while giving the Utah Department of Health (UDOH) administrative oversight for syringe exchange activities.

As the oversight body, the UDOH recognized the need to provide an educational resource to parties interested in engaging in syringe exchange activities that outlined the requirements of the legislation, provided guidance about establishing a syringe exchange operation, and offered a list of helpful resources for syringe exchange operating entities. This document serves as a comprehensive resource for organizations that wish to engage in syringe exchange operations in Utah.

The information contained in this handbook is the work of Heather Bush, UDOH Syringe Exchange Coordinator, and Kirsten Dodge, master of professional communication student at Westminster College. Ms. Bush developed the Glossary, the Administrative Rule, and the list of additional resources; Ms. Dodge created the Operating Entity Guide and designed the handbook layout. The UDOH will continue to update this handbook as necessary.

We hope organizations wishing to engage in syringe exchange activities find this handbook to be a valuable resource, which enables them to develop a syringe exchange operation that will provide great value to clients and the greater community, while serving the mission of the organization.

The Administrative Rule Guide provides an overview of the need for and reasoning behind syringe exchange programs, outlines Utah's approach to syringe exchange, and details state requirements for organizations interested in providing syringe exchange services in Utah.

Background

In the early 2000s, the nation began experiencing a growth in the use of illegal opioid drugs brought on by an increase in the number of prescription opioids prescribed to patients for pain management. Many patients became dependent on the prescription opioids and moved on to illegal opioid drugs when they were no longer able to legally

---

*Public document originally published as Utah Department of Health, "Utah Syringe Exchange Program," http://health.utah.gov/epi/prevention/syringeexchange/UTSEP_Handbook.pdf (November 2017).

obtain the prescription opioids. Illegal opioids are often injected into the blood stream; the increase in injection drug use has led to an increase in unsafe injection practices and has put people who inject drugs (PWID) at risk of contracting HIV and viral hepatitis. Recent surveys undertaken by the Centers for Disease Control and Prevention (CDC), indicate that approximately one-third of currently active PWID, ages 18–30 years, are infected with hepatitis C (HCV).

Older and/or former PWID typically have a much higher prevalence (approximately 70%–90%) of HCV infection, reflecting the increased risk of continued injection drug use. HCV is one of the most expensive diseases to treat, with costs ranging between $50,000 and $100,000 for twelve weeks of treatment.

In May 2016, the CDC released information indicating that in 2013 the annual HCV-related mortality rate surpassed the total combined number of deaths from 60 other infectious diseases, including HIV, pneumococcal disease, and tuberculosis. Further, since the studies used data from death certificates, which often underreport hepatitis C, there were likely even more HCV-related deaths than the reports suggest.

One means of preventing transmission of blood-borne infections, such as hepatitis C and HIV, is reducing the sharing of needles, syringes, and other drug injection equipment among PWID. Syringe exchange programs (SEP) allow PWID to exchange used syringes for sterile syringes. SEP are an effective component of a comprehensive approach to preventing the spread of HIV and viral hepatitis among PWID. A large number of scientific studies have found that SEP reduce HIV risk. In 2011, the U.S. Surgeon General determined that SEP are an effective way of reducing HIV transmission among PWID and that there is ample evidence that SEP promote entry to and retention in drug treatment and medical services. SEP are shown to provide a valuable service to PWID without increasing illegal drug use.

Furthermore, SEP support the overall health and well-being of PWID by providing links to substance abuse treatment, medical care, disease testing, overdose prevention, and other vital social services. SEP are based on respect and place value on prioritizing the rights and dignity of PWID people who use drugs.

Expanding the reach of SEP is part of a comprehensive approach to addressing the spread of HIV and viral hepatitis among PWID and supports the goals of the National HIV/AIDS Strategy and Viral Hepatitis Action Plan to reduce the number of new HIV and viral hepatitis infections. Additionally, SEP are an important tool in helping connect people to opiate overdose prevention services.

Drug poisoning deaths are a preventable public health problem. The numbers of drug poisoning deaths per year in Utah and in the U.S. have been rising steadily between 1999 and 2015 as described in "Health Indicator Report of Drug Overdose and Poisoning Incidents." Deaths from drug poisoning have outpaced deaths due to firearms, falls, and motor vehicle crashes in Utah. In 2015, Utah ranked 9th in the U.S. for drug poisoning deaths with a rate of 23.4 deaths per 100,000 population. Every month, 52 Utah adults die because of a drug poisoning. 83.8% of these deaths are accidental or of undetermined intent; 77.6% of these deaths involve opioids. The United States government recognizes the need to implement programs aimed at stopping the spread of disease and reducing overdose deaths across the country.

The U.S. Department of Health and Human Services (HHS) is committed to working with grantees and partners to reduce the spread of HIV and viral hepatitis in the U.S. In March 2016, HHS issued guidance for HHS-funded programs regarding the use of federal funds to implement or expand SEP. The guidance is the result of the bipartisan budget agreement that was signed into law in December 2015, which revised a previous Congressional ban on the use of federal funds for such programs. Communities that demonstrate a need may now use federal funds for the operational components of SEP.

The HHS guidance describes how health departments can request federal funds to start or expand SEP; it also outlines how the funds can be used. The guidance requires that state, local, tribal, and territorial health departments consult with the CDC and provide evidence that its jurisdiction is (1) experiencing, or (2) at risk for significant increases in viral hepatitis infections or an HIV outbreak due to injection drug use.

On behalf of the state of Utah, the UDOH submitted a "Determination of Need" (DON) to the CDC, identifying Utah as being at risk for significant increases in viral hepatitis infections or an HIV outbreak due to injection drug use. The DON was reviewed and approved by the CDC in June 2016.

The notice of approval to Utah from the CDC states:

> After careful review of the Utah Department of Health's submission, CDC concurs that Utah is at risk for an increase in viral hepatitis or HIV infections due to injection drug use. The submitted data provide sufficient evidence to determine a need for SEP within the jurisdiction. Specifically, the requestor presented statewide data on epidemiologic trends that indicate increases in unsafe injection of illicit drugs as well as data on statewide increases in HIV and acute HCV infections due to injection drug use. The increase in IDU-associated HIV infections, though small in number, is noteworthy insofar as nationally over the same period IDU-associated HIV infections have fallen and the fidelity with which HIV infection is diagnosed and transmission risk is determined is high. The narrative makes a compelling case that there are multiple counties within the state where these increases are focused. Increases in opioid-related deaths in the context of increasing seizure of heroin by law enforcement suggest the increase in heroin seizures represents a greater supply of drugs and consequent opioid deaths and does not necessarily reflect solely increased law enforcement activity.

Agencies within the state of Utah may now apply for or reallocate federal HHS funds for syringe exchange activities. Only HHS grantees that have direct HHS funding can request direct funding for SEP activities. For example, a direct grantee of CDC, HRSA, SAMHSA may apply for new funds or re-direct current funds within allowable funding announcements to be used to support SEP activities.

Utah Syringe Exchange Program Overview

On March 25, 2016, Governor Gary Herbert signed House Bill 308 into law, which legalized the development of a syringe exchange program in Utah. The Utah Syringe Exchange Statute, which went into effect May 10, 2016, states that agencies in Utah "may operate a syringe exchange program in the state to prevent the transmission of disease and reduce morbidity and mortality among individuals who inject drugs and those individuals' contacts." The law outlines required activities and reporting guidelines but does not provide funding or guidance for operating the Utah Syringe Exchange Program. An accompanying Administrative Rule was published on November 7, 2016. This rule provides guidelines for eligible agencies wishing to conduct a syringe exchange in Utah.

The following section describes the requirements of agencies conducting syringe exchange. For additional information, interested parties are encouraged to utilize the

UDOH Syringe Exchange Program Website and/or contact syringeexchange@utah.gov with any questions.

Syringe Exchange Program Enrollment

In accordance with the Utah Syringe Exchange Statute and the Utah Syringe Exchange Administrative Rule, agencies interested in providing syringe exchange services in Utah must meet the following conditions and requirements prior to being certified as a syringe exchange operator (SEO).

Eligible Agencies

The Utah Syringe Exchange Statute states that any of the following entities may operate syringe exchange services in the state:

- A government entity, including the Utah Department of Health, a local
- health department, the Division of Substance Abuse and Mental Health within the Department of Human Services, or a local substance abuse authority.
- A nongovernment entity, including a nonprofit organization or a for-profit organization.

Eligible agencies must enroll and meet certain requirements prior to beginning any syringe exchange activities.

Operating Entity

An operating entity is any eligible agency or program that has been approved to and is conducting syringe exchange activities as outlined in Administrative Rule 386–900.

Agencies that provide other related services, such as HIV/HCV testing, substance abuse treatment, etc., but DO NOT distribute or collect syringes are not considered an operating entity and do not need to enroll.

Enrollment Requirements

All eligible agencies interested in providing syringe services must enroll with the UDOH. Enrollment requires the submission of the following items: a completed agency enrollment form, a safety protocol plan, and a sharps disposal plan.

To request a Utah Syringe Exchange Program Agency Enrollment Form email syringeexchange@utah.gov with your agency's intent to become an operating entity. A link to the online enrollment form will be sent to the identified contact. The enrollment form provides written notice of intent to conduct syringe exchange activities and must be submitted to the UDOH 15 days prior to conducting syringe exchange activities.

The eligible agency's safety protocol plan must include details on how the agency will prevent needle sticks and sharps injuries for its workers, volunteers, and clients.

Additionally, the plan must include the agency's procedure for disposing of all spent or used needles it collects. Disposal of used and collected needles is the financial responsibility of the operating entity.

After the UDOH confirms receipt of an eligible agency's enrollment and safety protocol plan, the eligible agency will be notified of its status as an operating entity. The UDOH will provide the operating entity with a program number and a certificate of enrollment, as well as instructions on how to report information required by R386-900. Upon approval by UDOH and having met the requirements of R386-900, the operating entity may begin providing syringe exchange services in Utah.

Operating entities may request available supplies, materials, and training support from the UDOH. Agencies can submit requests using the UDOH Syringe Exchange Program Supplies Order Form. Completed forms should be sent to syringeexchange@utah.gov.

Termination of Syringe Exchange Operation

If an operating entity discontinues syringe exchange activities, written notice must be submitted to UDOH by sending an email of intent to terminate to syringe exchange@utah.gov and completing the online disenrollment form that is sent within 15 days of termination of activities.

An operating entity may choose to terminate services due to changes in management, agency priorities, funding, etc.

The Department can terminate an operating entity's status as a syringe exchange provider if the entity violates a provision of Administrative Rule R386. The Department can assess a penalty to an operating entity as provided in section 26-23-6 of the Administrative Rule.

Operating Entity Requirements

All operating entities must follow the requirements as outlined in the Utah Syringe Exchange Statute, the Utah Syringe Exchange Administrative Rule, and by the Department.

Program Element Requirements

The operating entity must include the following elements in its syringe exchange program:

- Facilitate the exchange of an individual's used syringes by providing a disposable, medical grade sharps container for the disposal of used syringes. Sharps disposal is the financial responsibility of the operating entity.
- Exchange one or more new syringes in sealed sterile packages with the individual free of charge.
- Provide and make available to all recipients of new syringe(s) verbal and written instruction on

- Methods for preventing the transmission of blood-borne pathogens, including HIV, HBV and HCV.
- Information and referral to drug and alcohol treatment.
- Information and referral for HIV and HCV testing.
- Instruction on how and where to obtain an opiate antagonist (naloxone).

Reporting Requirements

All operating entities must record and report aggregate data elements to the UDOH on a quarterly basis.

Required Data Elements

The following items are required data elements that must be reported quarterly to the UDOH:

- Number of individuals who have exchanged syringes
- A self-reported or approximated number of used syringes exchanged for new syringes
- Number of new syringes provided in exchange for used syringes
- Educational materials distributed
- Number of referrals provided

Optional Data Collection Elements

The following items are optional elements that an operating entity may wish to submit to the UDOH:

- Participant enrollment form
- Event activity log

Quarterly Reporting Information

In accordance with the Utah Syringe Exchange Statute, all entities engaging in syringe exchange services must submit a quarterly report to the UDOH.

Quarterly Report Form

Refer to the Online Database section found below for detailed information on reporting through the online database. Operating entities will be sent a report form to fill out at the end of the quarter. A paper version, Utah Syringe Exchange Program: Quarterly Report Form can be downloaded from the UDOH website. Operating entities engaging in syringe exchange services must return this form to the Department each quarter.

Online Database

The UDOH utilizes the browser-based Research Electronic Data Capture (REDCap) software to collect and analyze pertinent data on syringe exchange programs and participants. Within this software, the USEP utilizes both "surveys" and "forms" to collect data in REDCap. Surveys are initiated by an outside entity and do not require users to log into REDCap to enter data. For example, UDOH will send surveys to operating entities. However, users will not have access to the data that is entered into the survey.

Individual users from operating entities must log into REDCap in order to enter data. Users are able to see the data they collect and can generate statistics and reports within REDCap.

Agency Info and Login

The Agency Enrollment Form is available by sending an email to syringeexchange@utah.gov requesting interest in enrollment; the contact will be sent a link to an electronic form.

If an operating entity enrolls electronically through REDCap, it will receive an email from UDOH within 7 business days, indicating whether the agency has been enrolled as an SEP. If an operating entity seeking enrollment has not heard from the UDOH within this time, please email syringeexchange@utah.gov to inquire about enrollment status.

User Training

Operating entities that opt-in to using the online database, will be provided training on how to create a login, enter data, and run reports.

Additional Support

Technical assistance and capacity building is available for syringe exchange operating entities and program coordinators. For questions regarding syringe exchange, enrollment, operating procedures, or other program-related issues, please contact syringeexchange@utah.gov.

In an effort to provide ongoing support to the enrolled operating entities, the UDOH will provide educational materials, outreach supplies, and information on funding as these items become available.

In order to effectively conduct all of the elements of Administrative Rule 386-900, the UDOH will provide training on the following information to all operating entities upon request:

- Data Collection
- Harm Reduction and Syringe Exchange Basics
- HIV/HCV Basics
- Naloxone Administration
- Online Database
- Overdose Prevention

39. Arizona Declares Opioid Emergency, but Signals Are Mixed Over Best Response*

Will Stone

It's no secret why drug users come to George Patterson in a mall parking lot just outside Phoenix to get their clean needles, syringes and other supplies on Tuesday afternoons, instead of heading to the pharmacy down the street.

"It's really low-barrier the way we are doing it," Patterson said. "All you have to do is find us."

Patterson asks for no IDs, no signatures and no questions—all of which might dissuade IV drug users from seeking out clean needles or the overdose reversal drug naloxone, Patterson said. He's among the volunteers who run Central Arizona's only syringe exchange program; it's called Shot in the Dark.

"A lot of [the drug users he sees] have trust issues—understandably—with the health care industry, with what's going to be put on their record," Patterson said, as he handed out the medical supplies from the trunk of his car.

While many states have syringe exchanges, only some have laws that explicitly permit syringe exchanges—and Arizona isn't one of them. Shot in the Dark operates quietly, without public funding. The group sets up in different corners of the Phoenix metro area for a few hours at a time, Patterson said, and struggles to keep up with demand.

"There are still a lot of people that don't know even know about it," said one man who uses the service. "It shouldn't be so hidden." Kaiser Health News and NPR agreed not to use his name because his drug use is illegal.

States across the U.S. are pouring resources into fighting the opioid epidemic. According to state data from 2016, an average of two people died every day in Arizona from opioid-related overdoses. Deaths due to heroin more than tripled from 2012 to 2016.

"It's a problem that knows no bounds," Arizona's Republican governor, Doug Ducey, said in January during his State of the State address. "It affects men and women, young and old, rich and poor."

---

*Originally published as Will Stone, "Arizona Declares Opioid Emergency, but Signals Are Mixed Over Best Response," *Kaiser Health News*, https://khn.org/news/arizona-declares-opioid-emergency-but-signals-are-mixed-over-best-response/ (December 21, 2017). Reprinted with permission of the publisher. Kaiser Health News is a nonprofit news service covering health issues. It is an editorially independent program of the Kaiser Family Foundation that is not affiliated with Kaiser Permanente. This story is part of a partnership that includes KJZZ, NPR and Kaiser Health News.

Ducey has declared the opioid epidemic a public health emergency—a move that a handful of other states have made, too. In Arizona, the designation allowed public health officials to begin tracking overdose data in real time and set in motion a multiagency effort to combat the epidemic.

But some public health advocates, including Patterson, see the governor's declaration not necessarily translating into more help for people on the street using drugs.

"Instead of focusing on ways that you can connect with the IV-drug-using population—show them that their health matters, and prevent all the people who are likely never going to stop using IV drugs," Patterson said, "they, like, leave them out here to pick up dirty needles out of parks and give themselves diseases."

Needle exchanges are based on a concept known as harm reduction—they seek to reduce the negative consequences of drug use without forcing abstinence. The U.S. Surgeon General has determined such programs don't promote drug use and do improve health outcomes, including lower HIV rates.

But that hasn't convinced some of Arizona's most influential law enforcement figures.

"It's a well-intentioned, misguided program," Maricopa County Attorney Bill Montgomery said. "We don't have a free-case-of-beer-a-month program for alcoholics. It sends the wrong message—and it's not providing the treatment."

This is a common argument against syringe exchange programs—that they enable drug use. Proponents of harm reduction, however, point to research showing that people who use these programs are actually more likely than others to seek treatment.

Despite his lack of faith in needle exchange programs, Montgomery said he is sympathetic to people who are addicted to opioids—he is not out to prosecute drug users when he doesn't have to.

"Law enforcement really does look at 'treatment first' as an option for those who are addicted," Montgomery said. He pointed to a pretrial diversion program that is expanding statewide, and the Arizona Angel Initiative, which lets drug users turn to the police and opt for treatment.

Expanding those kinds of programs is part of the state's wide-ranging Opioid Action Plan, which treatment specialists helped craft.

Arizona's 100-page policy road map recommends improving access to treatment and naloxone, as well as enacting a Good Samaritan law that gives immunity to those who call 911 to report an overdose.

But the plan also proposes more regulation of doctors and their prescribing practices, including a five-day limit on initial opioid prescriptions for patients who are taking the drug for the first time.

That kind of focus on prescribers is "misguided," said Dr. Jeffrey Singer, an Arizona surgeon, and senior fellow at the libertarian Cato Institute.

"Our policies right now are aimed at the supply side," Singer said. "And all they are doing is driving the death rate up. They're not driving use down."

Opioid users are increasingly turning to heroin and fentanyl, Singer said. He points to research that shows the rate of opioid prescriptions has fallen in recent years while the deaths associated with illicit drugs continue to rise.

Singer believes even labeling the state's opioid crisis as a public health emergency could backfire.

"That tends to create a sense of panic," Singer said. "History has shown us every time we have a panic, we end up passing laws and doing things in haste that are not well thought out."

Singer thinks Arizona should embrace harm reduction strategies like syringe exchanges, instead of tamping down prescribing.

"My job is to save lives and to ease suffering," Singer said. "The law enforcement people need to have that same attitude. We've got to take personal biases out of it and just focus on the goal, which is less death and less disease."

Earlier this year, the Arizona Department of Health Services asked a group of treatment providers who were working on the state's action plan for their top recommendations. Legalizing syringe exchanges was one of the group's priorities, according to interviews and draft documents obtained by KJZZ News.

But that priority didn't make the final version of the plan; only a broad reference to using "harm reduction strategies" survived.

A spokesperson for the department said the recommendation was omitted because it "doesn't directly reduce opioid-related overdoses or deaths."

40. Unable to Arrest Opioid Epidemic, Red States Warm to Needle Exchanges*

Shefali Luthra

WILMINGTON, N.C.—Former heroin user Kendra Williams, 24, knows she's lucky. She recalls sharing dirty syringes to shoot up, risking hepatitis C and HIV. More than two years into recovery, she knows about 30 people who have died from drug overdoses—this year. Over the past five, she guesses, it's close to 50.

Against that grim backdrop, Williams has joined an unlikely coalition—composed of public health advocates, former addicts and the law enforcement officers who used to harass and arrest them—bent on battling sky-high rates of opioid abuse. With the goal of curbing the spread of disease and preventing overdose, the North Carolina Harm Reduction Coalition (NCHRC) has helped legalize needle exchanges, enabled safe disposal of used syringes and enacted protections for people who carry drug paraphernalia.

Such an approach might seem normal in liberal New York or California, and these strategies have long found support in public health and medical communities. Implementing them here—in a tough-on-drugs state with the help of a Republican-controlled statehouse—is no small task.

"Even five years ago, I wouldn't have seen this happening," said Williams, whose hometown is considered one of the worst in the country for opioid addiction. "We're in the Bible Belt. There are a lot of people that aren't very friendly to people who use drugs. They get grouped into, 'waste of time, waste of resources.'"

The shift is at odds with national rhetoric. U.S. Attorney General Jeff Sessions has instructed his state counterparts to take a hard line in the war on drugs, encouraging arrest and jail time for relatively low-level infractions. But even some of the most conservative corners of the country are moving in the other direction, often propelled by a growing awareness among veteran law enforcement officers that they can no longer try to arrest their way out of the problem.

Kentucky has already legalized needle swaps. Ohio and Indiana have loosened

---

*Originally published as Shefali Luthra, "Unable to Arrest Opioid Epidemic, Red States Warm to Needle Exchanges," *Kaiser Health News*, https://khn.org/news/unable-to-arrest-opioid-epidemic-red-states-warm-to-needle-exchanges/(June 14, 2017). Reprinted with permission of the publisher. Kaiser Health News is a nonprofit news service covering health issues. It is an editorially independent program of the Kaiser Family Foundation that is not affiliated with Kaiser Permanente.

restrictions on the practice. Georgia, South Carolina, Alabama, Tennessee, Mississippi and Louisiana are weighing it.

In North Carolina, NCHRC's message found a compelling voice with champions like Ronald Martin, a transplanted New York City police detective sergeant who moved here in 2012 and works to educate police departments on why harm-reduction strategies could benefit them. He points out that in states where needle possession has been decriminalized, or where exchanges are legal, officers conducting searches are less likely to get pricked by infected needles. Cops are often on the scene of drug overdoses. They see the toll addiction takes, and they count the bodies.

Support from law enforcement—notably, many well-known sheriffs—was the "golden ticket" for getting harm-reduction laws such as legalization of needle exchanges through the statehouse, said Tessie Castillo, who coordinates advocacy and communications for NCHRC. That flagship policy won approval in 2016.

There is no data yet indicating what effect the changes in North Carolina's laws have had on opioid deaths or associated infections. The federal Centers for Disease Control and Prevention, which tracks overdose deaths, found that in 2015—a year before syringe exchanges were legalized—heroin deaths in the state increased from the previous year by about 46 percent, and opioid deaths in general climbed by almost 15 percent. Rates of hepatitis C also climbed from 2014 to 2016, the state health department reports. Those numbers help explain the state's shift.

"If you had told me 10 years ago I was going to advocate for syringe exchanges, I'd have said you're crazy," said Donnie Varnell, an investigator with the Dare County Sheriff's Office, in eastern North Carolina.

Recruiting New Allies

Changing the mindset and culture among police and lawmakers in North Carolina was hardly simple. After all, harm-reduction advocates are asking the very people tasked with enforcing the law to permit illegal activity. Critics still worry that the new approach enables addiction and legitimizes crime.

Martin travels the state to teach officers about needle exchanges, syringe decriminalization and naloxone—a drug often sold in a nasal spray version as Narcan—that reverses overdoses. Despite his own background in narcotics, he wasn't originally a harm-reduction evangelist. But after hearing the case NCHRC laid out, he says, he was convinced. His efforts are a break from the traditional emphasis on arresting drug offenders. Martin's approach instead involves acknowledging that people use illicit drugs and then keeping them as safe as possible.

Martin, a burly 57-year-old, transports visual aids in a Wild Turkey bourbon box, eliciting jokes from fellow police. He peppers his speech with *Star Trek* jokes or, at a workshop, references to a *Guardians of the Galaxy* movie. He describes the course as a safety training: role-playing about de-escalation tactics so cops avoid needle pricks, while sharing his own New York stories. He doesn't mention the new harm-reduction laws until the presentation's end, framing them as an obvious precaution.

"I'm taking a needle off the street, so that little Johnny or little Betty doesn't find it in the parking lot, and I'm giving you a clean one back so you won't be exposed to HIV or hepatitis C," he said. "When you keep it relatively simplistic … there's not this tremendous resistance."

Cop-to-cop, many officers come around to thinking that harm reduction is logical. Take Brad Shirley, chief of police in Boiling Springs Lakes, a small town near the border with South Carolina. Shirley was initially skeptical, but his police department now keeps a biohazard waste bin outside headquarters, where people can drop off needles anonymously.

Jarryd Rauhoff, an officer with the Fayetteville Police Department, said the idea of syringe exchanges first crossed his radar maybe two years ago. Harm reduction doesn't match his crime-fighting philosophy, but he's come to think of the idea as a no-brainer.

"If we're able to improve the conditions of those people who have addiction—why would we not want to do that?" Rauhoff asked.

Changing a Culture

In Raleigh, officers are now generally on board with the changes, said Jesse Bennett, who coordinates Raleigh's exchange. He keeps needles, disposal kits, condoms and naloxone in his car. When meeting drug users unfamiliar with how needle swaps work, he explains cops generally understand the rules: Needle possession is legal if you have an exchange membership card.

He still advises members to call him if an officer seems skeptical. NCHRC will help navigate court proceedings that could follow.

"North Carolina shows that people's opinions can change. It's a big deal," said Corey Davis, a staff attorney at the National Health Law Program, a nonprofit that pushes for improved health care access for low-income people.

Still, advocates say they face challenges and resistance in fully implementing the strategy.

Chief is the awareness gap: Not all cops are as knowledgeable as the Raleigh squad is. When Martin spoke with 10 officers at a May event two hours outside of Raleigh, none knew needle exchanges were legal. And some maintain that, even with these laws on the books, they will not stop making drug arrests.

Plus, when North Carolina passed syringe exchanges, conservative lawmakers added a provision prohibiting public funds from paying for needles. This legislative session, NCHRC is pushing to get that ban reversed. Until that happens, meeting the demand for clean needles is harder and they must rely on private donations, said Robert Childs, NCHRC's executive director.

Meanwhile, the new push from the Justice Department could complicate efforts in states looking to push harm reduction, said Daniel Raymond, a policy analyst with the national Harm Reduction Coalition. But he argued that the surge in drug abuse and climbing rates of hepatitis C would still push lawmakers to rethink these kinds of policies.

And for people like Kendra Williams—where this sea change has already begun—the impact is tremendous.

Williams, who focused on getting clean after learning she was pregnant with her now-2-year-old son, Nathan, initially used money from working as a secretary, at a local diner and then at a day care center to buy clean needles from Walgreens for friends. And even after she stopped using, she habitually crossed the street to avoid police officers.

Now, she works with the police and can operate a syringe exchange in plain daylight, without worrying about the consequences. The friends she once worried about, who still use drugs, know where to find help. They can call organizers like her, or dial 911—something once inconceivable.

"I've had a friend go up to a cop and say, 'I know y'all are carrying Narcan now. I need to find help,'" she recalled. "That was pretty cool."

• *C. County and City* •

41. The Competing Views and a Way Forward*

ELISSA VELEZ *and* MICKEY P. MCGEE

This chapter provides an overview of the skeptical and optimistic views on syringe exchange approaches which inspired San Francisco's way forward—anchored on harm reduction, inclusion, and collaboration.

Skeptics

Syringe exchange is advancing as an HIV prevention strategy; however, there are several arguments as to why it should not be. The first argument against syringe exchange is based on the medical breakthrough that drug addiction is a complex disease. The argument claims that syringe exchange is well intended but ignores the soul-controlling darkness of addiction and the moral free fall that sustains it. "When addicts talk about enslavement, they're not exaggerating," says Terry Horton, medical director of Phoenix House, one of the nation's largest residential treatment centers. "It is their first and foremost priority. Heroin first, then breathing, then food" (Loconte, 1998)."

Christian groups and anti-syringe exchange proponents do not accept harm reduction efforts related to drug use. Archbishop Francis Chullikatt, Permanent Observer of the Holy See, referred to measures such as needle-exchange programs as "efforts that do not respect the dignity of those who are suffering from drug addiction as they do not treat or cure the sick person, but instead falsely suggest that they cannot break free from the cycle of addiction" (Catholic World News, 2011). Herbert Kleber, a psychiatrist and a leading addiction specialist, treated drug abusers for 30 years. He said needle exchange programs (NEPs), even those that offer education and health services, aren't likely to become beacons of behavior modification. "Addiction erodes your ability to change your behavior," he said. "And NEPs have no track record of changing risky sexual behavior."

Eric Voth, chairman of the International Drug Strategy Institute and one of the nation's leading addiction specialists, asked, "What makes anybody think they'll [drug addicts] make clean needles a priority?" By not talking much about drug abuse, NEP activists effectively sidestep the desperation created by addiction; a move that further amplifies risky sexual behavior. When drug users run out of money for their habit, for example, they often turn to prostitution no matter how many clean needles are in the

---

*Published with permission of the authors.

cupboard. And the most common way of contracting HIV is, of course, sexual intercourse. "Sex is a currency in the drug world," says Horton of Phoenix House. "It is a major mode of HIV infection. And you don't address that with needle exchange" (Loconte, 1998).

Along with the belief that dispersing clean needles does nothing for discouraging drug dependence, several other factors fuel the fight against needle exchange programs. Other arguments include the fact that drug addicts are still prone to death, perhaps not from HIV, but from overdose, collapsed veins, poisoned dope, or the violence and criminality that go along with the illicit drug trade; drug-addicted mothers will still deliver drug-addicted babies; sterile needles offer the path of least resistance rather than address underlying psychoses; and does nothing for broken homes, killings, and the harm created by drugs (Aaron, 2005).

Critics of needle exchange seem to acknowledge that there's a certain logic to the concept, at least in theory: Give enough clean needles to an IV drug user and he or she won't use a contaminated syringe when one is needed. However, concepts and theories are just that; the most relevant piece of the puzzle is data. Don Des Jarlais, a researcher at New York's Beth Israel Medical Center, writes in a 1996 report that "there has been no direct evidence that participation is associated with a lower risk" of HIV infection. Peter Lurie, writing in the American Journal of Epidemiology, says that "no one study, on its own, should be used to declare the programs effective" (Loconte, 1998).

According to a study published in 1993 by the University of California and funded by the Centers for Disease Control, a panel reviewed 21 studies on the impact of NEPs on HIV infection rates. But the best the authors could say for the programs was that none showed a higher prevalence of HIV among program clients. To further identify inefficacies panel members rated the scientific quality of the studies on a five-point scale: one meant "not valid," three "acceptable," and five "excellent." Only two of the studies earned ratings of three or higher. Of those, neither showed a reduction in HIV levels (Loconte, 1998).

Drug users face a myriad of challenges, according to a study conducted by the University of Pennsylvania which followed 415 IV drug users in Philadelphia over four years. Twenty-eight died during the study. Five died from causes associated with HIV and most died for other reasons: overdoses, homicide, heart disease, kidney failure, liver disease, and suicide (Loconte, 1998). In research from the *New England Journal of Medicine*, medical professors George Woody and David Metzger said that compared to the risk of HIV infection, the threat of death to drug abusers from other causes is "more imminent" (Loconte, 1998).

Optimists

Although arguments against needle exchange programs perceive the efforts of syringe distribution as facilitating and increasing illicit drug injection as well as doing nothing for the drug addiction disease, data says the answer is different. According to a study on the cessation of injection drug use and injection frequency between 1997 and 2002, 901 injection drug users (IDUs) were recruited from a NEP program or an area with no NEP in Chicago, Illinois, interviewed for drug use behaviors, tested for HIV and followed for three annual visits. All participants were exposed to prevention services targeting HIV and drug abuse. Injection cessation was defined as no injection drug use since the last interview, and changes in the number of injections in a typical month were examined. The findings showed that sixteen percent of study participants reported stopping injection for a median duration of 16 months, and most of them also ceased rather than initiated the use of non-injected drugs. Those who continued injecting reduced their injection frequency by 12% per year, on average. These results did not support the hypothesis that NEP use influences the frequency of injection over time. One-sixth of IDUs stopped injection for more than one year, providing a substantial window for relapse prevention interventions (Huo, 2005).

The World Health Organization concludes that there is reasonable evidence that needle syringe programs can increase recruitment into drug treatment and possibly also into primary health care. Additional research from WHO shows that overall, there is convincing evidence that NSPs, assessed conservatively, fulfill six of the nine Bradford Hill criteria (strength of association, replication of findings, temporal sequence, biological plausibility, coherence of the evidence and argument by analogy) and all of the five additional criteria (cost effectiveness, absence of negative consequences, feasibility of implementation, expansion and coverage, unanticipated benefits and special populations). Measured against any objective standards, the evidence to support the effectiveness of NSPs in substantially reducing HIV must be regarded as overwhelming (Wodak & Cooney, 2004).

Other compelling data indicates that many studies have demonstrated multiple health benefits of NSPs apart from a reduction in HIV infection. These additional benefits include improved entry to primary health care and drug treatment, prevention of other blood-borne viral infections, reduced proximal bacterial infection (e.g., abscess and cellulitis) and reduced distal bacterial infection (e.g., subacute bacterial endocarditis, brain abscess). NSPs offer a "package" of different services, including education about protection against other blood-borne viruses and sexually acquired HIV, overdose prevention, education about cleaning injection equipment and information about drug treatment. Reductions in risk behavior and HIV seroconversion could be the result of these other services (such as acquiring clean syringes from pharmacies, using condoms and other safer sexual practices) rather than the needle and syringe exchange, distribution or sale (Wodak & Cooney, 2004).

Needle exchange programs have operated for more than two decades as community-based interventions to reduce the spread of HIV and other blood-borne infectious diseases in IV drug users. Most of the studies reviewed have shown that NEPs are associated with impressive and generally consistent reductions in the lending, borrowing, and sharing of non-sterile syringes and related injection equipment, and with lower incidence of HIV seroconversion. Health care officials and program staff often fail to view NEPs and substance abuse treatment programs as complementary health care services that can provide a bidirectional continuum of services and support (Kidorf & King, 2008).

Many of the arguments against this harm reduction strategy discuss the reality that drug users are still prone to death due to overdose, drug related illness, or the violence and criminality that go along with the illicit drug trade. Arguments have been made about drug-addicted mothers delivering drug-addicted babies, broken homes, killings, and the harm created by drugs, yet needle exchange programs do not pledge to combat these issues. These are drug related problems that must be dealt with using social welfare programs and law enforcement initiatives. Needle exchange programs offer clients the ability to minimize the harm caused to their health by obtaining sterile syringes, education, drug treatment, and overdose prevention, providing referrals for health and social services, and giving clients more access to STI, hepatitis C, and HIV testing.

"Overall, HIV incidence among individuals exposed through IDU has decreased approximately 80% in the United States. Over that time, [people] exposed through IDU have reduced needle sharing by using sterile syringe available through needle exchange programs or pharmacies and have reduced the number of individuals with whom they share needles," the San Francisco Aids Foundation reports (SFAF, 2013). Mounting epidemiologic data point to an overall decline in new HIV infections among injection drug users (IDUs) over the past 20 years in the United States, with parallel but more modest decline in hepatitis C rates. Newly revised HIV incidence estimates from the CDC projected that in 2006, injection drug use accounted for 6,600 HIV infections in the U.S., with an additional 2,100 new infections among men who have sex with men (MSM) who also report injecting drugs (SFAF, 2013).

Studies (e.g., Normand, et al., 1995) have shown that a reduced HIV infection is not the only benefit of NEPs. The other benefits are less well documented and do not seem to be as powerful as the impact on HIV infection. For example, NEPs offer better access to HIV testing and treatment, addiction care, and most significantly, to general medical treatment for the many other health problems plaguing this marginal population (Drucker, 2012). The existence of these additional benefits is attractive from a public health and policy perspective, the effect of NEPs does not appear to be specific to HIV prevention (Wodak & Cooney, 2004). We found significant data through literature review indicating that NEPs exceed their intended purpose and contribute to the overall health and well-being of IDUs.

Because SAS is the nation's largest and most successful needle exchange program its unique and exceptional qualities can promote understanding and inform why harm reduction is effective, if at all. Needle distribution is based on a harm reduction philosophy which aims to curb the damage associated with drug use.

A Way Forward

It took decades of discussions and experimentation for San Francisco to develop a program that balances the views of both skeptics and optimists.

The advent of needle distribution emerged long before needle exchange became a formal process. According to a publication from Kaiser Forum, needle distribution in San Francisco can be remembered as far back as the 1970s at places like San Francisco State University.

Reggie Lyells of the Berkeley Police Department described the efforts of the time as "giving away needles was a way to deal with yellow jaundice and abscesses from shooting heroin" (Lane, 1991). As illness through blood borne pathogens increased, actions to curve the spread expanded as well. "Patricia Case, one of the early organizers of San Francisco's needle exchange program, remembers the early days of the HIV epidemic at San Francisco General Hospital. Doctors and nurses would leave a ten-pack of syringes in view of someone they knew was injecting drugs, then walk out of the room" (Lane, 1991).

On November 2, 1988, San Francisco's Prevention Point, the first ever San Francisco needle-exchange program was opened. This program was primarily volunteer. "Prevention Point started with two teams, one roving and one stationary; its approach involves five or six volunteers standing in a row; clients file past, exchanging needles and syringes, and collecting condoms, cotton, alcohol wipes, and bleach" (Lane, 1991).

Prevention Point program activities, although tolerated by the city remained illegal by state legislation. The AIDS epidemic continued to grow. AIDS case surveillance reported the highest number of new cases by date of diagnosis in 1993 (Osmond, 2003). The sobering increase of HIV/AIDS cases in San Francisco led then-Mayor Frank Jordon to declare a state of public-health emergency in San Francisco. Ultimately this declaration gave San Francisco the power to legalize needle distribution programs and provide funds to them. That year under Frank Jordon's leadership San Francisco committed $138,000 to Prevention Point.

"In the years that followed Mayor Jordan's emergency declaration, needle exchange became an integral part of HIV prevention in San Francisco. Eventually, Prevention Point became a part of San Francisco AIDS Foundation and has since grown into the nation's largest needle exchange program" (SFAF, 2012). In 1991 Prevention Point was distributing more than 8,000 syringes a week in San Francisco (Gross, 1991). Now, Syringe Access Services (formerly Prevention Point) distributes more than 2.4 million clean needles at nearly a dozen different sites across San Francisco (SFAF, 2012). These efforts continue to grow: Syringe Access Services (SAS) now collaborates with multiple other community partners to distribute clean needles across the city and is supported by a group of nearly 70 volunteers (SFAF, 2012).

Community collaboration is key for connecting with hard-to-reach populations. Public health experts have called attention on ways in which they can more effectively reach and influence injection drug users (IDUs) and intensify efforts to develop and carry out prevention and treatment strategies directed to IDUs and their sex partners and children (Gayle, 2000).

A coordinated and collaborative approach to serving IDUs, their sex partners, and their children is essential because no one provider or institution can or does deliver all required services.

In early 2010, the San Francisco Department of Public Health (SFDPH) convened a meeting of syringe providers at the San Francisco AIDS Foundation. The Department wanted to create a collaborative program that would reduce their administrative burden and be more cost-efficient. There was considerable resistance by the smaller providers to the SFDPH suggestion that they come under the umbrella of the San Francisco AIDS Foundation. A series of operational decisions were made by senior leadership that addressed these concerns and successfully led to the creation of a multifaceted collaborative called, Syringe Access Collaborative. This new entity both reduced the funder's monitoring expenses as well as created the opportunity to design a program that more effectively met the needs of a culturally diverse and geographically dispersed IDU population (SFAF, 2013).

IDUs are tremendously diverse. "They have different languages, cultures, sexual orientations, life circumstances, behaviors, and requirements for services. In planning and delivering interventions, programs and providers must take into account the factors that characterize IDUs—who they are, where they are, what they do, what motivates them, and with whom they socialize" (Gayle, 2000). The SAC allows several agencies in the city to work together under SFAF to provide clean needles to each agency's specific populations.

Monolingual Spanish communities seek out services in Spanish while women sex workers may feel comfortable at an organization that caters to their needs; as such, all HIV prevention organizations have made it a priority to have sterile syringes available to their constituents.

The introduction of San Francisco's needle exchange program has created an opportunity for thousands of individuals to be affected by HIV prevention efforts; however, this case study seeks to evaluate whether individuals are actually being helped by this program and if so, measure the extent of which the program increases well-being of the injection drug users.

Injection drug users are a marginalized population that keep hidden for fear of legal implications, shame, and drug users' stigma. Often confined to "shooting ranges" and "trap houses," drug users can find it difficult to leave, making access to clean needles limited and interactions with the outside world scarce. Most forms of injecting drug use are felony offenses in the United States. In addition, they are highly stigmatized, inherently dangerous, and harshly punished. These conditions contribute to a diminished sense of comfort, health, and happiness, essential components to an individual's well-being.

In the new context of the opioid crisis, San Francisco's syringe/needle exchange and safe injection program provides optimism to people who inject drugs (PWID), their families, caregivers, and the community at large.

References

Aaron, L. (2005). Why a Needle-Exchange Program is a Bad Idea. Retrieved from http://www.redorbit.com/news/health/221310/why_a_needleexchange_program_is_a_bad_idea/.

Catholic World News (2011). "Holy See opposes condoms, needle-exchange programs in fight against AIDS. http://www.catholicculture.org/news/headlines/index.cfm?storyid=10703 (June 17, 2011).

Drucker, E. (2012). Failed drug policies in the United States and the future of AIDS: A perfect storm. *Journal of Public Health Policy*, 33(3), 309–316.

Gayle, H. (2000). *A Comprehensive Approach Preventing Blood-Borne Infections Amonginjec Tion Preventing Blood-Borne Infections Among Injection Drug Users*. Washington, D.C.: Academy for Educational Development.

Gross, J. (1991). San Francisco Journal: Doing His Duty, Juror Finds a Cause. *The New York Times* (May 6, 1991).

Huo, D., Bailey, S.L., & Ouellet, L.J. (2006). Cessation of injection drug use and change in injection frequency: The Chicago Needle Exchange Evaluation Study. *Addiction*, 101(11), 1606–1613. doi:10.1111/j.1360-0443.2006.01577.x.

Kidorf, M., and King, Van L. (2008, August). Expanding the Public Health Benefits of Syringe Exchange Programs. *Canadian Journal of Psychiatry*, 53(8).

Lane, S.D. (1991). *Needle Exchange: A Brief History*. New Jersey: The Kaiser Forums.

Loconte, J. (1998). Killing them softly. *Policy Review*, 14–22. Retrieved from https://www.hoover.org/research/killing-them-softly.

Normand, J., Vlahov, D. and Moses, L.E. (eds.) (1995). Preventing HIV Transmission: The Role of Sterile Needles and Bleach. National Research Council/Institute of Medicine. Washington.

Osmond, Dennis H. (2003). *Epidemiology of HIV/AIDS in the United States*. San Francisco: University of California San Francisco.

SFAF. (2012). What We Do: http://www.sfaf.org/policy-center/what-we-do/. Retrieved April 7, 2012.

SFAF (2013). Syringe Access Program. Retrieved October 14, 2013, from http://www.sfaf.org/client-services/syringe-access/#.UlywGFBOPoc.

Wodak, A., and Cooney, A. (2004). Effectiveness of Sterile Needle and Syringe Programming in Reducing Hiv/Aids Among Injecting Drug Users. *World Health Organization Report*, Retrieved from http://www.who.int/hiv/pub/prev_care/effectivenesssterileneedle.pdf.

42. Harm Reduction Services in San Francisco

*Executive Summary**

SAN FRANCISCO DEPARTMENT OF PUBLIC HEALTH

Section I: Framing the Issue

There are an estimated 22,500 people who inject drugs (PWID) in San Francisco. Between 2006 and 2014, opioid overdose deaths in San Francisco remained relatively constant at between 110 to 120 per year. In 2015, saw a decline with 98 deaths due to opioids (prescription and heroin) and 81 deaths due to stimulants. Approximately 69 percent of PWID report living on the street, using homeless shelters or living in single room occupancy (SRO) hotels. The lack of stable housing opportunities has increased the public consumption of drugs and increased the nuisance of publicly discarded syringes.

Part of the continuum of harm reduction services for PWID, safe injection services (SIS) allow individuals to inject illicit drugs in a hygienic environment under the supervision of trained staff and have opportunities to engage in other health and social services. In April 2017, the Board of Supervisors passed resolution #123-17, introduced by Board President London Breed, urging the San Francisco Department of Public Health (SFDPH) to convene a Safe Injection Services (SIS) Task Force to make recommendations to the Mayor, the Board of Supervisors, and City departments regarding the potential opportunities and obstacles associated with safe injection facilities, the community need for such facilities, and the feasibility of opening and operating such facilities.

Section II: Information on People Who Inject Drugs in San Francisco

Demographics & Geography

SFDPH estimates the local population of PWID at approximately 22,500 individuals. In 2015, the majority of PWID were male (71.4%), ages 41–60 (55.1%), homeless

---

*Public document originally published as San Francisco Department of Public Health, "Harm Reduction Services in San Francisco: Executive Summary," https://www.sfdph.org/dph/files/SIStaskforce/IssueBrief-06202017.pdf (June 2017).

(68.6%), and primarily injecting heroin (49.5%) and methamphetamine (33.8%) The population most often resided in Tenderloin (31%), South of Market (24%), Mission (9%), and Bayview-Hunters Point (8%) neighborhoods.

Section III: Public Health Concerns Among PWID

PWID have multiple health needs that must be addressed in order to support their health and well-being, including how the use of drugs can lead to substance use disorder, transmission and acquisition to blood borne pathogens, exposure to communicable diseases and other unsanitary conditions, and overdose death.

Substance Use Disorder. Substance use disorder is a medical disorder that is: a primary, chronic disease of brain reward, motivation, memory and related circuitry; reflected in an individual pathologically; pursuing reward and/or relief by substance use and other behaviors; characterized by inability to consistently abstain, impairment in behavioral control, craving, diminished recognition of significant problems with one's behaviors and interpersonal relationships, and a dysfunctional emotional response; and often characterized by cycles of relapse and remission.

Human Immunodeficiency Virus (HIV). In San Francisco, PWID and PWID who are homeless: account for 21 percent of people living with HIV; report injecting drugs (8.1%) in the prior 12 months among patients receiving HIV care; are less likely to be virally suppressed and more likely to transmit HIV; and have the lowest five-year survival rate of those living with HIV.

Hepatitis C Virus (HCV). In San Francisco, there are an estimated 23,000 residents with antibodies to HCV, and, approximately, 70 percent of active HCV infections are among PWID. OVERDOSE Recently in San Francisco, deaths due to heroin and methamphetamine have been increasing, and the largest percentage of deaths (approximately 33%) occurred in Tenderloin and South of Market. Most deaths occurred in single room occupancy hotel units where people tend to use in isolated settings.

Section IV: Harm Reduction in San Francisco

San Francisco's continuum of substance use disorder services are based on the principles of harm reduction. Harm reduction is a public health philosophy that promotes methods of reducing the physical, social, emotional, and economic harms associated with drug and alcohol use and other harmful behaviors that impact individuals and their community. Harm reduction methods are free of judgment and directly involve clients in setting their own health goals. The City formally sanctioned syringe access in 1993 and began funding programs as an essential structural component of HIV prevention services. A local study showed that San Francisco syringe programs reduced drug use and drug-related harms without increasing drug use among PWIDs.

Additional studies have also found use of syringe services to be associated with reduced syringe sharing and other injection-related risk reduction behaviors. Today, methadone and buprenorphine (medication-assisted treatment for opioid addiction) are available on demand for people who want to stabilize their illness. Additionally, the Homeless Outreach Team has embedded street medicine specialists who initiate medication-assisted treatment and treat abscesses and injection wounds. All of these programs provide linkages to medical care and treatment services. In 2003, San Francisco was the first city in the U.S. to make Naloxone readily available to members of the public. This service has drastically reduced the number of overdose deaths from injection drug use, and 2016 saw 877 reported reversals of overdoses.

Section V: About Safe Injection Services Background

Safe injection services are a part of the continuum of harm reduction services that were developed to promote safer drug injection practices, enhance health-related behaviors among PWID, and connect PWID with external health and social services. Globally, these facilities are professionally supervised facilities where drug users can consume drugs in safer conditions.

Safe Injection Services Around the World

Data are available on 10 countries that provide SIS:

- Five countries (Spain, Switzerland, Germany, the Netherlands, and Denmark) reported having multiple locations (ranging from five to 37) with varying services at each. Spain and Denmark each reported having one mobile drug consumption room in addition to fixed sites.
- Five countries (Australia, Canada, Luxemburg, Norway, and France) reported having only one location. Australia, Luxemburg, and Norway restrict eligibility to person 18 years or older. All five are in fixed locations using an integrated model with a mix of services and linkages to other community services. In January 2017, officials in Seattle and King County, Washington approved opening safe consumption facilities sites in their jurisdiction and developed a document entitled Safe Consumption Facilities: Evidence and Models. The document reviews three different services delivery models (integrated, specialized, and mobile) that differ in staffing, size, and organizational structure with features and staffing levels based on local circumstances.

Section VI: Potential Benefits and Risks of Safe Injection Services Benefits

Studies indicate that SIS are associated with an array of benefits, including: attracting the most marginalized PWID; promoting safer injection conditions; enhancing access to primary health care and other services; reducing the overdose frequency; reducing public drug injections; and reducing dropped syringes and hazardous litter SIS are not found to increase drug injection, drug trafficking, or crime in the surrounding environments. Implementing SIS would not necessarily require any significant or fundamental changes in public policy or law. Additionally, they require the same working agreements with social service providers and the police that needle exchange, street-outreach, drug treatment and similar health programs for injectors already receive.

Cost Benefit. In 2017, Amos Irwin and colleagues published an article titled A Cost-Benefit Analysis of a Potential Supervised Injection Facility in San Francisco, California, USA. At an estimated cost of $2.6 million annually to operate a facility based on the Vancouver program InSITE, the researchers found that each dollar spent on SIS would generate $2.33 in savings, for total annual net savings of $3.5 million for a single 13-booth SIS site. They further found that a SIS site in San Francisco would not only be a cost-effective intervention but also a significant boost to the public health system.

Risks. Federal and State Controlled Substances Laws Currently, the possession of controlled substances, without the prescription of a licensed health professional, is prohibited by both state and federal law, in addition to prohibitions on building owners and operators from allowing the manufacturing, storing, or distributing controlled substances. On May 12, 2017, Attorney General Jeff Sessions directed all federal prosecutors to pursue the maximum penalties under the law for all crimes, including mandatory minimum sentences. Government Contracting Requirements Another risk is the standard boiler plate language used in federal, state and local funding agreements where contractors and subcontractors agree to maintain a drug-free workplace.

Section VII: Considerations for San Francisco Regarding Safe Injection Services Location

A key consideration for implementing SIS is identifying locations where PWID already access services. Research conducted in San Francisco in 2008 found that 85 percent of study participants reported they would use SIS if they were convenient for them. Focusing on existing locations already serving PWID increases the likelihood that PWID will use SIS. The survey further found that nearly three-quarters of respondents (72%) would be willing to walk up to 20 minutes to a SIS site.

Community. Engagement of the communities surrounding any proposed SIS location will be critical. One study that conducted in-depth interviews with 20 sampled stakeholders found concern about the implementation of SIS, including how they would impact a community struggling with safety and cleanliness, and the efficacy of harm reduction strategies to address drug use. Still, they were open to dialogue about how a SIS site might support neighborhood goals; and they stressed the importance of respect and collaboration between stakeholders and those potentially implementing SIS.

Program Design. The programmatic design of any contemplated SIS location would need to ensure acceptability by and support of PWID. Identifying locations where PWID are already being served, as noted above, is one key element of program design. Additionally, the presence of other onsite support services, the accessibility of services, and the structure of the rules governing the program would also be critical.

Legal. It will be important for any proposed SIS provider to fully understand the associated legal risks.

43. Syringe Access and Disposal Programs in San Francisco*

SAN FRANCISCO DEPARTMENT OF PUBLIC HEALTH

The San Francisco Department of Public Health (SFPH) strives to achieve its mission through the work of two Divisions—the San Francisco Health Network and Population Health and Prevention. The SF Health Network is the City's health system and has locations throughout the City including San Francisco General Hospital Medical Center, Laguna Honda Hospital and Rehabilitation Center, and over 15 primary care health centers. The Population Health and Prevention Division has a broad focus on the communities of San Francisco and is comprised of the Community Health and Safety Branch, Community Health Promotion and Prevention Branch, and the Community Health Services Branch.

San Francisco Syringe Access and Disposal History

- 1988: Underground "Needle Exchange" run by volunteers
- 1993: Mayor Frank Jordan declares State of Emergency
- 1993: Syringe programs formally sanctioned in SF
- 2010: Syringe Police Bulletin signed

Syringe Access & Disposal Programs follow DPH Program, Policies & Guidelines

Objective of Syringe Programs

- To reduce risk behaviors that may lead to the transmission of bloodborne pathogens among people who inject drugs and their sexual partners.

Strategies

- Provide access to sterile syringes and injection equipment and safer sex supplies.
- Promote safe disposal of syringes and injection equipment, including collection and disposal of used syringes.

---

*Public document originally published as San Francisco Department of Public Health, "Syringe Access and Disposal Programs in San Francisco," https://www.sfdph.org/dph/alerts/syringe.asp (2019).

- Develop and deliver education and health promotion activities relevant to the goal.
- Provide information about and referrals to other ancillary services.

Syringe Programs Are Evidence Based

- Research demonstrates that syringe programs that are needs based
- (or "distribution" models):
- have a larger impact on reducing syringe sharing and unsafe injection
- practices than one-for-one exchanges
- Reduce transmission of HIV and HCV
- Do not increase to syringe litter
- And one-for-one exchanges limit the number of syringes and make it
- more likely that people will end up re-using, or sharing, injection drug
- equipment.

Syringe Access Programs Are a Global Best Practice

- Research has shown that syringe access and disposal programs are the most effective, evidence-based HIV prevention tool for people who use drugs.
- In cities across the nation (including SF), people who inject drugs have reversed the course of the HIV epidemic by using sterile syringes and harm reduction practices.
- Harm reduction (including needle/syringe program and opioid substitution therapy) is an evidence-based approach to HIV prevention, treatment and care for people who inject drugs and is strongly supported by WHO and other UN agencies.

What Is San Francisco Doing to Control and Clean Up the Needles on the Streets?

The Health Department is committed to cleaner streets in San Francisco. This is an environmental health issue that affects everyone in the city, and it is a problem for cities all over the world. For the last five years we have made extra efforts to improve the pickup of needle litter. Here's what we're have in place to reduce the number of needles on the streets:

- A ten (10) person clean-up crew funded by SFDPH and operated through SF AIDS Foundation operates 12 hours per day, 7 days per week. They are mobile and are reachable by text at (415) 810–1337. They also work collaboratively with organizations including San Francisco Drug User's Union, Homeless Youth Alliance, St. James Infirmary, Glide Harm Reduction Services to expand needle cleanup. Community members can participate in volunteer cleanup events every Friday from 12–2 p.m. at 117 6th Street.
- The Healthy Streets Operation Center is a coordinated citywide effort to address

concerns about homelessness and street behaviors and includes 311, Public Works, Public Health, Homeless and Supportive Housing, Police, and Emergency Management working together to address complaints related to homelessness and street issues.
- The Health Department funds a collaborative of community-based syringe access and disposal programs. There are 13 sites that operate throughout the City. Each site provides an opportunity for disposal.
- A five (5) member Community Health Response Team works across SF to properly dispose needles, offer Narcan and engage with the community to offer resources and referrals to care including treatment.
- The City's Fix It Team, Downtown Streets, Community Benefits districts, and other City & community agencies address community concerns and conduct syringe clean up.
- There are 17 outdoor sharps containers for disposal located throughout the city.

Why Syringe Access?

- Syringe access is a public health intervention that is a global best practice to reduce the spread of HIV and hepatitis C. It saves lives, makes the community healthier, and is supported by the California Health Department, and the Centers for Disease Control.
- The Health Department continues to provide programs and care to help people who inject drugs to be as healthy as possible. This in turn protects the health of our community.
- The city of San Francisco has been providing syringe access since 1993. Data indicates that our early adoption of syringe access has contributed to the low level of HIV among San Franciscans who inject drugs.
- We practice harm reduction and disease prevention strategies such as syringe access, naloxone (Narcan) to reverse overdoses, and fentanyl testing. We also provide treatment on demand with same-day methadone, increased access to buprenorphine and a wide array of substance use services to help people with addiction to recover, and reduce their use of needles.

How Does Syringe Access Benefit the Community?

Research including studies from the CDC shows that syringe access programs improve public safety. Providing sterile needles and syringes and establishing appropriate disposal procedures substantially reduces the chances that people will share injection equipment and removes potentially HIV- and HCV-contaminated syringes from the community.

What Do I Do If I See Needles on the Street?

- If you see syringes on the street please call 311. Using 311 helps the city track the number of needles picked up and allows us to deploy the right teams to the area.
- You can also text 415-810-1337

Syringe Programs Are Provided by Community Partners

The SFDPH funds the San Francisco AIDS Foundation (SFAF) to provide syringe access and disposal. SFAF subcontracts with:

- San Francisco Drug User's Union
- Homeless Youth Alliance
- St. James Infirmary
- GLIDE
- Community services:
- Fixed Site
- Venue Based
- Pedestrian
- Satellite Syringe Access

Best Practice: Multiple Access Points, Multiple Disposal Options

Access Points

- 13 community sites
- For purchase at pharmacies

Disposal Options

- Disposal at every syringe program sites
- Syringe programs conduct regular community sweeps
- Community Health Response Team
- Walgreens Pharmacies
- Community Sharps Disposal Kiosks
- Citywide Hotline (311)
- DPW street cleaning and pit stops
- Residential biohazard pick-up
- Training of Community Partners
- 10 NEW Syringe Clean-up staff

44. Syringe Disposal Practices of Intravenous Drug Users in Monterey County*

JAIME TEETER HOUSEHOLDER
and MICKEY P. MCGEE

As defined by Des Jarlais, et al.'s 2006 study on the diffusion of the Drug Abuse Resistance Education program (commonly known as the D.A.R.E. program) and syringe exchange programs in the 1980s, "The defining characteristic of syringe exchange programs is the exchange of new, sterile needles and syringes to reduce HIV transmission among IDUs" (p. 1355). Many of today's syringe exchange programs have evolved to include other implements for safer intravenous drug injection with a focus on the prevention of transmission of blood borne pathogens such as hepatitis B and hepatitis C (HBV and HCV), referral services to drug treatment centers, referral services to housing and other social services programs, and free testing for HIV/AIDS, HBV and HCV.

Syringe exchange programs have had a controversial history in the United States since their inception in the late 1980s. Despite evidence that syringe exchange programs are effective in preventing infections associated with blood borne pathogens, the federal government has not financially supported syringe exchange programs as a part of a comprehensive program to reduce the transmission of HIV and viral hepatitis among IV drug users. Opponents of syringe exchange programs often cite that syringe exchange programs condone illegal activities, and they often express concern that syringe exchange programs may lead to increased drug use and increases in syringes being discarded publicly. In addition, opponents of syringe exchange programs question the validity of studies that state syringe exchange programs are effective and argue that even if the programs are effective in reducing the spread of disease that they still promote drug use, presenting a moral or ethical dilemma (Lee, 2014).

Monterey County's first syringe exchange program was a drop-in center in the city of Salinas called Street Outreach Services that was founded in the mid–1990s by a group of community activists in response to the high risk of HIV infection among local IDUs. While the County Board of Supervisors did not financially support the exchange, the Board allowed the syringe exchange program to operate legally in the County. This nonprofit exchange was privately funded, and after nearly 10 years of private sponsorship was unable to sustain itself financially and merged its services with the local HIV/AIDS

---

*Published with permission of the authors.

nonprofit group CCHAS. Public funding for syringe exchange has been limited throughout this time period. Funding for syringe exchange programs has been authorized for some facets, like outreach worker salaries, but never for the syringes or safer injection supplies. In 2009, the state of California's Office of AIDS budget was reduced by more than 50%, resulting in the inability of the state and local agencies, including Monterey County, to continue funding for many HIV/AIDS prevention programs. This has resulted in the complete dissolution of public funding for syringe exchange programs in Monterey County. Since 2010, CCHAS has operated the syringe exchange program without any public financial support. If the syringe exchange program is abandoned, the community will lose this resource for the proper disposal of syringes used by IDUs.

This chapter is based on a study designed to inform Monterey County public officials and stakeholders on the state of syringe exchange in Monterey County. The main research question examined by this study was: If the current Monterey County syringe exchange program offered by the nonprofit organization Central Coast HIV/AIDS Services (CCHAS) is abandoned, will there be an increase in the amount of syringes that are disposed of improperly, representing a public health risk? Key findings were determined based on the analysis of primary data collected and analyzed for this study. Four recommendations were provided to the Monterey County Board of Supervisors for their review and action in 2014.

Primary data was collected in three distinct ways and included key informant interviews with Public Health Officials, a survey questionnaire distributed to nine California county public health departments requesting information about the presence of syringe exchange programs in their counties and another survey questionnaire administered to syringe exchange program participants at each of CCHAS' syringe exchange sites regarding their syringe disposal habits (SEP Questionnaire). Key informants interviewed included: Dr. Ed Moreno and Amanda Mihalko, Health Officer & Director of Public Health and the HIV/AIDS Program Coordinator for Monterey County; Dr. Lisa Hernandez, Medical Services Director/County Health Officer for Santa Cruz County; and Kim Keefer, Executive Director of CCHAS. Additionally, analysis of secondary data was completed to help determine the likelihood of a public health risk that could be associated with improper disposal of syringes, namely secondary infection due to an increased risk of accidental needlestick injury that could be associated with increased improper syringe disposal.

Key Findings

The study resulted in three key findings. The first supports the main research assumption that the abandonment of the SEP would result in an increase in improper syringe disposal by IV drug users, but does not appear to support the assumption that improper disposal may pose a public health risk. Results from all of the key informant interviews, secondary data analysis, and questionnaire data support this finding.

Dr. Moreno and Ms. Mihalko of Monterey County Public Health Department both stated that they felt that the syringe exchange program administered by CCHAS is effective at preventing IDUs from disposing of used syringes improperly. Ms. Keefer, the syringe exchange program administrator, also reported that she feels the program is effective at keeping used syringes off the streets because the one-for-one exchange provides an incentive for IDUs to bring their syringes back to the program.

When asked "If this syringe/needle exchange site was not available, where would you be the most likely to dispose of used needles that you would normally bring for exchange?" nearly all (95%) of the respondents reported that they would dispose of used syringes improperly. The majority (60%) of respondents indicated that they would dispose of used syringes in the trash, 19% indicated that they would dispose of used needles in public spaces, 12% indicated that they would save and reuse syringes, and only 5% indicated that they would dispose of used syringes in a medical waste sharps container. The large number of respondents indicating that they would dispose of their used syringes in the trash would support an affirmative response to sub-question four that the dissolution of the syringe exchange program could create a public safety issue for employees who have to locate and/or remove syringes that are disposed of improperly. This could pose an increased risk of puncture wounds and secondary infection to waste management workers in Monterey County, and to law enforcement officials and community outreach workers who work with the IDU community.

The findings supported the assumption that the abandonment of the Monterey County SEP would result an increase in needles being disposed of improperly by IV drug users, these responses indicate that proper disposal options for IV drug users in Monterey County are limited, and that an increase in risk behaviors associated with an increase in HIV and viral hepatitis could also result from the lack of syringe access that the Monterey County SEP currently provides.

The second key finding is that proper disposal options for the IV drug using community that is served by the SEP are extremely limited and the abandonment of the Monterey County SEP would likely exacerbate this problem. When asked "Do you think that the syringe exchange program currently run by CCHAS is effective at preventing used syringes/needles from being disposed of improperly?" and, "Does the County take any additional measures to prevent used syringes from being disposed of improperly," Dr. Moreno replied that he feels that the Monterey County SEP is effective at reducing the amount of syringes disposed of improperly, however; there is no evidence to support this assertion. Additionally, Dr. Moreno stated that the County does not specifically offer any additional proper disposal opportunities targeted at the IDU community, but that some cities in Monterey County do offer medical waste sharps disposal containers in their facilities.

In contrast, additional proper disposal opportunities are provided for IDUs in neighboring Santa Cruz County. Dr. Hernandez, when asked "Can you tell me how the goal of decreasing the number of improperly disposed syringes is being met with the SSP's format? Which of the components of the program do you think contribute the most to this effort?," responded that providing more disposal opportunities through access to large sharps medical waste disposal kiosks that are available 24 hours a day for public use, in addition to having the syringe exchange program, is an important component of their syringe services program in decreasing improper syringe disposal. Dr. Hernandez provided that a third kiosk location is an expansion project for Santa Cruz County, and is planned to be installed in an area that is in close proximity to some of their County's government and social services and is in an area known to be frequented by the homeless IDU community. Additionally, the Santa Cruz "Syringe Services Program" offers syringe exchange five days a week, including some evening hours, and operates out of two locations.

The SEP Questionnaire was designed to answer the primary research questions of the study and were administered to syringe exchange program participants at the Central Coast HIV & AIDS Services syringe exchange program sites in Salinas and Seaside, California. The questionnaire was administered in the third week of July 2014 with 42 out of 87 people who used the syringe exchange program in Salinas and Seaside, California, participating in the study. Respondents of the study SEP Questionnaire also indicated a need for additional proper disposal options. When asked "When you don't dispose of needles at a syringe/needle exchange site where do you dispose of them," 40% of respondents reported that they either keep all other syringes not disposed of at the Monterey County SEP or that they only bring them to the SEP for disposal, 36% responded that they would dispose of used syringes in the trash, and 9% responded that they dispose of used syringes in public spaces, and only 5% of respondents reported disposing of used syringes in a medical waste sharps container. A large number of syringe exchange program users served by CCHAS are homeless. Respondents reported keeping or saving syringes and indicated the need for additional proper disposal opportunities and the need for additional syringe access. Respondents saving used syringes could be indicative that syringe coverage in the IDU community is not adequate, and if expanded could be more effective at meeting its prevention goals.

The third key finding is that an increase in the incidence of new HIV/AIDS or viral hepatitis infections is a greater public health risk than that posed by secondary infections as a result of needlestick injuries from improper syringe disposal. The risk of contracting HIV/AIDS or viral hepatitis that can be associated with accidental needlestick injuries is very small; therefore, the possibility of increased viral infections that could result from the abandonment of the SEP is a more critical public health risk. Results from questionnaire respondents, secondary data analysis and key informant data all support this finding.

The large percentage of questionnaire respondents (40%) who reported that they keep or do not dispose of syringes other than at the SEP could be an implication that they are already reusing syringes. In addition, 5% of respondents indicated that they give away syringes. Reusing and sharing syringes are risk behaviors associated with an increased incidence of HIV and viral hepatitis infection. The number of SEP questionnaire respondents that reported increased risk behaviors associated with viral infections implies that current syringe access levels are insufficient to meet the demand of the IDU community, and the abandonment of the syringe exchange program could lead to increased HIV and viral hepatitis infections, due to the lack of sterile syringe supplies. Those newly infected are then at risk of transmitting these infections to their sexual partners and family members, spreading these diseases to the general public. The costs associated with treating these diseases are significant and would pose a significant public health risk.

When asked "Do you feel that syringes/needles being disposed of improperly by IV drug users presents a public health risk in Monterey County to law enforcement officials, waste management workers and the community in general," Dr. Ed Moreno explained:

"There is probably a risk for injury from puncture wounds for needles in places where they aren't expecting them.... I'm not sure there is a public health risk in terms of acquiring a communicable disease or blood born disease, specifically HIV or hepatitis C because the viruses don't live very long on the needle.... The main reason communities would offer or make available SEP is to reduce the transmission of HCV and HIV in the substance abusing community."

Analysis of secondary data provides a greater depth of understanding regarding the increased risk to public health through needlestick injury secondary infections. In a study of community-acquired needlestick injuries treated at United States hospitals in 2001–2008, Dr. Janine Jason asserts that secondary infection such as HIV or viral hepatitis resulting from an accidental needlestick injury is "extraordinarily unlikely" given that worldwide only three cases of HBV and one case of HCV transmission of non-healthcare needlestick injuries have been reported, and no cases of HIV transmission from non-healthcare related needlestick injuries have been reported (Jason, 2013, p. 426). The CDC reports that the average risk of contracting an HIV infection from a needlestick or other sharp instrument contaminated with HIV positive blood is only 0.3%, and the average risk of contracting HCV from a needlestick or other sharp instrument contaminated with blood from an HCV positive person is about 1.8% (CDC, Infection Control in Dental Settings, 2013). The public health risk that could be posed by the number of syringes disposed of improperly should the Monterey County SEP be abandoned would represent a limited public health risk.

In relation to the Syringe Service Program in Santa Cruz County, Dr. Hernandez was asked if she felt that the abandonment of their program would cause an increase in HIV infections, viral hepatitis infections and syringes being disposed of improperly in public. Dr. Hernandez responded emphatically: "Yes, yes, and yes!" indicating that the syringe exchange program is effective at preventing all three of these consequences. In Santa Cruz County, public health officials believe that their syringe services program has contributed to the decrease of the incidence of HIV in IDUs, and statistics from Santa Cruz HIV/AIDS surveillance show that in 2012 and 2013 Santa Cruz had no new HIV infections with IDU as a risk factor.

The study concluded that the key findings supported the assumption that if the Monterey County syringe exchange program is abandoned, there will be an increase in the amount of needles disposed of improperly by IV drug users, representing a public health risk. As demonstrated by the study results, 95% of SEP Questionnaire respondents stated they would dispose of used syringes improperly if the syringe exchange program was not available. Supporting data from the study indicate that the closure of the syringe exchange program would lead to an increase in improper disposal. Should the CCHAS syringe exchange program be abandoned, it is likely that IDUs who frequent the syringe exchange program will engage in risk behaviors that increase their chances of contracting HIV and viral hepatitis. Further research on the syringe coverage levels and program components that would be needed to make the Monterey County syringe exchange program optimally effective at preventing new HIV and viral hepatitis infections should be analyzed and implemented.

The following recommendations were provided to Monterey County to improve the effectiveness of the syringe exchange program at encouraging proper syringe disposal and enhancing current HIV and viral hepatitis prevention programming.

Recommendation #1: Provide Funding to CCHAS to Expand the Current Syringe Exchange Program

It is recommended that the Monterey County Board of Supervisors should immediately provide funding to CCHAS to bring the level of syringes exchanged to meet the demands of the IDU community that uses the exchange. An increase funding level for the CCHAS program provide for a realistic exchange syringe coverage by providing funds for additional staff and supplies, expanding the hours and number of sterile syringes that could be provided by the syringe exchange program. Approving and funding this proposal could prevent new HIV and viral hepatitis infections in the IDU community served by the exchange.

Recommendation #2: Provide Additional Proper Syringe Disposal Options

The Monterey County Health Department and Environmental Health Departments should expand opportunities for proper disposal options. This can be accomplished through providing disposal opportunities in addition to syringe exchange. In addition, Monterey County should consider forming collaborative agreements with local pharmacies to provide proper syringe disposal collection sites. Enlisting pharmacies in the collection of syringes can provide proper disposal opportunities to both prescription medication injectors and IDUs.

Recommendation #3: Implement a Community Education and Outreach Campaign

The Monterey County Public Health Department should implement a community education and outreach campaign that provides policy makers and the general public with the evidence needed to understand the public health benefits of syringe access services to IDUs. An educational campaign should provide evidence demonstrating the low risk of secondary infection associated with needlestick injuries, and supporting evidence that syringe exchange programs do not cause the unintended consequences commonly referred to by opponents of syringe exchange: increased drug use, increased frequency of drug use, and an increase in syringes disposed of in public.

Recommendation #4: Develop a Task Force to Develop and Implement a Comprehensive Syringe Services Program for Idus

The Monterey County Board of Supervisors should convene a task force to develop and implement a comprehensive syringe services program. This program should include increased investment in syringe exchange and the development of a task force made up of stakeholders that will devise and implement a comprehensive syringe services plan that is effective at preventing blood borne infections, preventing improper syringe disposal, and capitalizes on opportunities for additional community outreach services to the IDU community in Monterey County.

REFERENCES

American Foundation for AIDS Research. (2013, March). Federal funding for syringe services programs: saving money, promoting public safety, and improving public health. *Issue Brief*. Retrieved from http://www.amfar.org/uploadedFiles/_amfarorg/Articles/On_The_Hill/2013/IB%20SSPs%20031413.pdf.

AVERT. (2013, February 20). "Needle Exchange & HIV Prevention," Accessed on June 20, 2014. http://www.avert.org/needle-exchange.htm.

Bowen, E.A. (2012, June). Clean Needles and bad blood: needle exchange as morality policy. *Journal of Sociology and Social Welfare*, 39(2), 121–141. Retrieved from http://www.wmich.edu/hhs/newsletters_journals/jssw_institutional/institutional_subscribers/39.2.Bowen.pdf.

Broadhead, R.S., Van Hulst, Y., Heckathorn, D.D. (1999, September/October). The impact of a needle exchange's closure. *Public Health Reports*, 114, 439–447.

Burris, S., Welsh, J., Ng, M., Li, M., Ditzler, A. (2002, November/December). State syringe and drug possession laws potentially influencing safe syringe disposal by injection drug users. *Journal of the American Pharmaceutical Association*, 42(6), S94-S97. Retrieved from: http://japha.org on June 13, 2014.

Burrow, D., Walsh, N. (2007). *Guide to Starting and Managing Needle and Syringe Programs*. Geneva: WHO Press.

Centers for Disease Control and Prevention. (2013, April 16). HIV Cost-effectiveness. Retrieved from http://www.cdc.gov/hiv/prevention/ongoing/costeffectiveness/.

Centers for Disease Control and Prevention. (2013, October 25). Infection Control: Frequently asked questions – blood borne pathogens – occupational exposure. Retrieved from http://www.cdc.gov/OralHealth/infectioncontrol/faq/bloodborne_exposures.htm#a3.

Coffin, P.O., Latka, M.H., Latkin, C., Wu, Y., Purcell, D. W., Metsch, L., ... Gourevitch, M. N. (2007). Safe syringe disposal is related to safe syringe access among HIV-positive injection drug users. *AIDS and Behavior*, 11(5), 652–62. doi:http://dx.doi.org/10.1007/s10461-006-9171-x.

Committee on the Prevention of HIV Infection Among Injecting Drug Users in High Risk Countries. (2007). *Preventing HIV Infection among Injecting Drug Users in High Risk Countries: An Assessment of the Evidence*. Washington D.C.: National Academies Press.

Deo, Len. (n.d.). *No Reason to Fund Needle Exchanges*. Retrieved from http://www.njfpc.org/no-reason-to-fund-needle-exchanges.

Des Jarlais, D.C., Sloboda, Z., Friedman, S.R., Tempalski, B., McKnight, C., Braine, N. (2006, August). Diffusion of the D.A.R.E and syringe exchange programs. *American Journal of Public Health*, 96(8), 1354–1358.

Des Jarlais, D.C., McKnight, C., Goldblatt, C., Purchase, D. (2009, September). Doing harm reduction better: syringe exchange in the United States. *Addiction*, 104(9), 1441–6. doi: 10.1111/j.1360-0443.2008.02465.x.

Doherty, M.C., Junge, B., Rathouz, P., Garfein, R.S., Riley, E, Vlahov, D. (2000, June). The effect of a needle exchange program on numbers of discarded needles: a 2-year follow-up. *American Journal of Public Health*, 90(6), 936–939.

Drucker, E. (2012, August). Failed drug policies in the United States and the future of AIDS: a perfect storm. *Journal of Public Health Policy*, 33, 309–316. doi:10.1057/jphp.2012.16.

Hernandez, L.B., (2014, April 15). Syringe Services Program Annual Report 2014. Retrieved from: http://www.santacruzhealth.org/pdf/SSP%20Annual%20Report%202014.pdf.

Jason, J. (2013, April). Community-Acquired, non-occupational needlestick injuries treated in US emergency departments. *Journal of Public Health*, 35(3), 422–430.

Lee, M., (2014). Needle Exchange Programs: An Overview. *Points of View: Needle Exchange Programs*, 1.

Lorentz, J., Hill, L., Samimi, B. (2000 February). Occupational needlestick injuries in a metropolitan police force. *American Journal of Preventive Medicine*, 18(2), 1460150. DOI: 10.1016/S0749-3797(99)00137-3.

Pearson, J., Sprague, N. (2014 April). Point: Needle Exchange Programs Promote Drug Addiction. In *Points of View: Needle Exchange Programs* (pp2–2). Toledo, OH: Great Neck Publishing.

Tempalski, B., Flom, R.L., Friedman, S.R., Des Jarlais, D.C., Friedman, J.J., McKnight, C., Friedman, R. (2007, March). Social and political factors predicting the presence of syringe exchange programs in 96 US metropolitan areas. *American Journal of Public Health*, 97(3), 437–447.

Tempalski, B. (2007, June). Placing the dynamics of syringe exchange programs in the United States. *Health Place*, 13(2), 417–431. Retrieved from http://europepmc.org/articles/PMC2169509.

Tookes, H.E., Kral, A.H., Wenger, L.D., Cardenas, G.A., Martinez, A.N., Sherman, R.L,... Metsch, L.R. (2012, June). A comparison of syringe disposal practices among injection drug users in a city with versus a city without needle and syringe programs. *Drug and Alcohol Dependence*, 255–259. doi:10.1016/j.drugalcdep.2011.12.001.

White House National Office of AIDS Policy. (July 13, 2010). *National HIV/AIDS Strategy for the Unites States*. Retrieved from http://www.whitehouse.gov/administration/eop/onap/nhas.

45. How Did Ohio Local Government Leaders Dramatically Reduce Opioid Deaths?*

GERALD YOUNG

One of the biggest challenges facing local government leaders is attracting and retaining employees to deliver essential taxpayer services. While virtually all services delivered by city employees are aimed at improving the lives of citizens, few services more directly touch those lives than the work of public health professionals like physicians, nurses, and mental health professionals.

But these health and human services (HHS) jobs are some of the most difficult positions to fill at a time when unemployment levels across the country are at a historic low, according to a recent survey of public sector human resource professionals. Further complicating this workforce challenge is pressure on city governments to constrain spending when the demand for public health services is growing.

Take for example the opioid crisis. Nationwide, 70,200 Americans died of drug overdoses in 2017, with more than half attributed to opioid overdoses according to the National Institute on Drug Abuse. This public health emergency is putting increased stress on local governments, and that pressure comes at a cost. The Society of Actuaries and actuarial consulting firm Milliman released a report last month that calculated the one-year cost of opioid crisis in 2018 was $179 billion. Of that cost, about one-third is borne by governments providing taxpayer-funded services.

So how are local governments coping with growing public health demands like the opioid crisis amid workforce shortages? In short, they are innovating, collaborating, and making data-driven decisions.

One such example is in Montgomery County and Dayton, Ohio—jurisdictions overwhelmed by an alarming number of opioid overdoses. Sharing a sense of urgency to take action, leaders established an innovative and highly collaborative Community Overdose Action Team (COAT) to break down silos and foster productivity between agencies, while also instituting a data-driven decision process.

There were many challenges in bringing together such diverse partners to address complicated public health issues, including data-sharing barriers. COAT, led by

---

*Originally published as Gerald Young, "How Did Ohio Local Government Leaders Dramatically Reduce Opioid Deaths?," in the November 2019 issue of *Public Management (PM)* magazine, https://icma.org/blog-posts/how-did-ohio-local-government-leaders-dramatically-reduce-opioid-deaths-innovation, and copyrighted by ICMA, the International City/County Management Association (icma.org). Reprinted with permission.

Montgomery County, Ohio, public health officials, includes Dayton community police officers, judges, hospital administrators, and leaders from the coroner's office, chamber of commerce, faith-based organizations, the nonprofit community, law enforcement, and fire and emergency services from multiple jurisdictions.

This cross-jurisdictional and collaborative approach, coupled with data-driven processes, made dramatic progress in reducing opioid overdose deaths by nearly half. The deaths went from a high of 566 in 2017 down to 289 in 2018. And this decline continues into 2019. Importantly, there has been little staff turnover, with the leadership at COAT remaining intact since launching in 2016.

This case study is detailed in a new report from the Center for State and Local Government Excellence (SLGE) and Kronos, Innovations in the Health and Human Services Workforce: State and Local Governments Prepare for the Future. This report provides additional case studies and outlines strategies jurisdictions are deploying to more effectively compete for talent, while also combating the stress of HHS jobs:

1. Establish good relationships. Candidates considering a social work job in a rural community like Butte County, California, are more likely to accept the job and stay in the organization if they meet people who can help them acclimate, such as peers in other social service agencies.

2. Provide learning and growth opportunities. Often a top priority for employees, professional development also helps build a pipeline of candidates who are prepared to take on more responsibility as vacancies occur.

3. Ask employees what is important to them. The Bureau of Working Families in Wisconsin's Department of Children and Families began to survey employees annually in 2015. The leadership team committed to analyze the survey results and take action on targeted areas for improvement.

4. Stay focused on the mission. People drawn to health and human services jobs are passionate about their work and drawn to a public sector mission. To retain people who are motivated by a desire to help others, leaders can tell stories that remind employees to picture the person in need who is counting on their best efforts.

46. How Lowell Is Fighting the Opioid Crisis*

Audrey Fraizer

You name it, the city of Lowell, in Middlesex County, Massachusetts, has tried it in its fight against opioid use and abuse. And it's a war where more and more battles are being won. The overall strategy—one that garnered a grant from the U.S. Department of Justice and extensive community support—presents a major departure from punitive approaches to opioid use and abuse.

The approach is called collaborative compassion and involves developing a stronger understanding of opioid use and connecting overdose victims to treatment, according to Robin Toof, director of the two-year funded Lowell Opioid Overdose Project.[1]

The project inspired communitywide involvement backed by data gathering to lend greater insight into the nature of the opioid crisis. Among the initiatives funded through the grant is a robust database that leads to evidence-based solutions for local government to better tailor their responses, including intervention, education, prevention, and enforcement.

Jon Kelley, director of operations, communication, and IT for Trinity EMS, Inc., a private ambulance provider with roots in Lowell, is a data person. He understands the importance of collecting and applying data to identify and solve problems. As an emergency medical technician (EMT), he recognized the devastation of opioid abuse and recognized that it doesn't discriminate by ZIP Code. He wanted to do something about it.

"This can happen to anyone," he said. "It's everywhere. People get hurt, get a prescription for opioids, and, in some, an addiction develops. As a data person, I knew the data was there. Data gives us the opportunity to do some good. We can do so much to turn the tide."

Steps Taken

Statistics show the tide is turning, but first, a little about Lowell's history in coming to terms with its the opioid crisis.

---

*Originally published as Audrey Fraizer, "How Lowell Is Fighting the Opioid Crisis," in the August 2019 issue of *Public Management (PM)* magazine, https://icma.org/articles/pm-magazine/opioids-how-city-lowell-massachusetts-fighting-crisis and copyrighted by ICMA, the International City/County Management Association (icma.org). Reprinted with permission.

While information varies depending on the source, overlapping reasons for high numbers of fatal and non-fatal opioid overdoses in Lowell include demographics not unlike those of any large urban center. Lowell is the fourth most populous city in Massachusetts (111,670 according to a 2018 census estimate) and, according to a 2017 Community Needs Assessment,[2] housing and homelessness emerged at the top of the list of unmet needs in the Lowell community, with substance abuse resources identified as second, and jobs as third.

Lowell and neighboring Lawrence are reportedly regional hubs of the opioid trade, and fentanyl has featured prominently in that trade.[3]

Data is a big factor in curbing fatal and non-fatal opioid use. The Massachusetts Ambulance Trip Reporting Information System (MATRIS), originally created to collect and maintain standardized EMS patient data and information based on trip records, was enhanced statewide to accurately identify ambulance trips that are opioid related—for example, that a trip was listed as a poisoning, that the trip included administration of naloxone, or that the patient admitted to drug use.

As mentioned, Trinity EMS is committed to data collection to better frame the issue within its expanded service area. Collection starts at the communication center. Since 2015, Joseph Breen, a Trinity EMS dispatcher and quality assurance supervisor, has reviewed every single patient care report that indicates an opioid-related call. He monitors volume to identify spikes and tracks demographics such as age and gender of the patients, time of day and day of the week, and location of fatal and non-fatal overdoses within each community.

In 2016, Trinity EMS added FirstWatch (www.firstwatch. net) to instantly notify community leaders when a call involving an overdose comes into the communication center. The software speeds up notifications into real-time data in a format compliant with HIPAA (the Health Insurance Portability and Accountability Act of 1996). A FirstWatch app displays the data as pinpoints on a map—the what and the where—to hasten response to the scene. The same call also triggers an email to the Lowell Community Opioid Outreach Program (CO-OP, www.lowellma.gov/1193/ CO-OP), which follows up with the individual regarding treatment options. The faster the response, the better the outcome.

"Any time we can help someone, it's one more opportunity for that person to change [his or her] path," Kelley said.

Data Show Progress

Data shows that programs such as CO-OP and Lowell House (lowellhouseinc.org, an addiction recovery service) are helping to lessen the problem. From 2015 through 2018, Lowell had one of the highest numbers of opioid overdoses and fatalities in the state, with 63 deaths and 579 confirmed nonfatal overdoses in 2015, 68 deaths and 687 confirmed nonfatal cases in 2016, 53 overdose deaths in 2017, and 64 overdose deaths in 2018.[4] (Statistics are unavailable for nonfatal cases in 2017 and 2018.) Numbers for the first quarter of 2019 show a dramatic increase of 30 percent in nonfatal overdoses. Success is a matter of reaching people before the overdose becomes fatal; fewer people are dying.

Kelley said Trinity's approach and its continued positive results have attracted attention statewide. Everybody wants to be on the winning end of the opioid fight, although reasons may vary. In Lowell, it's a matter of taking responsibility. "These are our people. These are our citizens," he said. "Let's own this. Let's figure out how we can help."

FirstWatch has partnered with more than 200 medical and police agencies nationwide interested in opioid abuse prevention and suppression. Agencies can contact FirstWatch to configure a controlled drug trigger based on key words (e.g., opioid, Narcan) to identify potential overdoses at the 911 level. The data's application is also agency-specific, such as mapping areas of particularly high overdoses—which could indicate a surge in fentanyl.

The task is much more difficult than you might expect, said Sylvia Verdugo, FirstWatch clinical solutions specialist. For example, callers might not come right out and admit an "opioid overdose" when talking to the emergency medical dispatcher. Many lack awareness of Good Samaritan laws that protect victims and those who call 911 for help from charge and prosecution. Massachusetts passed its Good Samaritan Law in 2007.

Often, it's a matter of gathering clues. Did the caller mention physical symptoms (altered status, respiration rate)? A medical protocol software—Medical Priority Dispatch System (MPDS)—simplifies the collection through the targeted keywords picked up during the emergency dispatcher's questioning of the caller. The scripted questions direct the emergency dispatcher to the specific chief complaint (the patient's medical situation) to coordinate medical response.

Verdugo recommends that agencies develop standardized definitions of opioid overdose to clarify what exactly they want in a data surveillance program. She also encourages agencies to work together—share information—to develop best practices.

Why does it matter?

"FirstWatch gives you the evidence," she said. "But what absolutely matters is the story behind a number, and the face that goes with the story. Knowing what we can do to help someone."

Notes

1. Lowell Opioid Overdose Project, Prescription Drug Monitoring Program (PDMP) October 1, 2016–September 30, 2018 (grant period), http://www. pdmpassist.org/content/lowell-opioidoverdose-project (accessed May 21, 2019).

2. 2017 Community Needs Assessment, http://www.commteam.org/wpcontent/uploads/2017/06/2017-Community-Needs-Assessment.pdf (accessed June 14, 2019).

3. Vance, A., Schuster, L. "Opioid Addiction Is a National Crisis. And It's Twice as Bad in Massachusetts," Boston Indicators, https://www.bostonindicators. org/reports/report-website-pages/ opioids-2018 (accessed May 31, 2019).

4. Massachusetts Department of Public Health. Number of Opioid Related Overdose Deaths, All Intents by City/Town 2014–2018, May 2019, https://www.mass.gov/files/ documents/2019/05/15/Opioidrelated-Overdose-Deaths-by-City-TownMay-2019.pdf (accessed June 3, 2019).

47. How One City Went "All In" to Fight the Opioid Epidemic*

INTERNATIONAL CITY/COUNTY MANAGEMENT ASSOCIATION

In 2014, the city of Worcester, Massachusetts (population approximately 182,000), confronted this reality: nine deaths from opioid overdoses over the course of six days. The overdoses, explains City Manager Edward Augustus, "were an issue that had been rippling through the community for some time." The city of Worcester isn't alone. *The New York Times* reports that in 2014, nationally, 125 people a day died from drug overdoses, 78 of them from heroin and painkillers, otherwise known as opioids. Small towns, big cities, and rural communities are seeing the tragic effects of this addiction in the most public of places, and there's no sign of the trend slowing down.

Augustus was ready to do anything to keep people alive and determined to slow down the epidemic in his community. After the nine deaths, the city convened a town hall meeting with local service providers and the substance abuse advocacy community, and together they created a game plan that municipal government could run with.

As a result, the city instantly began implementing strategies—from public education and awareness programs to unwanted prescription medication drop-off kiosks—to counter the opioid epidemic. ICMA recently interviewed Augustus about those tactics. Here's what we learned:

It takes collaboration and coordination.

You can't fight this epidemic alone. It takes collaboration from all parts of local government as well as working with other services to explore options for programs, policy, and funding to reduce opioid use, abuse, and overdose.

The city of Worcester collaborates on several initiatives, including:

The Regional Response to Addiction Partnership Coalition, coordinated by the Worcester Division of Public Health, consists of many individuals, organizations, and municipal partners from the Central Massachusetts Regional Public Health Alliance (Worcester's public health district) and hosts Substance Abuse Awareness and Resource fairs as well as other initiatives to raise awareness about substance abuse, especially among youth and parent populations.

To assess the reach of substance abuse, the Worcester Division of Public Health has

---

*Originally published as International City/County Management Association, "How One City Went 'All In' to Fight the Opioid Epidemic" in the March 2016 issue of *Public Management (PM)* magazine, https://icma.org/articles/article/how-one-city-went-%E2%80%9Call-%E2%80%9D-fight-opioid-epidemic, and copyrighted by ICMA, the International City/County Management Association (icma.org). Reprinted with permission.

agreements with Worcester Public Schools and with member communities of the Central Massachusetts Regional Public Health Alliance to survey high school and middle school students on perceptions and health behaviors, which will help identify trends and program needs for this population.

AIDS Project Worcester, in partnership with the city, has hired staff to conduct outreach across Worcester to engage with homeless individuals to collect used syringes that these staff have found in parks, on streets, and in other public locations—in other words, in places where the used syringes pose a danger to public safety.

Another benefit of collaboration can be mutual funding and sharing of resources. You might, for example, locate partners willing and able to donate services or resources. Finding ways to use existing resources in creative ways or "cobbling together," as Augustus put it, additional resources can be a collective effort. Like any new endeavor, it takes innovative thinking and, of course, some risk taking.

Massachusetts FY2016 Substance Abuse Service Expansion Awards

On March 11, Health and Human Services announced $94 million in Affordable Care Act funding to 271 health centers in 45 states, the District of Columbia, and Puerto Rico to improve and expand the delivery of substance abuse services in health centers, with a specific focus on treatment of opioid use disorders in underserved populations. The city of Worcester has been awarded $352,083 from the $94 million investment.

"Anything and everything we thought we could do to keep people alive," is what Augustus says he and his team decided would be the best approach in combating the epidemic. The city started by training and supplying its police and fire departments with the opioid overdose reversal drug, naloxone (Narcan). The Massachusetts Department of Public Health Bureau of Substance Abuse Services awarded the city of Worcester police and fire departments a "First Responder Naloxone Grant." The funding (applied to those municipalities that met a certain criteria) is for the prevention of overdose and supports facilitating the purchasing, carrying, and administering of Narcan. The funds also support components of community outreach and training.

To take it a step further, the city provided front-line employees who work in municipal buildings and who are most impacted by opioid overdoses with training on how to recognize and respond to an overdose, including how to administer Narcan. "Having trained employees who themselves have and can administer Narcan expands the safety net," explains Augustus. This training applies to local government staff whose jobs put them in contact with the public on a regular basis—for example, employees at senior centers and libraries and people who are doing code enforcements to inspect homes and businesses, as well as employees in city hall.

According to a 2010 study by researchers at the University of Buffalo, opioid prescription drugs are the most common type of gateway drug for illicit drug addicts. The study's researchers noted that more than half of the opioid-addicted patients reported that legal prescription drugs were their first drug of abuse. To prevent drugs from homes in the community from becoming gateway drugs to illicit drugs, Worcester created two initiatives that lead to the collection of unwanted prescription drugs.

First, the city worked with police departments in adding kiosks that collect unwanted prescription medications from community members who simply need a place to get rid of them. Our directive, says Augustus, is "Don't throw it in the trash can, don't flush it down the toilet, drop it off at the police station, no questions asked." In addition, Augustus noted, a benefit of having the kiosk at the police station is that it's open 24 hours a day, seven days a week.

Second, through Neighborhood Watch programs, certain individuals are authorized to collect unwanted prescription drugs from people who attend those meetings. Again, no questions asked.

Ultimately, the steady rise of opioid abuse and overdose is a nationwide public health crisis. According to a tracking poll from the Kaiser Family Foundation, more than 56 percent of the public has been personally affected by opioid abuse, and 50 percent of the public believes that state officials should make combating the problem of opioid abuse one of their top priorities. In the same poll, large majorities of the public say that policies to reduce prescription painkiller abuse would be at least somewhat or very effective.

Augustus and the city of Worcester have effectively figured out a way to create programs and policies that work to reduce prescription painkiller abuse in their community. The prescription drug take-back initiative has collected 450 pounds of prescription drugs and over-the-counter medications. In addition, Worcester police and fire department personnel have reversed more than 200 overdoses with the use of Narcan. In a report developed by Augustus written to the Worcester city council, he states: "Addressing the stigma while working together at the federal, state, and local level to address substance abuse prevention, intervention, treatment, and recovery will continue to reduce the numbers of people being lost to the epidemic. This is an all hands on deck, all of the above approach to saving lives. From prescription take-back days to our public safety personnel carrying lifesaving Narcan—there is a space for everyone to get involved, get educated, and save a life."

When asked whether he would do anything differently, Augustus quickly replied, "Start earlier." The words of someone determined to make a difference.

48. The High Cost of Opioid Abuse in Your Community*

MARTY HARDING

These are difficult times for many communities. Budgets are being cut, resources are dwindling. Law enforcement personnel, county officials, social services agencies, and health care providers are struggling to do more with less. At the same time, the opioid epidemic is devastating families and communities throughout America.

According to the Centers for Disease Control and Prevention (CDC), more people in the United States died from drug overdoses in 2014 than in any previous recorded year. In that same year, there were about one and a half times more deaths from drug overdose than from car crashes, and 61 percent of all overdose deaths involved opioids. It is for these reasons and more that the CDC has classified the rise in opioid overdose as an epidemic.

For the past year, I've had the opportunity to work in six states to mobilize communities to address this epidemic: Massachusetts, Minnesota, Wisconsin, Kentucky, Florida, and Arkansas. In each state, people from every community sector have shared devastating stories of how they have been affected by opioid use. People who work in emergency rooms of their local hospitals are seeing a flood of overdose patients (from young teens to older adults), and first responders tell of the role they are now playing in saving lives by administering Narcan.

Law enforcement officers talk about their struggle to crack down on dealers and distribution networks. Employers are worried about lost productivity in the workplace due to opioid use. Faith leaders are overwhelmed by the number of deaths in their congregations. Community leaders are concerned about public safety. Educators ask if they're doing enough to prevent opioid use among adolescents and how to intervene. And probably the most heartbreaking of all the stories are those told by parents who have lost a child to an opioid overdose.

As a local government administrator, you've seen and heard it all. Opioid use affects all of the departments you administer: public safety, facility management, transportation, fire and emergency services, and community and economic development. People turn to you for guidance about public policy.

---

*Originally published as Marty Harding, "The High Cost of Opioid Abuse in Your Community," in the August 2016 issue of *Public Management (PM)* magazine, https://icma.org/articles/high-cost-opioid-abuse-your-community, and copyrighted by ICMA, the International City/County Management Association (icma.org). Reprinted with permission.

Fortunately, communities are finding solutions to these concerns, and working together across sectors to prevent opioid use, intervene, and provide resources for those who are affected by opioid use. This is a critical time for cities and counties to mobilize and provide their communities with vital information and tools to combat heroin and prescription painkiller abuse with the goal of minimizing its social and economic impact.

There is hope! Communities can successfully mobilize and take action.

On August 31, 2016, ICMA conducted a webinar on solutions that cities and counties are implementing to respond to the opioid epidemic. Lee Feldman, 2016–2017 ICMA president, and city manager of Fort Lauderdale, Florida, joined me for this webinar, and we explored these ideas that counties and cities have explored:

1. Creating community coalitions to work together across sectors. Managers have joined or started community coalitions that focus directly on the opioid crisis. They have recruited members from such diverse sectors of the community as employers, youth workers, faith community leaders, school administrators, teachers and counselors, public health and human services personnel, treatment professionals, law enforcement and county court services personnel, local pharmacists, and doctors, as well as other committed individuals, including people from the recovering community. These coalitions have joined forces and disseminated relevant information, conducted visioning sessions, developed and implemented action plans, and conducted educational sessions and informational campaigns throughout their communities.

2. Developing ordinances and places for safe drug disposal. Generally, these safe disposal sites are located in city halls under the supervision of law enforcement. Although drug take-back days are effective in increasing public awareness of the problem of unwanted prescriptions, a consistent, 24–7 lockbox for safe drug disposal dramatically increases the pounds of unwanted prescriptions that are collected, keeping them out of the hands of children and out of our water and landfills.

3. Establishing drug diversion task forces. Dedicated to sharing information and investigations to combat prescription fraud and illegal trafficking of prescription painkillers.

4. Providing training for first responders in the use of naloxone (Narcan) for reducing opioid overdoses. This strategy has been successfully implemented in many communities throughout the country, saving countless lives. New intranasal Narcan makes administration easier for both law enforcement and emergency personnel. Stigma about using Narcan still abounds, however, and city/county administrators must be armed with a strong rationale for counteracting negativity toward this approach.

5. Using drug courts to fight opioid addiction and trafficking. This approach reduces recidivism, encourages compliance with treatment, and supports families of drug court participants. It also reduces some of the burden on jails by creating an effective diversion program.

6. Creating referral programs through law enforcement agencies. Some communities are trying innovative programs that allow people to voluntarily obtain help by going to the local sheriff's office and requesting assistance. The community, county, or individual donors often cover the cost of treatment in these instances.

7. Disseminating information about state laws that encourage intervention.

Good Samaritan laws protect citizens when they intervene to save a life due to an opioid overdose. Drug overdose amnesty laws allow people to call 911 when a friend or family member is overdosing without fear of being arrested themselves for opioid use or possession.

    8. Building awareness about their state's prescription drug monitoring program (PDMP). These efforts are critical to cutting down on "doctor shopping" and preventing opioid overdoses, but they are underused for a variety of reasons. Cities and counties are involving local doctors and pharmacies to build awareness of PDMPs and remove barriers to implementing them fully.

    9. Hosting community mobilization events to put tools into the hands of every community sector. Community mobilization events, using Hazelden's "Toolkit for Community Action," have reached more than a 1,000 people in the past six months. We'll share what we've learned from these events, and let you know how you can plan and launch an event in your community.

Mobilizing your community doesn't happen overnight, and it requires hard work. But the return on your investment of time, money, and effort is worth it. Imagine… If hospital admissions for overdose death decrease. If law enforcement costs are reduced. If employers in your community see a rise in productivity. If violence, theft, and other crimes in your community decrease. If schools are a safer place for your children. If one life is saved. It's worth it.

49. Boston's Heroin Users Will Soon Get a Safer Place to Be High*

Martha Bebinger

A Boston nonprofit plans to soon test a new way of addressing the city's heroin epidemic. The idea is simple: Starting in March, along a stretch of road that has come to be called Boston's "Methadone Mile," the program will open a room with a nurse, some soft chairs and basic life-saving equipment—a place where heroin users can ride out their high, under medical supervision.

Dr. Jessie Gaeta, chief medical officer at the Boston Health Care for the Homeless Program, which initiated the project, walks the avenue several times a day on her way to and from work. The path takes her past the city's needle exchange program and a methadone clinic, as well as past one of the city's busiest emergency rooms, at Boston Medical Center.

"There are people—just in the few blocks around our building and hospital—that we're watching overdose on our way from the parking lot," Gaeta said.

Addiction treatment providers in the area have had conversations for many months about creating a safe place where heroin users could get high. At least eight countries around the world have some sort of supervised injection facilities, monitored by nurses, where patients can both use drugs and rest or sleep off the effects.

With state statistics indicating that roughly four Massachusetts residents die every day from an overdose, the need for some sort of new approach seems more urgent than ever, Gaeta said. Still, her organization plans only a limited version of the "safe place" other countries offer. In Boston, patients will not be allowed to take drugs in the room.

"It's not a place where people would be injecting," Gaeta said. "But it's a place where people would come if they're high and they need a safe place to be that's not a street corner, and not a bathroom by themselves, where they're at high risk of dying if they do overdose."

All the funding isn't yet secured, she said, but the plan is to convert a conference room for this purpose. A nurse and outreach worker would move among 10 or so users to check breathing, other vitals and general health. If patients in the room need more than nursing care, there's a hospital across the street.

---

*Originally published as Martha Bebinger, "Boston's Heroin Users Will Soon Get a Safer Place to Be High," Kaiser Health News, https://khn.org/news/bostons-heroin-users-will-soon-get-a-safer-place-to-be-high/ (March 3, 2016). Reprinted with permission of the publisher. Kaiser Health News is a nonprofit news service covering health issues. It is an editorially independent program of the Kaiser Family Foundation that is not affiliated with Kaiser Permanente. This story is part of a partnership that includes WBUR, NPR and Kaiser Health News.

Gaeta says staff in the room will "try like heck" to get patients coming off a high into treatment.

Ray Tamasi, the CEO at Gosnold, an addiction treatment network on Cape Cod, says his staff tried a similar approach with alcohol addiction about 15 years ago.

It was marginally successful, Tamasi said, "but it was taxing, very labor intensive and difficult. You have to have the resources to be able to do it."

The Boston organizers say they are desperate to try something new. Overdoses have become the leading cause of death among Boston's homeless men and women. But will users who inject drugs or take a cocktail of pills find their way to this room?

"I could say, for myself, I would use it just to be safe," said Nicole, who currently is getting treatment with methadone for her heroin addiction. She asked to be identified by only her first name because some family members don't know about her heroin use.

"A lot of addicts are homeless or by themselves," Nicole said. "So, to have somebody—especially a nurse—keep an eye on you, and have a place to go when you're under the influence or high ... and somebody monitors you ... that's an awesome idea."

A review in 2014 of 75 research articles found that supervised injection facilities—the type of "safe room" offered outside the United States—reduced the rate of overdose. And a 2008 study found that patients in Vancouver, British Columbia, and Sydney, Australia, who were monitored by a nurse while they used heroin were more likely to end up in treatment than patients who were not monitored.

The use—or lack of use—of these safe rooms in various countries highlights a divide in addiction treatment, said Dr. Barbara Herbert, president of the Massachusetts chapter of the American Society of Addiction Medicine.

"The controversy," Herbert said, "is, does it encourage people to keep using if we make their lives less dangerous and less miserable, or can we scare people into care?"

Herbert said many health care providers in the field of addiction medicine have moved away from the "tough love/abstinence-or-nothing" approach and instead now favor options like the "safe-use room."

"It's not that we don't want people to be drug free," Herbert said. "But dead people don't recover."

The safe-use room is part of what's known in the world of addiction treatment as "harm reduction." The approach includes needle exchange programs so that users don't spread infections, training in the use of naloxone, the opioid reversal drug, and more education about the dangers of opioid prescriptions and use. Some addiction experts say Massachusetts must focus more on reducing the dangers of drug use and stop expecting users to just stop.

"We're having problems reducing people's involvement with drugs," said Vaughan Rees, an addiction expert at the Harvard School of Public Health. "Short of being able to implement treatment, we need to think about how we can reduce the risk of drug use."

The idea is still widely controversial among both elected leaders and those in public health. But Charlie Baker, the state's Republican governor, says he's open to hearing what Boston Health Care for the Homeless has planned.

"I have tremendous faith in them," Baker said, "and think because they are on the ground and because they are closer, most of the time, than practically anybody else who's working with the homeless population, they tend to be a pretty good bellwether about good ideas."

And Boston Mayor Marty Walsh, who speaks openly about his own past alcohol addiction and his recovery, says creating a space that's supervised in this way could be an effective method of bringing heroin users into short-term care.

"I'm up for trying anything when it comes to addiction and active using," Walsh said. "If we can help some folks—homeless folks in particular—we should try anything."

Boston police say they have no concerns about the program's "safe room" as planned. They would not support allowing injections inside.

"We can't allow the illicit distribution or sale or transfer of narcotics to be happening and not take action against that," said Lt. Detective Michael McCarthy, a spokesman for Boston's police department.

Some in the addiction community say a room where heroin users who are high would get care, not criticism, is another sign that attitudes about addiction are shifting.

"I think we've come a long way," said Joanne Peterson, who started a parent support network in Massachusetts called Learn to Cope. "There's a lot more talk and a lot more compassion and understanding because there's been so many deaths. This is an enormous epidemic."

In just the past month, EMTs revived six people after overdoses in the neighborhood where Boston Health Care for the Homeless plans to open its safe-use space for heroin users.

50. In Boston's "Safe Space," Surprising Insights into Drug Highs*

MARTHA BEBINGER

Some arrive on their own, worried about what was really in that bag of heroin. Some are carried in, slumped between two friends. Others are lifted off the sidewalk or asphalt of a nearby alley and rolled in a wheelchair to what's known as SPOT, or the Supportive Place for Observation and Treatment, at the Boston Health Care for the Homeless Program.

Nine reclining chairs have been full most days, especially during peak midday hours. It may be the only room in the country where patients can ride out a heroin or other high under medical supervision.

"It's a safe place to be," said Tommy, 39, who's been using heroin for at least 21 years. "It's a lot safer than being out on the street, possibly walking into traffic. I might OD if I was alone out there."

Tommy is looking for a job and housing, and we've agreed not to use his full name. He's one of 180 people who've come to this former conference room to ride out an opioid or other drug high since SPOT opened in late April. Nurses have logged almost 900 visits. At least half of the patients have come more than once.

If the person can speak, a nurse will ask what they took before settling them in a chair, wrapping a blood pressure cuff around one arm and placing an oxygen monitor over a finger.

"The monitors are really convenient," Dr. Jessie Gaeta, chief medical officer for BHCHP, said as she pulled the Velcro edges of a blood pressure cuff apart. "It takes a lot of the guessing out of understanding how far someone is into an overdose syndrome."

Gaeta coined the term "overdose syndrome" to describe what's happening to patients in this room. In many cases, she is surprised by what she's seeing.

"A classic opiate overdose is characterized by a person who stops breathing," Gaeta said. "They have central nervous system depression. So it's mostly respiratory depression and respiratory arrest."

But Gaeta says about 75 percent of her SPOT room patients show something different. "What we're seeing in this room is more depression of heart rates and blood pressures

---

*Originally published as Martha Bebinger, "In Boston's 'Safe Space,' Surprising Insights into Drug Highs," *Kaiser Health News*, https://khn.org/news/in-bostons-safe-space-surprising-insights-into-drug-highs/(August 26, 2016). Reprinted with permission of the publisher. Kaiser Health News is a nonprofit news service covering health issues. It is an editorially independent program of the Kaiser Family Foundation that is not affiliated with Kaiser Permanente. This story is part of a partnership that includes WBUR, NPR and Kaiser Health News.

as actually the primary—sometimes the only—abnormalities," Gaeta said. So the patient may be unconscious with low blood pressure, but have nearly normal breathing.

Patients tell Gaeta they may start the day with heroin or another opioid and then, a few hours later, take pills that will enhance the high.

"People are talking about that a lot here," Gaeta said, "about the layering of this cocktail of medications, and that's really reflected in the vital signs that we're seeing, which is not indicative of pure opiate overdoses. I'm not sure that we'd have seen that without doing this kind of monitoring."

Gaeta described a typical combination or cocktail of four drugs: heroin or another opioid, clonidine (which lowers blood pressure), Klonopin (to control for anxiety) and gabapentin (used to treat seizures or nausea).

The observations are just a snapshot based on a small number of addiction patients in one area of Boston. But what Gaeta is seeing is reflected in overdose death reports and is changing the way she and her staff respond to these patients who look like they are falling into a deep sleep. To boost sinking blood pressures, for example, they've brought IV fluid equipment into the room. They are going through many more tanks of oxygen than expected.

Dr. Barbara Herbert, president of the Massachusetts chapter of the American Society of Addiction Medicine, said she's never heard anyone use the term "overdose syndrome."

"But I think it's a great phrase, and I suspect it will move into more conversations. Because we created a safe space, we can now think about what's in front of us with more science than we could before we had this," she said. "So, while all of us knew this cocktail could produce overdose, few of us have ever had the opportunity of seeing people after they use and monitoring their blood pressure or their heart rate. So, this is an unexpected positive for us, coming to understand the disease better from that safe space."

SPOT nurse April Donahue said some patients in the room appear so sedated that they don't respond when she speaks loudly in their ear or raps on their sternum. But, she says, some of those people "have rock-solid vital signs, better than mine." So, she said, "What you see subjectively looking at someone and what their vital signs are don't always match up."

If Donahue weren't monitoring the vital signs, she says, she'd be racing to inject naloxone, the drug that reverses the effects of opioids. But Donahue found she can sometimes avoid using naloxone, which is very harsh on the body, by giving patients oxygen or fluids to keep them alive.

The nurses speak to each patient about addiction treatment. Getting patients into treatment is their top priority after keeping people safe while high.

"I think what's struck me the most is the gratitude—just to get out of that environment, even for a little while, to get off the street and be cared for," Donahue said. "I mean, so many of our participants don't have anyone who's caring for them."

It's one reason Tommy is becoming a repeat client. "This is just a great start," Tommy said. "I think it will slow down a lot of overdoses and could save a lot of lives. It will save a lot of lives in the long run."

And Tommy knows. He went into respiratory failure a few weeks ago while at SPOT and was brought back with naloxone.

51. What's Next for "Safe Injection" Sites in Philadelphia?*

ELANA GORDON

Philadelphia is a step closer to opening what could be the nation's first supervised site for safe drug injection. But turning the idea into reality won't be easy.

City officials gave the proposition the green light Tuesday. They were armed with feasibility studies, harrowing overdose statistics and the backing of key leaders, including the mayor and a newly elected district attorney.

"There are many people who are hesitant to go into treatment, despite their addiction, and we don't want them to die," said Dr. Thomas Farley, Philadelphia's health commissioner and co-chair of the city's opioid task force. Supervised safe-injection sites, he said, save lives by preventing overdose deaths and connecting people with treatment.

While one big hurdle is now cleared, the details of how safe-injection sites would actually work in Philadelphia have yet to be figured out. Who will actually fund and operate a site? Where will it be located? Will users really be safe there?

"We have a long way to go," said Brian Abernathy, first deputy managing director for the city.

Neither city council approval nor special zoning ordinances would be required to proceed, Abernathy said, but the city doesn't plan to operate or pay for any sites. Instead, Philadelphia officials would play the roles of facilitator and connector with providers of addiction services.

In that way, Tuesday's announcement by the city was more like an open call to potential investors and operators than it was the rollout of a specific plan.

"We took a really, really big first step," said Jose Benitez, executive director of Prevention Point Philadelphia, a large, nonprofit needle exchange. "It's early to talk about our involvement at this particular point. As the city officials said, there's a lot to consider."

Broadly, the city envisions a place where people would be allowed to bring in drugs and inject them using clean equipment. If someone overdosed, trained staff would respond to prevent death. The sites could save lives and money otherwise lost to hospitalizations and emergency response efforts. Advocates say the sites also could reduce neighborhood problems associated with addiction, like people injecting in public and discarding needles.

---

*Originally published as Elana Gordon, "What's Next for 'Safe Injection' Sites in Philadelphia?," *Kaiser Health News*, https://khn.org/news/whats-next-for-safe-injection-sites-in-philadelphia/(January 26, 2018). Reprinted with permission of the publisher. Kaiser Health News is a nonprofit news service covering health issues. It is an editorially independent program of the Kaiser Family Foundation that is not affiliated with Kaiser Permanente. This story is part of a partnership that includes WHYY, NPR and Kaiser Health News.

A safe, supervised site wouldn't just be about a spot to inject, Farley stressed, but also somewhere people could connect with other services and treatment.

Still, the effort to open a site will likely face additional hurdles and unknowns, from community buy-in to legal concerns.

For one, Councilwoman Maria Quiñones-Sánchez, who has voiced opposition to a safe-injection site in her district (one at the heart of the crisis), is wary of the city's plan.

"This notion of letting a private developer or a private person come tell us how this could be done, we're not paying for it, we'll do wrap-around services, so much of that is just up in the air," Quiñones-Sánchez said. "So why make an announcement with no answers?"

Another question: Could such a site be immune from federal prosecution? Realistically no, said Philadelphia official Abernathy, though some legal scholars are exploring potential safeguards.

The city's police commissioner, Richard Ross, has gone from "adamantly against" any injection site to having an open mind. Whether police will take a hands-off approach remains to be seen. So would what the department's role would be, what police officers would be asked to do, and how that would affect the policing of narcotics?

"I don't have a lot of answers," he said.

One point of clarity: Philadelphia District Attorney Larry Krasner has no plans to prosecute.

"What will we do? We will allow God's work to go on," Krasner said, citing state laws as justification that allow the committing of minor violations in the interest of preventing greater harms. "We will make sure that idealistic medical students don't get busted for saving lives and that other people who are trying to stop the spread of disease don't get busted."

After all this, it should come as no surprise that the timeline is really unclear, too. Rollout will take months, at least, leaders have said. Though if it were up to Krasner, one would have opened years ago.

"My biggest concern moving forward with harm reduction is that government takes forever," he said. "When we have three or four people dying every day, nobody can afford to wait."

52. "Crackhouse" or "Safehouse"?*

Nina Feldman

Philadelphia could become the first U.S. city to offer opioid users a place to inject drugs under medical supervision. But lawyers for the Trump administration are trying to block the effort, citing a 1980s-era law known as "the crackhouse statute."

Justice Department lawyers argued in federal court against the nonprofit, Safehouse, which wants to open the site.

U.S. Attorney William McSwain, in a rare move, argued the case himself. He said Safehouse's intended activities would clearly violate a portion of the federal Controlled Substances Act that makes it illegal to manage any site for the purpose of unlawfully using a controlled substance. The statute was added to the broader legislation in the mid-1980s at the height of the crack cocaine epidemic in American cities.

Safehouse argued the law does not apply because the nonprofit's main purpose is saving lives, not providing illegal drugs. Its board members said that the so-called crackhouse statute was not designed to be applied in the face of a public health emergency.

"Do you think that Congress would want to send volunteer nurses and doctors to prison?" Ed Rendell, the former Philadelphia mayor and Pennsylvania governor who serves on Safehouse's board, asked after the hearing. "Do you think that's a legitimate result of this statute? Of course not, no one could have ever contemplated that, ever!"

Safehouse earned the backing of Philadelphia's current mayor, Jim Kenney, the health department and district attorney, who announced they would support a supervised injection site in January 2018 as another tool to combat the city's dire overdose crisis.

More than 1,100 people died of overdoses in Philadelphia in 2018—an average of three people a day and triple the city's homicide rate.

In response, various harm-reduction advocates and medical professionals founded Safehouse, created a plan for its operations and began scouting a location.

But the Trump administration sued the nonprofit in February to block it from opening.

In June, the Justice Department filed a request for motion on the pleadings—essentially asking the judge to rule on the case based on the arguments that had already been submitted. Since then, a range of parties have filed amicus briefs in support of and

*Originally published as Nina Feldman, "'Crackhouse' or 'Safehouse'? U.S. Officials Try to Block Philly's Supervised Injection Site," *Kaiser Health News,* https://khn.org/news/crackhouse-or-safehouse-u-s-officials-try-to-block-phillys-supervised-injection-site/ (September 9, 2019). Reprinted with permission of the publisher. Kaiser Health News is a nonprofit news service covering health issues. It is an editorially independent program of the Kaiser Family Foundation that is not affiliated with Kaiser Permanente. This story is part of a partnership that includes WHYY, NPR and Kaiser Health News.

opposition to the site. Attorneys general, mayors and governors from across the country filed briefs backing Safehouse, while several neighborhood associations in Philadelphia's Kensington section and the police union filed against it.

U.S. District Judge Gerald McHugh requested an evidentiary hearing to learn more about the nuts and bolts of how the facility would work were it to open. At that hearing, in August, Safehouse's legal team, led by Ilana Eisenstein, explained that Safehouse would not provide drugs but people could bring their own to inject while medical professionals stood by with naloxone, the overdose reversal drug. They said Safehouse would also be an opportunity for people to access treatment, if they were ready.

Safehouse vice president Ronda Goldfein said the only difference between what Safehouse would do and what's already happening at federally sanctioned needle exchanges and the city's emergency departments is that the injection would happen in a safe, comfortable place.

"If the law allows for the provision of clean equipment, and the law allows for the provision of naloxone to save your life, does the law really not allow you to provide support in that thin sliver in between those federal permissible activities?" she said.

McSwain contended that operating in that "sliver" is exactly what makes Safehouse illegal.

Much of the debate at the hearing revolved around interpreting the word "purpose." The statute in the Controlled Substances Act makes it illegal for anyone to "knowingly open … use or maintain any place … for the purpose of … using any controlled substance."

The government said it's simple: Safehouse's purpose is for people to use drugs. McSwain conceded it will also provide access to treatment, but so does Prevention Point, the city's only syringe exchange. Effectively, he argued, the only difference between Safehouse and what's already going on elsewhere would be that people could inject drugs at Safehouse, which is prohibited by the statute.

"If this opens up, the whole point of its existing is for addicts to come and use drugs," McSwain said.

Safehouse said its purpose is to keep those at risk of overdose safe from dying.

"I dispute the idea that we're inviting people for drug use," Eisenstein argued.

"We're inviting people to stay to be proximal to medical support."

McSwain conceded that if Safehouse were to offer the medical support without opening up a space specifically for people to use drugs, the statute would not apply.

"If Safehouse pulled an emergency truck up to the park where people are shooting up, I don't think [the statute] would reach that. If they had people come into the unit, that would be different," he said. Mobile units and tents in parks are supervised injection models that other cities have implemented.

Safehouse has also said it hasn't ruled out the idea that it might incorporate a supervised injection site into another medical facility or community center, which would indisputably have other purposes.

McSwain ultimately argued that Safehouse had come to the "steps of the wrong institution," and that if it wanted to change the law, it should appeal to Congress. He accused Safehouse's board of hubris, pointing to Safehouse president Jose Benitez's testimony at the August hearing, where he acknowledged that they hadn't tried to open a site until now because they feared the federal government would think it was illegal and might shut it down.

"What's changed?" asked McSwain. "Safehouse just got to the point where they thought they knew better."

"Either that, or it's the death toll," Judge McHugh replied.

San Francisco, Seattle, New York City, Pittsburgh and Ithaca, N.Y., are among other U.S. cities that have expressed interest in opening a site and are watching the Philadelphia case closely. In 2016, a nonprofit in Boston opened a room where people could go after injecting drugs to ride out their high, with nurses equipped with naloxone standing by.

The Justice Department's motion for the judge to rule on the pleadings is pending. McHugh could decide he now has enough information to issue a ruling, or he might request more hearings, arguments or a full-fledged trial.

Safehouse's legal team said that if the judge ruled in its favor, it might request a preliminary injunction in the form of relief to allow the facility to open early.

"We recognize there's a crisis here," said Safehouse's Goldfein. "The goal would be to open as soon as possible."

• *D. Nonprofits and Associations* •

53. Offering Syringes Along with Prayers, Churches Help IV Drug Users*

TAYLOR SISK

FAYETTEVILLE, N.C.—When Gov. Pat McCrory signed legislation in July legalizing syringe exchange programs in North Carolina, James Sizemore rejoiced.

The pastor of a small church, Sizemore had—with the tacit approval of some, but not all, local law enforcement—been offering clean syringes to drug users to help them avoid contracting HIV and hepatitis C. Now he could do so without fear of arrest.

Sizemore, who in 2007 launched Radiant Church, an affiliate of the Church of God of Prophecy, has sought to alleviate the effects of drug addiction, work that he sees as a natural extension of his other pursuits: feeding, clothing and otherwise offering sustenance to his parishioners and others in need.

"It was never an issue of, 'Is this the right thing to do spiritually, scripturally?'" Sizemore said of his efforts. "For us, it was the right thing to do.... You can't save somebody's soul if they're dead."

Churches and other faith-based organizations have increasingly voiced approval of syringe exchange programs, sometimes launching their own. Their efforts have contributed to growing support for the programs, which the federal Centers for Disease Control and other health organizations see as a valuable tool in combating the opioid epidemic. Most programs include components such as education, treatment and testing for HIV and hepatitis C, which can be spread by sharing needles. Some also distribute naloxone to reverse overdoses.

The CDC offered further encouragement November 29, reporting greater use of syringe exchanges by people who inject drugs. Even so, one-third of users cited in the CDC analysis reported in 2015 that they had shared a needle within the past year. Exchange programs allow drug users to turn in used syringes and get sterile ones.

While more than half of states have not explicitly authorized syringe exchange, Corey Davis with the Network for Public Health Law said that most have at minimum

---

*Originally published as Taylor Sisk, "Offering Syringes Along with Prayers, Churches Help IV Drug Users," *Kaiser Health News*, https://khn.org/news/offering-syringes-along-with-prayers-churches-help-iv-drug-users/ (January 3, 2017). Reprinted with permission of the publisher. Kaiser Health News is a nonprofit news service covering health issues. It is an editorially independent program of the Kaiser Family Foundation that is not affiliated with Kaiser Permanente.

removed the prescription requirement for syringes. A number have "patchworks" of what's permitted in terms of exchange and what's not.

The North American Syringe Exchange Network, or NASEN, reports 228 syringe exchange programs operating in 35 states and Washington, D.C. But the number of programs is growing weekly in response to the rise in heroin overdose deaths across the country.

Neither NASEN nor the Harm Reduction Coalition has an estimate of the number of faith-based churches and organizations directly involved in syringe exchange, but momentum is clearly gathering. Church-based programs are operating in communities across the country, including Seattle; Cincinnati; Albany, N.Y.; and even in traditionally conservative southern states.

Institutions such as the United Methodist Church, Presbyterian Church (U.S.A.), United Church of Christ and National Council on Jewish Women have issued statements of support for syringe exchange.

"Ultimately, we want people to live without the burdens of addiction, but for many people the road to recovery is long and arduous, and protecting public health in the meantime is fundamental," said Kara Gotsch, who until recently was director of advocacy for the Interfaith Criminal Justice Coalition.

Hillary Brownsmith researches and writes about faith-based harm reduction initiatives and helps run the Steady Collective, a mobile syringe exchange program in Asheville, N.C. The program is based at the Haywood Street Congregation, a United Methodist Church ministry, and has received funding from three other congregations.

Brownsmith has engaged ministers and churchgoers in theological conversations about reaching out to drug users, and said she's received only positive feedback.

"I think the tide is definitely shifting," she said, with church officials and congregants recognizing that syringe exchange is in keeping with soup kitchens, temporary shelters and other outreach ministries.

St. Paul's Episcopal Church in Fayetteville, Arkansas, launched its syringe exchange program last November. Shelby Carrothers, a church member, saw the need for one while offering HIV testing during a weekly free hot meal. She discovered that most of the people being tested identified as IV drug users.

Carrothers said that while providing clean syringes is a critical service, "Almost equally important is that we provide a nonjudgmental space to talk about what they're going through and answer questions that they might otherwise be afraid to ask."

Sherman Terry, 40, is among those who've found help at St. Paul's. A former IV drug user, he came for a hot meal and has received a lot more.

"Shelby, bless her heart," Terry said during a recent Wednesday lunch at the church, recounting how Carrothers had introduced him to a variety of support services. No longer an IV drug user, Terry now advocates in the community for safe sex, clean needles, healthy living in general.

Carrothers distributes some 300 to 400 syringes each week. But the need to help IV drug users continues to mount. She's now talking with a Lutheran church in Fayetteville and Episcopal churches in Little Rock about hosting exchanges.

In North Carolina, James Sizemore tells of his own circuitous route to harm-reduction advocacy.

President of his high school's "Just Say No" club, Sizemore went from being a Duke Divinity School student to a cocaine mule, transporting kilos from Miami to North

Carolina. For five years, he struggled with addiction. Once free of drugs, he found his way back to the pulpit.

Disenchanted with mainstream churches—which, he perceives, too often fail to embrace the marginalized members of their communities—Sizemore started his own, in a section of Fayetteville marked by poverty and drug use.

Syringe exchange fits into his church's primary mission, tending to an array of immediate needs.

You can't "preach salvation" to someone who's in the throes of addiction, battling for their life, or turning tricks to feed their kids, Sizemore said. "They're not interested in hearing anything about the spirit because they're concerned about these issues first."

"Slowly, but surely," he said, "we established a good enough relationship in the neighborhood that they trusted us enough to care for them spiritually."

54. San Francisco AIDS Foundation's Syringe Access Services Evaluation Results*

ELISSA VELEZ *and* MICKEY P. MCGEE

This chapter provides an in-depth look at the efficacy of the San Francisco AIDS Foundation (SFAF)'s Syringe Access Services (SAS) program and evaluates whether syringe exchange (also known as needle exchange) has had a positive effect on San Francisco's community of injection drug users.

Primary and secondary data were collected and evaluated to examine the efficacy of the SAS program. Statistics from the literature review reveal substantial evidence that NEPs decrease HIV rates; however, the data collected in this case study will evaluate additional benefits of NEPs. The following data provided below first analyses the secondary data set from SAS's annual Client Satisfaction surveys from years 2012 and 2013. The primary data was collected by key informant interviews from experts in the field of HIV, substance use, and behavioral health. Other key informants were Syringe Access Services clients discussing the impact the program has had on them. Both data sets are analyzed for trends and compared to each other for a deeper understanding of how SAS services affect the well-being of clients.

2012 and 2013 Client Satisfaction Surveys

- 59% completely agree with the statement "because of SAS, I know how to use drugs more safely." 18% somewhat agree, 9% disagree, 1% disagree completely, 11% reported not applicable and 4% left the question blank.
- 67% completely agree with the statement "because of SAS, I use drugs more safely." 18% somewhat agree, 5% somewhat disagree, 8% reported not applicable and 4% left the question blank.
- 37% completely agree with the statement "because of SAS, I reduced the amount I use." 16% somewhat agree, 22% somewhat disagree, 15% disagree completely, 9% reported not applicable and 3% left the question blank.
- 35% completely agree with the statement "because of SAS, I have better access

---

*Published with permission of the authors.

to substance use services." 20% somewhat agree, 14% somewhat disagree, 7% disagree completely, 21% reported not applicable and 5% left the question blank.
- 38% completely agree with the statement "because of SAS, I have better access to health services." 23% somewhat agree, 17% somewhat disagree, 3% disagree completely, 18% reported not applicable and 3% left the question blank.
- 55% completely agree with the statement "because of SAS, I have better access to HIV testing services." 21% somewhat agree, 5% somewhat disagree, 1% disagree completely, 17% reported not applicable and 3% left the question blank.
- 55% completely agree with the statement "because of SAS, I have better access to Hep C testing services." 17% somewhat agree, 8% somewhat disagree, 2% disagree completely, 25% reported not applicable and 3% left the question blank.

Key Informant Interviews

Interview questions were sent to key informants through e-mail. The first key informant interview was conducted with Katie Bouche, the SAS program manager. Katie was asked eight questions about the SAS program at SFAF. First revealing the other services provided by staff other than needle exchange. The medical/health related list included: "Hep C and HIV testing, Hep C support group, new women's support group starting this month, nurse practitioner once per week and people can get basic medical care, referrals to other medical care, abscesses lanced and drained and antibiotics for abscesses, get basic over the counter meds." Katie discussed how SAS provides a large number of referrals to "tons of things like safer injection information, drug and alcohol treatment referrals/linkage, public bathrooms, free eats in the city, shower services, safer injection materials, HIV and Hep C materials, and referrals to shelters."

The city's new initiative is to provide crack pipes to users. SAS has been participating in the endeavor to move this initiative along. For many years SAS provides "Pipe covers so people don't burn their lips and spread blood when sharing pipes with each other, chore boy to use as a pipe filter. Chore boy is an engagement tool to get folks in the door for testing and other services; over the past few years that we have been handing out safer smoking supplies, we are seeing hundreds of people that otherwise would not be seeking services." Katie also spoke to the emotional connection that SAS provides to clients "we also offer peer counseling, care and compassion. A stigma free environment where people will not be judged."

When asked what Katie thought was the most important aspect of needle exchange, she said, "I think the stigma and judgment-free environment is the foundation for a successful program." She further discussed how staff build connections and how building relationships increase the services provided.

While conducting the literature review other health related issues were revealed as plaguing the IDU community; such as overdoses, homicide, heart disease, kidney failure, liver disease, and suicide. Katie was asked whether SAS does anything to address these issues. "In IDU's liver disease is often a result of Hep C, so we offer the support group, rapid Hep C testing, information about Hep C, we really try to stress Hep C and HIV prevention through all of the supplies and information we hand out."

Katie was asked what she thought is working well in the needle exchange program.

In the last two years the city of San Francisco has made the San Francisco AIDS Foundation's SAS program the hub for needle exchange; these partnerships are referred to as the Syringe Access Collaborative (SAC). In response to this question, Katie talked about the success of the SAC. "I think the role we have within the SAC is working out pretty well. All of the supplies for all of the needle exchanges in the city come through us and get distributed that way. The agencies include St. James Infirmary, catering to sex workers, Homeless Youth Alliance which caters to homeless youth, API Wellness who cater to the Trans community and Glide who mainly serves folks that live in the Tenderloin. The SF Drug User's Union is not an official member of the SAC, but we supply all their syringes and supplies as well. By working closer together than we did before we were the SAC is great for referring people to each other's programs and allows for each agency to really reach their target audience. It also allows us to collaborate on issues and make some programmatic decisions together. I think it's great that we are beginning a support group for women, who really can't get too many other services at SFAF besides the needle exchange. Our staff is passionate about the work we do and that leads to people staying in the job for a while and getting to know the participants pretty well."

Syringe Access Service's most meaningful contribution to the IDU community comes from the social, emotional, and interpersonal connections that arise from needle exchange.

Injection drug users are a marginalized population, dealing with stigma, discrimination, shame, isolation and the internal struggle of addiction. Dr. Siever, former director of Behavioral Health Services at the San Francisco AIDS Foundation, describes how discrimination perpetuates self-loathing and addiction. "The people who come to SAS sites [and other SAC sites] are treated mostly with impatience and disdain if not outright banishment by other agencies and programs." Society and media demonizes people who uses drugs. The taboo association with drug use is so widespread that even many people who support drug policy reform hold negative assumptions about people whose drug use they consider abusive.

Grace Ricco-Penca, an HIV care coordinator from San Francisco General Hospital's HIV Ward, was asked her opinion about the most important part of needle exchange and parallel to the other interviewees she expressed the interpersonal communication that produces relationships. "First, principles of Harm Reduction must be strictly adhered to; clients will not participate if there is any trace of judgment from the staffers, or at the location. Next, it is crucial that the staff are open, friendly and welcoming. It is useful as a positive health reinforcement when the staff express sincere gratitude that the client is exchanging their 'sharps.' It gives the staff opportunities to 'hang out' and talk about upcoming events in the community."

Dr. Siever and Katie Bouche, the SAS program manager, both regard the stigma and judgment-free environment as the foundation for a successful needle exchange program. Bouche recognizes the population that SAS serves as largely stigmatized "and when you add poverty or homelessness, mental health issues, or physical illnesses to it, the stigma is that much worse. We find sometimes that when people come into exchange and we ask them how they're doing, we are the only people that day who cared to ask how they were doing." Staff and volunteers are trained on how to establish boundaries, reframe from imposing personal judgments, and hopes onto participants. This consciousness is built by acknowledging that everyone is different.

At SAS, "We look at substance use on a continuum. At one end there is abstinence and at the other end there is chaotic use, and every place in between. Not all people's drug use looks the same. We meet people as individuals, learn from them (because they often know the social service system/ medical care systems and safer injection techniques better than we know it ourselves), offer information, but not advice, and we offer straight up compassion and a listening ear. Building trusting relationships with participants ensures that they feel safe enough to return and continue to use our services." This approach is different from more formal and conservative views of substance use, addiction, and social services. Services are often provided with the intention to "help" people while providers bring their own personal philosophies, values, morals, and beliefs to their clients with the hopes to change his or her behavior. This approach can be counterproductive, cause judgment, and manifest a disconnect between the service provider and the client.

SAS works to adhere to the principles of harm reduction and create a welcoming environment for their clients. Dr. Siever explained, "by treating them the way all humans should be treated, they are more likely to let down their walls and defenses and open up about whatever issues are going on in their lives, be they about physical, emotional, or spiritual health. From that, hopefully we're able to provide information, education, and referrals that point them in the right direction to get their needs met if we're not able to." This is a philosophy that is felt by the clients.

The author interviewed with two needle exchange clients; these interviewees are referred to as client A and client B. Interviews were conducted at the needle exchange site on 6th Street in San Francisco. During the first interview client A was asked "In which way(s) has SAS helped improve your health?" Client A responded that the most significant way that SAS has helped him is by not judging him.

The judgment free environment was the "first step to realizing my time was worth something." Client A was asked to speak more about what SAS meant to him. Client A presented as nostalgic; he spoke about a time long ago when "his people [injection drug users]" were viewed at mysterious. "Before we had lost our teeth, before we lost 40 pounds, and looked like demons, we were mysterious. Then we fell apart and were left in the dust until a program like SAS comes along, it makes me proud." He remarked that SAS is a program that's there to remember people like him and to serve the people that have been forgotten. "SAS helped me realize that I am human and that I deserve to be happy." After this interview it was clear to the author that needle exchange is more than a means for sterile syringes, it's a portal to a better way of life, whether that means safer injection practices or accessing a gateway to better self-esteem.

Client A was asked if SAS has improved his HIV risk behavior. Client A reported that SAS has improved his HIV risk behavior through "slamming less, smaller gauges, new rigs, and safe disposal—I don't put myself in powerless conditions anymore and they helped me go to the doctors more often." Client A was asked to talk more about how SAS helped reengage him with primary care. He said that through the encouragement of SAS staff he was able to break a period of two years in which he did not attend the doctor. "I'm still dealing with the consequences of not seeing the doctor during that time."

Client B was asked if SAS was able to help him see his doctor more frequently. He responded "No, I have coverage with a private doctor." Client B described that he is both HIV positive (30 years) and Hep C positive and already sees his doctor regularly. He was asked if he felt supported in his health by SAS. He responded that indeed he does feel supported because although he has not used the nurse service at SAS he knows he can go to a site to see a nurse for wound care and related issues.

Grace was asked the same question and responded "People who use needle exchange programs do so for a variety of reasons. For some, they are proud of themselves for injecting with clean syringes because it means they are taking good care of themselves despite their situation. This allows the primary care team to expand on the client's belief and utilize it to explain how medication adherence, staying active in primary care, etc. are also taking good care of themselves." As expressed many times throughout the collection of primary data, the staff of needle exchange must first connect with participants in order to initiate and build on increasing overall well-being.

Grace also acknowledged that "These programs allow many who fear or disdain the 'healthcare system' to meet healthcare professionals [educators, case managers, nurses, NPs, MDs] who frequently staff the exchanges in a non-traditional setting. This often allows for the development of a trust relationship which can become a bridge to potential future health care and treatment." Through the use of SAS services, in 2013 38% of clients have reported that they completely agree to having better access to health services and 23% somewhat agree. In the 2013 client satisfaction survey data, one client reported that he could not make wound care hours and "liked it better when there were more doctors and nurses." Grace also expressed the need for SAS to educate "how to recognize injection site abscess or infiltration and when to seek help for it, what is Hep C (HCV) and where to go for testing / info." The author's assumption is that if there were available resources clients would use additional services such as onsite doctors and nurses.

When asked what other areas that the needle exchange should focus on Grace not only remarked with abscess care and Hep C education she indicated that it "would be wonderful if all needle exchanges had mini-education sessions (3 min or so) on each of the following: safe injection practices, how to use of naloxone in OD situations, and how not to contaminate drugs and equipment."

According to the literature review, other arguments against needle exchange include the circumstance that drug addicts are still prone to death, perhaps not from HIV, but from overdose, collapsed veins, and poisoned dope. The San Francisco needle exchange is deeply rooted in harm reduction and continually seeks ways to minimize harm cause to their clients by working very closely with the Drug Overdose Prevention Education (DOPE) Project.

The SAS program gives people the opportunity to get trained in overdose prevention skills such as recognizing the signs of an overdose, how to do rescue breathing, and how to administer naloxone (Narcan) with a legal prescription for the drug. Katie, SAS's program manager further describes how overdose prevention is critical to well-being of the IDU community. "Naloxone is an opiate antagonist that reverses the effects of an overdose. It is what the paramedics use when they respond to an overdose. There is a fairly new law, I think from last year or two years ago, that says when police respond to an overdose, they cannot use the drugs that they find on the premises as evidence. This is called the Good Samaritan law. It helps ensure that people won't be too scared to call the paramedics since the police show up at the same time. There have been hundreds of lives saved in San Francisco, or overdoses reversed, since the DOPE project started years ago. 1184 is the most recent number of overdoses reversed in SF since the DOPE Project started in SF. When people have access to naloxone, it literally empowers them to save lives and it's cool to acknowledge that when someone comes back with a story of how they used the Narcan in an overdose situation. We also offer refills whenever folks use it or lose it." During an interview with Client B, he stated that due to SAS he has become a mentor in his building. He provides clean needles for the whole facility and knows how to handle situations such as overdose.

When Dr. Michael Siever was asked what aspect of the needle exchange he thought was the most important, he responded: "At this point in history [25 years of syringe access in San Francisco], we've been successful enough that the prevalence of HIV among folks who inject is quite low, probably among the lowest in the country, and because of the DOPE Project distributing and training people in the use of naloxone, we have dramatically cut down on fatal overdoes, so the importance now is more I think the things I talked about in my first two answers—making a connection, gaining trust, helping folks navigate what are usually not very friendly systems whether we're talking about healthcare systems, housing bureaucracies, food distribution systems, or any other of the bureaucratic systems that the poor and marginalized have to deal with." This statement speaks to the gains and the progress the needle exchange is making in the community. Like with so many other struggles, each juncture and each bound that the needle exchange makes allows for ground to be broken, more lives to be saved, and more community to serve.

Summary

Illicit drug use is fundamentally dangerous; it's an activity that often costs drug users their families, homes and jobs, while exposing them to risk of disease, arrest, and violence. Well-being equates to a better life condition in the form of happiness, health, and success. The interviews conducted with key informants explores the extent to which the program affects the well-being of SAS clients.

Among the five interviews conducted, three trends emerged: interpersonal connections/emotional support, access and support for engagement in primary care, and overdose prevention. These trends were reported as the most prevalent SAS services to show an increase in well-being. Interviews with HIV service providers concede that the most important piece of needle exchange is the ability to connect with the IDU community; Katie remarked the stigma and judgment-free environment as the foundation for a successful program. SAS client interviewees note that the personal connections with staff have made the biggest impact on their lives. Other than rating how friendly, approachable, knowledgeable, capable, and respectful the staff of SAS is with clients there is little secondary data that was collected regarding interpersonal relationships with SAS staff and building trust. However, other than providing sterile needles the primary data showed this to be the most important aspect of needle exchange across the board.

Secondary data shows an increase in client satisfaction with the program staff. The evaluation of this data indicates the program is increasing efficacy through the development of personal relationships. By improving on staff's friendliness and approachability, knowledge and capability, and ability to respect and treat all clients with dignity, the program gains the trust of its constituents and increases successful interactions.

The second area of needle exchange that induces well-being among IDUs is the use of doctors and nurses at the needle exchange sites. SAS Client A revealed how he underwent a two-year period in which he did not access medical care or treatment. SAS encouraged and supported Client A into seeing a doctor. Primary data finds the value of these programs which allow many who fear or disdain the "healthcare system" to meet healthcare professionals. Just having medical professionals available to staff the exchanges in a non-traditional setting makes the clients feel support in their health and gives them the opportunity to seek assistance if needed. Ricco-Penca points out that "These interactions allows for the development of a trusting relationship which can become a bridge to potential future health care and treatment."

According to 2013 client satisfaction data, 59% of SAS clients have a regular doctor and 57% have had a doctor's visit in less than three months. The data does not indicate how many SAS participants were reengaged into the health care system due to SAS services, encouragement, or influence; however, the number of clients accessing health care services is high compared to the national average. These numbers are interesting considering the level of marginalization this population faces.

The third area that SAS has improved the well-being of IDUs is through their work is with the DOPE Project, providing training in overdose prevention skills. Fatal overdose and infection with HIV and other blood-borne viruses transmitted through shared needles are the most common causes of death for IDUs (Mathers, Degenhardt & Bucello, 2012). SAS works to address both these issues via sterile syringes and through overdose prevention education. In San Francisco, needle exchange is often credited as one of the main reasons HIV/AIDS isn't prevalent in the general heterosexual population of the city. The prevalence of HIV among IDUs in San Francisco has drastically been reduced leaving overdose as one of the leading health risks of IV drug use. However, according to the collection of primary data SAS has been able to train a number of its constituents on how to use naloxone (Narcan) in the case of an overdose. The education in overdose prevention and the development of these skills not only contributes to the well-being of the individual, it contributes to the well-being of the larger IDU community. Often times individuals will come together to get high, in the case that an overdose were to occur the education one person has can save the lives of the people around them.

Conclusion

Did the introduction of NEPs lead to other unintended and welcome benefits (such as referral to drug treatment, decreased drug use, engagement in primary care, HIV testing, etc.)? An analysis of the findings show positivity in the health and wellness of injection drug users by means of the needle exchange. Both primary and secondary data show a link between the needle exchange and increased well-being. The findings support the authors' hypothesis that the introduction of the Syringe Access Services (SAS) program has increased overall well-being for injection drug users within the city of San Francisco.

Primary data identifies three specific areas of support for SAS clients: (1) emotional support; (2) doctor and nurse practitioner presence; and (3) overdose prevention.

Interviews with HIV service providers concede that the most important aspect of needle exchange is the ability to build human connections with participants. Additionally, increasing access to primary care and providing onsite doctors and nurses allows for clients to take care of their otherwise overlooked health issues while overdose prevention efforts are credited with saving 1184 lives in San Francisco. The conclusion that can be drawn from these findings reveal that clean needles serve as a baseline for better health; however, unintended benefits are found in many of the services SAS provides. These services are not limited to just the San Francisco needle exchange program. Many other

NEPs provide judgment free environments, doctor and nurse presences, as well as overdose prevention training which leads to the conclusion that NEPs are gateways to a better life condition.

At the most basic level needle exchange programs are said to promote a healthier existence. Providing clean syringes increases the likelihood that intravenous drug users are going to lessen needle sharing and increase a sense of personal value. "Because of the fact that needle exchange programs do not attempt to force people to change in ways which they do not choose for themselves, these programs are often very successful in engaging hard-to-reach individuals in services which they have traditionally refused to receive from other agencies" (Anderson, 2013). Studies have established that NEPs, when implemented as part of a comprehensive HIV/AIDS prevention strategy, are an effective HIV prevention intervention and do not promote drug use.

There has been a longstanding ban on most Federal funding for needle exchange programs. In 2009 the ban was lifted and shortly thereafter Congress reinstated the ban (The White House, 2012). The Administration continues to support a consistent policy that would allow Federal funds to be used in locations where local authorities deem needle exchange programs to be effective and appropriate. Surveys done in the late 1990s as well as a Kaiser Family Foundation Survey from 1996 found that 66% of Americans support such programs.

Recommendation 1: Help lift the current ban on federal funding for needle exchange programs. This study confirmed the increased well-being and health needs for and of SAS participants. This policy recommendation advocates legislative action to appeal the current ban for federally funding needle exchange programs. The initial step to take is to form an action committee by April 1, 2014. This committee will be led by Ernest Hopkins, director of Legislative Affairs at the San Francisco AIDS Foundation. Committee members will include representatives with an interest or "stake" in lifting the ban initiative. The committee is to analyze needs, design legislation and work with House Minority Leader Pelosi's staff to introduce the bill to life regarding the current federal funding ban. Further, the committee will find advocates who support the bill, and build alliances with stakeholders such as harm reduction, AIDS, and diabetes advocates that support the efforts of needle exchange.

By October 1, 2014, the committee will develop a campaign strategy to introduce the bill by January 2015. During the six months of development the committee formulates support for when the 2015 national HIV/AIDS statistics are releases. The National HIV/AIDS Strategy (NHAS) goals were to significantly decrease annual HIV infections, increase the proportion of HIV-positive people in care, and reduce HIV-related health disparities by 2015. If by 2015 the data shows no significant HIV reduction in IDUs in areas that don't have NEPs, or shows maintenance or increase in IDU health in areas that do have NEPs the committee will begin campaigning the new bill. By January 1, 2015, the committee is to develop next steps on a campaign to lift the funding ban.

Success for this recommendation is viewed as the passing of legislation that lifts the funding ban—first imposed in the late 1980s. The passing of a bill for federally funding needle exchange holds a mission that supports the National HIV/AIDS Strategy and would be ground-breaking for the elimination of the discriminatory barriers of stigma, homophobia, racism, poverty and the marginalization of drug users in our society.

Recommendation 2: Develop state and local guidelines on how to address the issue of wide-spread disease through injection drug use. Recognizing that NEPs are valid forms of disease prevention and pose additional benefits to participants receiving services, each state will develop guidelines on how to address the issue of wide-spread disease through injection drug use regardless of congresses decision to not support the bill.

Currently SFAF works with partners from throughout the state to ensure that the governor and legislature provide state funding to augment federal support of essential HIV prevention and care efforts. In response to the recommendation this core group of individuals will expand these efforts and develop guidelines to be used across the United States.

The ad hoc group will be formed by April 1, 2014, and contain members from the Office of National AIDS Policy, SFAF, and other key stakeholders. This group will have six months to develop and present the report to Dr. Grant Colfax, MD. Dr. Colfax is the Director of the Office of National AIDS Policy, the president's lead advisor on domestic HIV/AIDS and is responsible for overseeing implementation of the National HIV/AIDS Strategy. By October 1, 2014, the ad hoc group is to develop and present the draft of state and local guidelines report to Dr. Grant Colfax. By December 31, 2014, ad hoc group will complete the final report for submission to The Office of National AIDS Policy for implementation.

The hope is that the report created by the ad hoc group will be able to guide the administration's HIV/AIDS policies across state agencies and address how states that do not support NEPs can curb the spread of disease through injection drug use regardless of congresses decision on federal funding for NEP. Success for this recommendation is viewed as full support by Dr. Colfax in the implementation of guidelines for each state to deal with IDU risk reduction.

Summary

Primary data identifies three specific areas of support for SAS clients; these included: (1) emotional support; (2) doctor and nurse practitioner presence; and (3) overdose prevention. The conclusion that can be drawn from these findings reveal that clean needles serve as a baseline for better health; however, unintended benefits are found in many of the services SAS provides.

These services are not limited to just the San Francisco needle exchange program. Many other NEPs provide judgment free environments, doctor and nurse presences, as well as overdose prevention training which leads to the conclusion that NEPs are gateways to a better life condition.

Because of the benefits associated with NEPs the authors' recommendation is to (1) lift the ban on federal funding for needle exchange programs and (2) develop state and local guidelines on how to address the issue of widespread disease through injection drug use. In order to achieve the goals of reducing blood borne diseases, operational plans must address the issue of funding and have mechanisms to regularly monitor and publicly report on the outcome of the nation's HIV/AIDS investments. Funding allocation is essential to the success of national reduction of disease among IDUs and increased well-being. The second recommendation is a contingency plan created to address the issue of IDU health regardless of funding availability for NEP. State and local guidelines on how to address IDU health are needed to ensure high risk populations are minimizing risk and addressing the stigma and criminalization associated with IDU discrimination.

Further, case study findings reveal a new public health interest in providing crack pipes to the public; this initiative is said to decrease HIV risk. Very little research has been conducted on this subject and the authors recommend further research be conducted regarding free and available crack pipes in the city of San Francisco.

References

Anderson, K. (2013). Why Needle Exchange Is Good for Your Community. *Psychology Today* (July 2013).

Mathers, B. M., Degenhardt, L., & Bucello, C. (2012). Mortality among people who inject drugs: a systematic review and meta-analysis. *Bulletin of the World Health Organization*, 2013(91), 102–123.

The White House. (2012). Federal Funding Ban on Needle Exchange Programs. Retrieved from http://www.whitehouse.gov/blog/2012/01/05/federal-funding-ban-needle-exchange-programs.

55. Leading the Fight Against the Opioid Crisis*

GEOFF BECKWITH

Our nation is in the midst of an unprecedented opioid epidemic. This epidemic transcends locality, income level, gender, and race. In 2014, more Americans died from drug overdoses—47,055—than in any year since 1968 when the federal government began tracking this data.

The majority of those drug overdose deaths (more than six out of 10) involved an opioid—a category of drugs that includes heroin and prescription pain medicines like morphine, codeine, oxycodone, hydrocodone, methadone, and fentanyl. Since 1999, the rate of overdose deaths involving opioids has nearly quadrupled, from 4,030 in 1999 to 18,893 in 2014.

Among new heroin users, approximately three out of four report abusing prescription opioids prior to using heroin. The increased availability, lower price, and increased purity of heroin in the U.S. have been identified as possible contributors to rising rates of heroin use.

Because of managers' unique position in the heart of our communities, they have an obligation to lead the fight to prevent opioid abuse and overdoses. Local government leaders and their employees have the resources, tools, and credibility to take the lead on this incredibly complex public health crisis.

While cities and counties have long provided a variety of essential services to residents, the opioid epidemic stands out as a unique challenge because it demands immediate action on multiple fronts. Local governments are actively seeking ways to effectively marshal and deploy local resources to assist residents who are directly and indirectly impacted.

In the summer of 2014, recognizing the opioid abuse crisis as a major public health issue, the Massachusetts Municipal Association (MMA) Board of Directors created a special Municipal Opioid Addiction and Overdose Prevention Task Force to assist local officials as they take action to combat the epidemic in their communities.

To ensure broad representation of cities and towns and local officials, 11 members were appointed by the board, including seven officers of MMA along with affiliate

---

*Originally published as Geoff Beckwith, "Leading the Fight Against the Opioid Crisis," in the October 2016 issue of *Public Management (PM)* magazine, https://icma.org/articles/article/pm-article-leading-fight-against-opioid-crisis, and copyrighted by ICMA, the International City/County Management Association (icma.org). Reprinted with permission.

organizations, the executive director, and three municipal leaders from communities particularly hard hit by the opioid crisis.

The task force focused its efforts in several key areas, including identifying opportunities for leadership at home and across the state, enhancing intra- and inter-community information sharing, increasing public education and awareness, and ensuring the effective coordination of resources between federal, state, and local agencies.

Its 11 members met regularly for more than a year, seeking input from a wide range of partners, including service providers, advocates, experts, and organizations, to gather the broadest possible perspective. They reached out and surveyed the chief municipal officials in communities across the state to gauge the level of current and planned initiatives.

As task force members gathered information, assessed strategies, met with people who had lost loved ones, and learned from a wide range of professionals who are nearly overwhelmed by the scale of the problem, their sense of urgency grew. MMA's final report, "An Obligation to Lead," was issued in January 2016 and broadcast a call to action to local leaders, focusing on leading practices and immediate steps that local officials could take to combat this public health crisis and save lives.

Local Leadership Initiatives

Here are 10 opportunities and recommendations the task force identified for local leadership:

Take the lead to increase public awareness and engagement. Local leaders can work every day to disseminate information, enhance public awareness, reduce the stigma associated with addiction, and engage the community as a whole in a dialogue on the issue of substance abuse prevention.

Through the use of social media, information on local websites, and convening forums and events, local officials can facilitate connecting residents with valuable resources.

Local officials should act as a central clearinghouse for information, resources, and referrals in their cities and counties. They also should take the lead in reducing the stigma of substance abuse by providing a "safe space" for residents struggling with abuse as well as for family members and groups forming to support prevention and recovery efforts.

Increasing public awareness means recognizing the existence of a problem and being willing to have difficult and sometimes uncomfortable conversations. By publicly acknowledging victims and families and frequently publicizing municipal efforts, local leaders can become role models and encourage others to recognize the crisis in their communities.

MMA's report identified specific examples of community-based initiatives, including a vigil organized by Medford, Massachusetts, to honor residents who have died from addiction-related overdoses. Brockton, Massachusetts, has an excellent website that is rich with information and can serve as a model for other local governments.

Designate a municipal point person on substance abuse prevention. In MMA's municipal opioid response survey, many cities and towns responded that a designated staff member has been assigned to lead their community's efforts to respond to the opioid crisis.

The designees worked in a variety of departments, including health, police, human services, youth outreach, and fire. In some cases, the board of selectmen or mayor serve in this capacity. Some communities created a new staff or department-level position to act as the local lead.

Communities may want to consider developing a cross-functional internal working group, whose members could include these designees

- Town manager/administrator
- Mayor's office
- Councilmember/selectman
- Police
- Fire
- Emergency medical services
- Public health
- Schools (school nurse, health and physical education teachers, school committee)
- Library.

Encourage intracommunity, regional, and statewide collaboration. A number of coalitions have been funded through Drug-Free Communities grants

The federal Substance Abuse and Mental Health Service Administration (SAMHSA) oversees the program, which provides grants up to $125,000 per year for up to 10 years. SAMHSA is an agency within the U.S. Department of Health and Human Services that leads national public health efforts on substance abuse. These grants require that these 12 distinct sectors of the community be engaged in the coalition:

- Youth
- Parents
- Law enforcement
- Clergy and faith-based groups
- Schools
- Health care
- Media
- Business
- Civic or volunteer groups
- Youth-serving organizations
- Government agencies with expertise in the field of substance abuse
- Organizations involved in reducing substance abuse.

In MMA's survey, local governments indicated that the coalitions included representatives of these sectors, and also mentioned specifically engaging concerned residents, district attorney's offices, and recovery high schools—public schools where students can earn a high school diploma and are supported in their recovery from alcohol and drug use (www.massrecoveryhs.org).

They also included intervention and treatment agencies, ambulance services, judges, state and regional government, chambers of commerce and economic development agencies, pharmacies, jails, mental health services, and support groups.

Develop a one-page resource guide for families and those seeking treatment or assistance. Localities can develop a community-specific resource guide that is made available to family or community members seeking help for a neighbor or loved one. This one-pager should provide a checklist of action items and a list of available resources in the areas of prevention, intervention, and support.

It will be important to gather input from all sectors of the community, including local government departments, nonprofit service organizations, health care providers, support groups, and others to ensure that the resource guide is both comprehensive and appropriately customized for each community. It's important for this guide to be available as a physical document in government buildings, posted on the local government website with links to resources, and distributed at community meetings and events.

The Massachusetts Department of Public Health website provides an array of information and links that may be helpful as local officials customize their own resource guides for residents and families.

Pilot innovative programs based on local needs. Local officials have the opportunity to think outside the box and implement innovative solutions based on local needs and available resources.

These programs will be most effective when they are intended to de-stigmatize opioid addiction and transition the community away from a criminal justice approach to a more holistic focus on education and prevention, intervention, and support.

The Gloucester, Massachusetts, Police Department, for example, gained national attention when the police chief announced that any addict turning to the police department for help and willing to turn in any remainder of his or her drugs would not face criminal drug charges.

Instead, the person would be connected to appropriate treatment and recovery resources. This was in response to a community forum on what the city could do to help. The police department also indicated that it would pay for nasal Narcan for anyone who wanted it but could not afford it, using funds seized during drug dealer arrests.

Naloxone, also known as Narcan, can swiftly reverse the effects of an opioid overdose. When administered in a timely manner, it can dispel opioids that have bound to the body's nervous system receptors and restore breathing to a normal rate.

Attleboro, Massachusetts, has implemented a problem-oriented police (P.O.P.) team to help address the opioid crisis. This innovative community-policing method relies heavily on preventative measures instead of traditional criminal justice tactics. It engages directly with community stakeholders, taking proactive steps to reach out to those struggling with opioid addiction issues.

The department regularly monitors the outcomes from the use of preventative measures and reports on its findings. The city's website at https://attleboropolice.org/attleboro-police-p-o-p-team-action provides information on the P.O.P. team.

Arlington, Massachusetts, has added an Arlington Police Mental Health Clinician to the police force to reach out to drug addicts, residents who have previously overdosed, affected family members, and the community as a whole.

This expert provides valuable resources and information, teaches about the administration of potentially lifesaving Narcan, and works with members of the department to reduce the stigma associated with substance abuse.

Publicize the Good Samaritan Law. Local officials can encourage individuals to take action to intervene immediately when they are with overdose victims by publicizing that the Good Samaritan Law provides protection from prosecution.

Witnesses, friends, and bystanders can contact emergency personnel to convey that someone is not breathing, with a clear address and location. The Massachusetts

Department of Public Health has identified personal fear of police involvement by bystanders as a leading cause of inaction in overdose situations.

Survival rates dramatically improve when medical intervention is quickly administered. The Good Samaritan Law is intended to add lifesaving measures to prevent overdose deaths, and can also help to break down barriers around the stigma of substance abuse. Most states have Good Samaritan laws in place. For information on states with drug overdose immunity and Good Samaritan laws, go to https://bit.ly/1rHABM8.

Partner with schools to implement programs aimed at prevention. The adolescent brain, which continues to develop until age 25, is profoundly susceptible to the influence of drugs and alcohol. Early substance use greatly increases the risk of addiction.

It is crucial to engage students in education and prevention as early as is appropriate, and municipal and school departments and officials should collaborate to make sure that initiatives are in place locally.

Local officials can consider working with their state education and public health agencies to identify effective programs and models to implement, especially such evidence-based programs as screening, brief intervention, and referral to treatment (SBIRT), which is a practice used to identify, reduce, and prevent problematic abuse and dependence on alcohol and illicit drugs.

More information on SBIRT is available from SAMHSA at https://www.samhsa.gov/sbirt.

Create prevention curriculum and education programs. It's good for schools to implement prevention curriculum and education programs for students at the earliest possible age. Local officials are encouraged to work with their school departments to make sure that prevention education programs are in place.

There are many evidence-based prevention education programs available. Evidence-based programs are those that have been evaluated and found to be effective in reducing unwanted behaviors in students. Some prevention education programs are targeted to specific demographic subsets of students, and other programs are universal, meaning that any student can benefit from participation.

Federal agencies and other entities maintain lists of evidence-based prevention education programs, including Department of Education, Department of Justice, National Institute on Drug Abuse, Center for Substance Abuse Prevention, American Medical Association, Office of National Drug Control.

56. Statement of Policy
*Opioid Epidemic**

NATIONAL ASSOCIATION OF COUNTY
AND CITY HEALTH OFFICIALS

Policy

The National Association of County and City Health Officials (NACCHO) recognizes prescription and illicit opioid misuse as a significant public health threat and national emergency, and the critical role of local health departments in responding to the nation's opioid epidemic.

NACCHO urges local jurisdictions, states, and the federal government to appropriately fund efforts to respond to the opioid epidemic and to implement evidence-based policies and programs for the prevention and treatment of opioid use disorder and its related health consequences.

NACCHO supports the following strategies:

- **Improve Monitoring and Surveillance**
    ◊ Increase local and state capacity for expanded opioid surveillance, including surveillance of fatal and non-fatal overdoses and reversals, illicit drug use, and neonatal abstinence syndrome.
    ◊ Promote universal use of state prescription drug monitoring programs (PDMPs) that track all prescriptions within states and across jurisdictions to better monitor patient-specific prescription data and healthcare provider prescribing activities.
    ◊ Increase coordination of data collection and sharing among members from multiple sectors (e.g., state and local health departments, first responders, hospitals, law enforcement, treatment providers, behavioral health services, judicial system, and social services.)
- **Increase Prevention and Education**
    ◊ Expand and promote education for healthcare providers, first responders, law enforcement, judicial system, correctional facilities, schools, social services, nonprofit organizations, the general public, and other key partners

---

*Originally published as National Association of County and City Health Officials, "Statement of Policy: Opioid Epidemic," https://www.naccho.org/uploads/downloadable-resources/18–01-Opioid-Epidemic.pdf (March 2018). Reprinted with permission of the publisher and author.

and stakeholders about opioid misuse and addiction to reduce stigma and improve access to prevention, treatment, and recovery support services.
- ◊ Make access to life-saving overdose reversal medications, such as naloxone, widely available to first responders, people who use opioids or are prescribed opioids, family members, companions and caregivers of people who use or are prescribed opioids, and the public.
- ◊ Expand and promote education on how to recognize signs of overdose and to administer naloxone or similar drugs, especially among first responders, law enforcement, people who use or are prescribed opioids, and family members, companions and caregivers of people who use or are prescribed opioids.
- ◊ Expand and promote education on the safe storage and proper disposal of prescription opioids.
- ◊ Encourage adoption of local guidelines or legislation to lower barriers to report a potential overdose, such as Good Samaritan amnesty laws.
- ◊ Increase implementation of syringe services programs to reduce harms from injection drug use and opioid use disorder, such as the spread of human immunodeficiency virus (HIV) and viral hepatitis, and to increase access to substance use disorder treatment and other medical, mental health, and social services.
- ◊ Explore implementation of other evidence-based and practice-informed harm reduction services, such as safe consumption sites (also referred to as safe injection facilities.)

- **Promote Appropriate Opioid Prescribing Practices**
    - ◊ Expand and improve mandatory education for healthcare providers who prescribe prescription pain medication about prescription drug misuse and overdose, including risk factors, prevention strategies, and prescription security.
    - ◊ Encourage healthcare providers and pharmacists to educate patients, their families, caregivers, friends, and the public about prescription drug misuse and overdose, including risk factors and prevention strategies.
    - ◊ Promote use of guidelines for appropriate opioid prescribing, such as the Centers for Disease Control and Prevention (CDC) Guideline for Prescribing Opioids for Chronic Pain.

- **Improve Treatment and Recovery**
    - ◊ Increase availability of and access to effective opioid use disorder treatment, including medication-assisted treatment (MAT).
    - ◊ Increase capacity of and access to inpatient and outpatient recovery support services.
    - ◊ Improve insurance coverage and reimbursement for opioid use disorder treatment and recovery services.
    - ◊ Encourage healthcare providers to link people with substance use disorders to appropriate and accessible treatment and recovery support services.
    - ◊ Promote exploration of options to bulk-purchase naloxone for distribution to state and local health departments and/or negotiate deep discounts and rebates to bring down the cost of naloxone across delivery modalities.

The opioid epidemic requires an increased and sustained investment by Congress and the Administration to state and local health departments to support and inform the development, evaluation, and promotion of programs and policies to prevent opioid misuse and overdose. Furthermore, NACCHO urges Congress to completely remove the ban on the use of federal funds to support syringe service programs. Additionally, NACCHO would like to highlight the critical role that local health departments and their partners play in supporting the prevention of prescription and illicit opioid overdose and ensuring appropriate prescribing.

Justification

Deaths from drug overdose have risen steadily and are now the leading cause of injury death in the United States, with opioids in particular killing 42,000 people in 2016.[1] The majority of these drug overdose deaths involve an opioid, including both prescription and illicit opioids, with the latest estimates reporting 91 Americans dying each day from an opioid overdose in 2015.[2] In 2016, 62,000 Americans died from a drug overdose, surpassing the peak yearly death counts for HIV, car crashes, and guns.[3] Contributing to an estimated $183 billion in healthcare costs related to addiction, opioid use has emerged as a national emergency.[4] Aside from the increasing rates of fatal drug overdoses, 2.5 million emergency department visits in 2011 were attributed to drug misuse, with a 183% increase in visits that involved drugs classified as opioids.[5]

Overdose deaths that involve prescription opioids have quadrupled since 1999 and are responsible for nearly half of all U.S. opioid overdose deaths today. In 2015, more than 15,000 people died of overdoses involving prescription painkillers. Although there have been recent declines in opioid prescribing in the U.S., prescribing rates remain inconsistent and high, with three times higher amounts of opioids prescribed per person in 2015 than in 1999.[6] In 2013, providers wrote almost a quarter of a billion opioid prescriptions, which is enough for every American adult to have their own bottle of prescription opioid pills.[7] Taking too many prescription opioids can lead to death, and anyone who takes prescription opioids can become addicted. In 2014, almost two million Americans were either dependent on or abusing prescription opioids.[8]

Rates of prescription painkiller misuse and overdose death are highest among persons aged 25–54 years, and non–Hispanic white and American Indian or Alaskan Natives. Although women are more likely to use prescription opioids than men, men are still more likely to die from a prescription opioid overdose. Deaths of prescription painkiller overdoses in women have increased more than 400% since 1999. Those with mental illness are more often prescribed opioids and more often overdose. Additionally, people who obtain multiple prescription medications from multiple healthcare providers (also known as "doctor shopping"), and people who take high daily dosages of prescriptions and misuse multiple abuse-prone prescription drugs are at highest risk for prescription drug overdose.[9] Drug overdose deaths are highest in the Southwest and Appalachian regions of the U.S., while the Northeast and Southern regions have seen significant increases in death rates from 2014 to 2015.[10] Cases of neonatal abstinence syndrome, which is a group of problems that can occur to newborns exposed to opioids, grew by nearly 300% between 2000 and 2009. This may be fueled by the fact that women (1) are prescribed prescription painkillers at higher doses and for longer time periods than men; (2) become dependent on prescription painkillers more quickly than men; and (3) are more likely to engage in "doctor shopping" than men.[8]

Although prescription opioids have been a major contributing factor in the increase in opioid overdose deaths over the past two decades, recent opioid-involved death rate increases have been largely driven by increases in the deaths involving heroin and synthetic opioids other than methadone. Since 2010, heroin-related deaths have more than quadrupled. Heroin overdose death rates increased by 20.6% from 2014 to 2015, when almost 13,000 people died from a heroin overdose.[11] Death rates from synthetic opioid overdoses, which include fentanyl and other fentanyl analogues, increased 72.2% from 2014 to 2015, likely due to an increase in illicitly manufactured fentanyl.

Role of Local Health Departments in Addressing the Epidemic

Local health departments protect individuals, families, and communities from the devastating impact of opioid misuse and overdose through the ongoing collaboration of local, state, and national agencies. Local surveillance committees are valuable tools for identifying overdose trends, risk factors, and points of intervention. For instance, local poison death review committees are instrumental in determining the prevalence of overdoses due to prescription opioids, heroin, and other synthetic opioids, and are key contributors to state Health Burden of Injury reports.

Moreover, national surveillance is integral in tracking the growing opioid epidemic. PDMPs address prescription drug diversion (i.e., illicit drug trafficking of legitimately made controlled substances) and inappropriate prescribing or use in a number of ways, including helping healthcare providers identify drug-seeking behaviors or "doctor shopping," and aiding professional licensing boards to identify clinicians with patterns of inappropriate prescribing and dispensing. They can also assist clinicians in practicing appropriate prescribing practices, such as providing reminders to co-prescribe naloxone with an opioid prescription. A total of 49 states have active PDMPs with the capacity to receive and distribute controlled substance prescription information to authorized users; however, just 16 states require mandatory use of PDMPs. Studies indicate that PDMPs are a promising intervention at the state level, and that expansion of interstate PDMPs bolstered by federal support and funding could positively contribute to improved prescribing practices and better surveillance of opioid prescriptions across jurisdictions.

The coordination and collaboration of federal, state, local, and tribal partners and the engagement of policymakers, parents, youth and youth-serving agencies, healthcare professionals, concerned citizens, and persons in recovery are imperative to implementing strategies that target persons most at risk of opioid misuse, overdose, and diversion.[9] Local health departments are skilled conveners of cross-cutting community partners, such as physicians, pharmacists, first responders, law enforcement, correctional systems, substance use treatment providers, behavioral health services, regulatory agencies, and public health systems. The benefits of collaboration at the local level are essential to address this multifaceted epidemic. Together, these groups work to raise awareness through community-based outreach; identify points of prevention; analyze data from multiple sources to increase knowledge of local opioid misuse and overdose trends; and encourage professional licensing boards to take action against inappropriate prescribing and dispensing of prescription opioids. Local health departments are critical in providing increased access to opioid overdose prevention education, as well as improved access to medical, mental health, and social services for people who use or misuse opioids.

Substance Use Disorder Treatment Accessibility

Accessible and effective substance use disorder treatment programs can reduce drug overdose among people with dependence and addiction.[10,11] Unfortunately, in 2015, while 21.7 million Americans ages 12 and older needed treatment for substance use disorders, only 2.3 million (10.8%) actually received treatment at a substance use disorder facility.[12] The availability of accessible, effective treatment is essential. It is integral for local health departments to work with healthcare systems to identify patients in need of treatment and to link them to care. Local health departments can encourage healthcare providers to play an integral role in this process by promoting the healthcare provider's role in linking a person experiencing opioid use disorder to appropriate treatment or recovery support services.

Additionally, overdose drug reversal medications, such as naloxone, save lives in the event of overdose. In April 2014, the U.S. Food and Drug Administration (FDA) approved Evzio, a naloxone auto-injector that provides verbal instruction to the user describing how to use the medication for emergency treatment of known or suspected opioid overdose.[13] In November 2015, the FDA then approved Narcan, a nasal spray version of naloxone, which performs the same function as Evzio.[14] These innovative treatments have the potential to save millions of lives by stopping or reversing the effects of an opioid overdose. In the event of an overdose, first responders, such as law enforcement and emergency medical services (EMS), should be trained to administer naloxone and have access to this life-saving medication. Additionally, family and friends of people who use or are prescribed opioids, along with other members of the public, can also be trained on how to administer naloxone to someone experiencing an opioid overdose.

Healthcare providers and pharmacists can increase the co-prescribing of naloxone with an opioid prescription. Federal agencies can also explore options to bulk purchase naloxone, in order to distribute the reversal drug at deep discounts or rebates to local health departments to strengthen naloxone distribution across the delivery modalities.

Heroin Use and Increase in HIV, HCV, and HBV

There is increasingly more research that suggests non-medical use of prescription pain relievers may raise the risk of turning to heroin use. In a recent study, people aged 12 to 49 who had used prescription pain relievers for non-medical use were 19 times more likely to have initiated heroin use recently (within the past 12 months of being interviewed) than others in that age group (0.39 percent versus 0.02 percent).[15] The report also shows that four out of five recent heroin initiates (79.5 percent) had previously used prescription pain relievers for non-medical use.15 Research indicates that opioid misuse may be a precursor to heroin misuse with individuals making the "switch" to heroin because of cheaper costs, greater availability, and ease of use.[16,17,18] Opioid use disorder treatment programs must address the risk of heroin initiation in opioid-dependent clients, and provide safeguards to prevent heroin initiation.

Additionally, increases in opioid use has led to increases in HIV, hepatitis C virus (HCV), and hepatitis B virus (HBV). More than 50% of states report HCV cases are more than twice the national goal set by Healthy People 2020, with an overall national increase in acute HCV by 133% from 2004 to 2014.[19,20] The most dramatic increases in rates of opioid injection and acute HCV infections from 2004 to 2014 were among younger Americans (ages 18–39), while increases in HCV among pregnant women have also raised concern about the potential trajectory of HCV risk among a new generation of Americans.[20,21] Injection drug use is the primary risk factor for the spread of HCV, and a person who injects drugs represents one in ten new HIV diagnoses nationwide.[22] In 2015, injection drug use was the primary cause of the HIV outbreak that occurred in Scott County, Indiana.[23] More than 90% of those diagnosed with HIV during the outbreak were co-infected with HCV. In response to the HIV outbreak in Scott County, CDC conducted an assessment to identify counties that might be particularly vulnerable to the rapid spread of HIV and HCV among people who inject drugs. The analysis identified 220 in 26 states as being most vulnerable to new HIV, HCV, or HBV infections due to unsafe injection drug use.[24] Given the relationship between increased opioid use and increased injection drug use, not surprisingly, many of the locations identified in the vulnerability assessment are in states heavily impacted by the opioid epidemic, such as those in the Appalachian region.

Comprehensive Approaches to Harm Reduction Services

As local health departments develop plans to combat opioid use, the inclusion of comprehensive harm reduction services to prevent the spread of infectious disease, as well as to provide other prevention, screening, and linkage to care services, is critically important. For example, syringe service programs (SSPs) have proven to be highly effective at reducing HIV transmission among people who inject drugs and are an essential strategy to prevent HCV infection. Local health departments have a long history of addressing HCV and HIV prevention needs of persons who inject drugs, and are critical to the implementation and scale-up of comprehensive harm reduction services for people who use drugs. In 2015, the ban on federal funding for SSPs was lifted. While the legislation still prohibits the use of federal funds to purchase sterile needles or syringes for the purpose of injection of illegal drugs, it allows for federal funds to be used for other aspects of SSPs, based on evidence of a demonstrated need.[25] Local health departments are essential to scaling-up the availability of SSPs in response to increased vulnerability to the spread of infectious diseases that is being fueled by the opioid epidemic.

In addition to SSPs, supervised consumption sites, also referred to as safe injection facilities, are gaining increased attention for their role in harm reduction. A number of cities, including Baltimore, Denver, Seattle, San Francisco, New York City, and Philadelphia, are actively exploring opening such facilities and healthcare provider groups, such as the Massachusetts Medical Society, have expressed support for this public health intervention.[26] Supervised consumption services are a public health intervention that provide a hygienic space for people to use illicit drugs under the supervision of a trained staff. Such services are designed to reduce the risk of HIV, HCV, and HBV transmission, prevent overdose fatalities, and connect persons who inject or use drugs with addiction treatment and other social services. Additionally, they may decrease drug use in public places, reduce improperly discarded syringes, and diminish crime sometimes associated with open-air drug use. There is no persuasive data to support the idea that they increase drug use or frequency of injecting drugs.[27,28]

Appropriate Prescribing Practices

Over the past decade, healthcare providers have struggled to treat patients' pain appropriately without overprescribing painkillers, which is reflected in a quadrupling of opioid prescriptions since 1999 without a similar change in the reported amount of patients' pain. In 2010, enough prescription painkillers were prescribed to medicate every American adult around the clock for a month.[29] With national support, local health departments can provide education to healthcare providers that encourages them to identify alternate treatment options prior to prescribing opiates. Additionally, providers who do prescribe opioids for non-cancer chronic pain can utilize guidelines such as the CDC "Guideline for Prescribing Opioids for Chronic Pain."[30]

The general public is in need of accurate information about the risks associated with prescription drugs. According to the Partnership Attitude Tracking Study, 27% of teens believe it is safer to misuse prescription drugs than illegal drugs, while 30% believe prescription painkillers are not addictive.[31] Local health departments are well-suited to tailor public health campaigns to their communities to educate the general public and those most at risk of the dangers of prescription drug misuse.

There are multiple laws that states can implement in an effort to prevent drug misuse, overdose, and diversion. As of April 2017, 50 states and the District of Columbia have state-wide prescription drug monitoring programs; 36 states have regulations mandating or allowing pharmacists to check ID before dispensing prescriptions; and 18 states require continuing medical education for clinicians prescribing controlled substances.[32,33,34] Additionally, as of March 2015, 47 states and the District of Columbia have prescription drug limit laws.[35] Other laws and regulations that states have implemented include requiring physical examinations of patients by a healthcare provider prior to prescribing certain medications, requiring tamper-resistant forms of prescription drugs, limiting an individual's ability to "doctor shop" for prescription opioids, and regulating pain clinics.[36] These laws and regulations offer a strategy for mitigating the effects of prescription drugs on the opioid epidemic. Additionally, a handful of states provide immunity from prosecution or mitigation in prosecution or at sentencing for people who call 911 in the case of an overdose emergency.[37] These types of Good Samaritan amnesty laws can also improve overdose outcomes, since they lower barriers for a bystander to call 911 by reducing their fear about arrest for drug charges.

While there are increasing examples of promising practices, more research is needed to expand the evidence base to evaluate the impact of current strategies on reducing opioid misuse and overdose, and to inform the development and promotion of effective strategies in the future. The 56 recommendations provided in the final report of the President's Commission on Combating Drug Addiction and the Opioid Crisis can act as a starting block for federal funding and activity around the opioid epidemic.[38] Local health departments play critical roles in the ongoing prevention of opioid overdose, and require a renewed federal investment in the form of increased and sustained funding to support the development and evaluation of programs and policies to improve prevention, treatment, and recovery support services.

References

1. Centers for Disease Control and Prevention. (2017). Opioid overdose webpage. Retrieved January 8, 2018, from https://www.cdc.gov/drugoverdose/index.html.
2. Rudd, R. A., Aleshire, N., Zibbell, J. E., & Gladden, R.M. (2016, January). Increases in drug and opioid overdose deaths—United States, 2000–2014. *Morbidity and Mortality Weekly Report, 64*, 1378–82. Retrieved January 8, 2018, from https://www.cdc.gov/mmwr/preview/mmwrhtml/mm6450a3.htm.
3. Katz, J. (2017, June). Drug deaths in America are rising faster than ever. *The New York Times*. Retrieved January 8, 2018, from https://www.nytimes.com/interactive/2017/06/05/upshot/opioid-epidemic-drug-overdose-deaths-are-rising-faster-than-ever.html.
4. Frank, R.G. (2017, June). Ending Medicaid expansion will leave people struggling with addiction without care. *The Hill*. Retrieved January 8, 2018, from http://thehill.com/blogs/pundits-blog/healthcare/338579-endingmedicaid-expansion-will-leave-people-struggling-with.
5. Substance Abuse and Mental Health Services Administration. (2013). The DAWN report: Highlights of the 2011 Drug Abuse Warning Network (DAWN) findings on drug-related emergency department visits. Retrieved January 8, 2018, from http://www.samhsa.gov/data/2k13/dawn127/sr127-dawn-highlights.htm.
6. Automation of Reports and Consolidated Orders System (ARCOS) of the Drug Enforcement Administration. (2015). *QuintilesIMS Transactional Data Warehouse*. Retrieved January 8, 2018, from https://www.cdc.gov/vitalsigns/opioids/index.html.
7. Centers for Disease Control and Prevention. (2014). Opioid painkiller prescribing: where you live makes a difference webpage. Retrieved January 8, 2018, from https://www.cdc.gov/vitalsigns/opioid-prescribing/.
8. Centers for Disease Control and Prevention. (2013). Prescription painkiller overdoses: A growing epidemic, especially among women webpage. Retrieved January 8, 2018, from http://www.cdc.gov/vitalsigns/prescriptionpainkilleroverdoses/.
9. Centers for Disease Control and Prevention. (2012). CDC Grand rounds: Prescription drug overdoses—a U.S. epidemic. *Morbidity and Mortality Weekly Report, 61*(01). Retrieved January 8, 2018, from http://www.cdc.gov/mmwr/preview/mmwrhtml/mm6101a3.htm.
10. Hedegaard, H., Warner. M., & Miniño, A.M. (2017, December). Drug overdose deaths in the United States, 1999–2016. *NCHS Data Brief, 294*. Retrieved January 8, 2018, fromhttps://www.cdc.gov/nchs/products/databriefs/db294.htm.
11. Rudd, R. A., Seth, P., David, F., & Scholl, L. (2016). Increases in drug and opioid-involved overdose deaths—United States, 2010–2015. *Morbidity and Mortality Weekly Report, 65*, 1445–52. Retrieved January 8, 2018, from https://www.cdc.gov/mmwr/volumes/65/wr/mm655051e1.htm.
12. Trust for America's Health. (2013). Prescription drug abuse: Strategies to stop the epidemic. Retrieved January 8, 2018, from http://healthyamericans.org/assets/files/TFAH2013RxDrugAbuseRptFINAL.pdf.
13. U.S. Food and Drug Administration (2014). FDA approves new hand-held auto-injector to reverse opioid overdose. Retrieved January 8, 2017, from https://wayback.archive-it.org/7993/20170112032835/http://www.fda.gov/NewsEvents/Newsroom/PressAnnouncements/ucm391465.htm.
14. U.S. Food and Drug Administration (2015). FDA moves to quickly approve easy-to-use nasal spray to treat opioid overdose. Retrieved January 8, 2018, from https://www.fda.gov/NewsEvents/Newsroom/PressAnnouncements/ucm473505.htm.
15. Muhuri, P., Grfoerer, J., & Davies, M. (2013, August). Associations of nonmedical pain reliever use and initiation of heroin use in the United States. *Substance Abuse and Mental Health Services Administration*. Retrieved on January 8, 2018, from http://www.samhsa.gov/data/2k13/DataReview/DR006/nonmedical-pain-reliever-use-2013.pdf.
16. Pollini, R. A., Banta-Green, C. J., Cuevas-Mota, J., Metzner, M., Teshale, E., & Garfein, R.S. (2011, October). Problematic use of prescription-type opioids prior to heroin use among young heroin injectors. *Substance Abuse and Rehabilitation 2*(1), 173–180. Retrieved January 8, 2018, from https://www.ncbi.nlm.nih.gov/pubmed/23293547#.
17. National Institute on Drug Abuse. (2012). Epidemiologic trends in drug abuse: Proceedings of the community epidemiology work group. Retrieved on January 8, 2018 from http://www.drugabuse.gov/sites/default/files/files/cewg_january_2013_vol1_508.pdf.
18. Cicero, T. J., Ellis, M. S., & Surrat, H.L. (2012, July). Effect of abuse-deterrent formulation of Oxycontin. *New England Journal of Medicine, 367*(2), 187–189. Retrieved on January 8, 2018 from https://www.ncbi.nlm.nih.gov/pubmed/22784140.
19. Boschma, J. (2017, October). Opioid epidemic triggers hepatitis C outbreak. *Politico*. Retrieved January 8, 2018, from https://www.politico.com/story/2017/11/01/opioid-crisis-next-steps-politico-working-group-244439.
20. National Center for HIV/AIDS, Viral Hepatitis, STD, and TB Prevention. (2017, December). Increase in hepatitis C infections linked to worsening opioid crisis. *Centers for Disease Control and Prevention*. Retrieved January 8, 2018, from https://www.cdc.gov/nchhstp/newsroom/2017/hepatitis-c-and-opioid-injection-press-release.html.
21. Patrick, S. W., Bauer, A. M., Warren, M. D., Jones, T. F., & Wester, C. (2017, May). Hepatitis C virus

infection among women giving birth—Tennessee and United States, 2009–2014. *Morbidity and Mortality Weekly Report, 66*(18), 470–473. Retrieved January 8, 2018, from https://www.cdc.gov/mmwr/volumes/66/wr/mm6618a3.htm.

22. Vital Signs. (2016, December). Syringe services programs for HIV prevention. *Centers for Disease Control and Prevention.* Retrieved January 8, 2018, from https://www.cdc.gov/hiv/images/risk/Syringe-Services-Programs-for-HIV-Prevention.jpg.

23. Peters, P. J., Pontones, P., Hoover, K. W., Patel, M. R., Galang, R. R., Shields, J., … Duwve, J.M. (2016, July 21). HIV infection linked to injection use of oxymorphone in Indiana, 2014–2015. *New England Journal of Medicine, 375,* 229–239. Retrieved January 29, 2018, from http://www.nejm.org/doi/full/10.1056/NEJMoa1515195.

24. Whalen, J., & Campo-Flores, A. (2018, January). Jump in HIV cases among drug users seen in Northern Kentucky. *The Wall Street Journal.* Retrieved January 10, 2018, from https://www.wsj.com/articles/jump-in-hiv-cases-among-drug-users-seen-in-northern-kentucky-1515544558.

25. Centers for Disease Control and Prevention. (2017). Syringe services programs webpage. Retrieved January 29, 2018, from https://www.cdc.gov/hiv/risk/ssps.html.

26. Fitzgerald, T.C. (2017, April). Establishment of a pilot medically supervised injection facility in Massachusetts. *Massachusetts Medical Society.* Retrieved January 29, 2018, from http://www.massmed.org/advocacy/state-advocacy/sif-report-2017/.

27. Hodel, D. (2017, June). Issue brief: The case for supervised consumption Services. *The Foundation for AIDS Research (amfAR).* Retrieved January 8, 2018, from http://www.amfar.org/uploadedFiles/_amfarorg/Articles/On_The_Hill/2017/IB-Supervised-Consumption-Services-061217.pdf.

28. Project Inform. (2016, September). Safer consumption spaces in the United States: Uniting for a national movement. Baltimore, MD. Retrieved January 29, 2018, from https://www.projectinform.org/wp-content/uploads/2017/06/SCS-Think-Tank-Report.pdf.

29. Centers for Disease Control and Prevention. (2011). Prescription painkiller overdoses in the U.S. webpage. Retrieved January 8, 2018, from http://www.cdc.gov/vitalsigns/painkilleroverdoses/index.html.

30. Dowell, D., Haegerich, T. M., & Chou, R. (2016). CDC guideline for prescribing opioids for chronic pain—United States, 2016. *MMWR Recommendations and Reports, 65*(1), 1–49. Retrieved on January 8, 2018 from https://www.cdc.gov/mmwr/volumes/65/rr/rr6501e1.htm.

31. Partnership for Drug-Free Kids (2013). Partnership attitude tracking study. Retrieved January 8, 2018, from https://drugfree.org/wp-content/uploads/2014/07/PATS-2013-FULL-REPORT.pdf.

32. The Prescription Drug Monitoring Program Training and Technical Assistance Center. (2017, August). Status of prescription drug monitoring programs (PDMPs). Retrieved January 8, 2018, from http://pdmpassist.org/pdf/PDMP_Program_Status_20170824.pdf.

33. The National Alliance for Model State Drug Laws (NAMSDL). (2016, March). Overview of state pain management and prescribing policies. Retrieved January 8, 2018, from http://www.namsdl.org/library/052D1242-E158-6B44-A6E69A0729BCDF0C/.

34. Shopov, V.L. (2017, April). State-by-state breakdown of opioid regulations. *AthenaInsight.* Retrieved January 8, 2018, from https://www.athenahealth.com/insight/infographic-opioid-regulations-state-by-state.

35. Public Health Law. (2015, March). Prescription drug time and dosage limit laws. Retrieved January 8, 2018, from https://www.cdc.gov/phlp/docs/menu_prescriptionlimits.pdf.

36. Centers for Disease Control and Prevention. (2015, August). Prescription drugs: State laws on prescription drug misuse and abuse webpage. Retrieved January 8, 2018, from https://www.cdc.gov/phlp/publications/topic/prescription.html.

37. Public Health Law. (2012, September). Menu of state laws related to prescription drug overdose emergencies. Retrieved January 8, 2018 from https://www.cdc.gov/phlp/docs/menu-pdoe.pdf.

38. Christie, C., Baker, C., Cooper, R., Kennedy, P. J., Madras, B., & Bondi, P. (2017, November). Final report. *The President's Commission on Combating Drug Addiction and the Opioid Crisis.* Retrieved January 8, 2018, from https://www.whitehouse.gov/sites/whitehouse.gov/files/images/Final_Report_Draft_11-15-2017_0.pdf.

57. Statement of Policy

*Syringe Services Programs**

NATIONAL ASSOCIATION OF COUNTY
AND CITY HEALTH OFFICIALS

Policy

The National Association of County and City Health Officials (NACCHO) supports a comprehensive, evidence-based approach to syringe services programs, also known as syringe or needle exchange programs, in order to support the health of people who inject drugs and to curb transmission of HIV, viral hepatitis, and other blood-borne diseases. NACCHO urges state and local policy makers to do the following:

- Support syringe services program development and operation in accordance with the peer-reviewed evidence base, best practices, and local health department and other expert recommendations;
- Remove legal barriers to accessing and safely disposing sterile needles, syringes, and other injecting equipment;
- Modify state and local statutes to permit over-the-counter pharmacy sales and purchase of syringes;
- Revise paraphernalia laws to decriminalize syringe possession;
- Increase the availability of drug treatment and overdose prevention, including Medication-Assisted Treatment and naloxone training and distribution;
- Ensure education of law enforcement, criminal justice personnel, health department staff, healthcare providers, pharmacists, and other relevant professional and community partners regarding the benefit of syringe services programs, as well as other harm reduction strategies, and relevant laws, policies, and processes; and
- Assure adequate resources to support health department surveillance, program planning, and program evaluation capacity to assess disease and risk behavior trends and the impact of syringe services programs, as well as other disease prevention and health promotion interventions for persons who inject drugs, on local health outcomes.

---

*Originally published as National Association of County and City Health Officials, https://www.naccho.org/uploads/downloadable-resources/Policy-and-Advocacy/05-09-Syringe-Services-Programs.pdf (June 2015). Reprinted with permission of the publisher and author.

Furthermore, NACCHO urges Congress to remove the ban on the use of federal funds to support syringe services programs.

Justification

Injection drug use is a major route of transmission for HIV, viral hepatitis, and other blood-borne pathogens. Over the past 25 years, syringe services programs have proven to be highly effective at reducing HIV transmission among people who inject drugs and are an essential strategy to prevent hepatitis C virus (HCV) infection. In addition to providing sterile syringes and other injecting equipment, many syringe service programs also provide medical and social services, including HIV and viral hepatitis testing, overdose prevention training, referrals to social services and housing, and linkages to medical care, mental health care, and substance use treatment, to individuals who are not often served by traditional healthcare providers.[1]

In the United States, HIV incidence among people who inject drugs declined by approximately 80% from 1988 to 2006 following the adoption of syringe service programs in a number of states.[2] Despite that overall decline, people who inject drugs continue to represent a substantial proportion of persons with new HIV diagnoses, accounting for approximately 8% of new HIV infections in 2010 and 15% of those living with HIV in 2011.[3] Since the epidemic began, approximately 186,728 people with AIDS who inject drugs have died.[4]

The sharing of drug injection paraphernalia is the primary risk factor for HCV infection. The rate of reported new hepatitis C infections has risen rapidly nationwide, more than doubling from 2010 to 2013.[5] An estimated 3 million to 4 million people in the United States are living with chronic hepatitis C, which is at least 10 times more infectious than HIV. In 2007, the number of U.S. deaths associated with hepatitis C surpassed those from HIV for the first time. After receiving reports of approximately 800 to 1,000 cases of acute hepatitis C each year from 2006 to 2010, there was a significant increase of 151.5% in reported cases of acute hepatitis C infection from 2010 to 2013. Based on surveillance data and epidemiologic studies, new cases of HCV are highest among young persons who are white, live in non-urban areas, and have a history of injection drug use.[6] The number of cases reported represent only a fraction of the total number of new hepatitis C infections. Additional capacity for surveillance to detect these new infections and additional prevention capacity to link persons to services and medical care that can stop transmission are needed, particularly for states already reporting increases in transmission. A comprehensive public health response that includes expanded syringe access is necessary to reduce the transmission of HCV, HIV, and other blood-borne pathogens.

Numerous federally funded studies, including studies conducted by the Centers for Disease Control and Prevention (CDC) and the Institute of Medicine (IOM), have established that syringe exchange is an effective HIV prevention intervention and does not promote drug use.[7-10] Rather, studies show that people who inject drugs who participate in syringe services programs are more likely to enroll and complete substance use treatment. A study in Seattle found that new syringe services program participants are five times more likely to enter a drug treatment program than nonparticipants.[11] Drug treatment programs, such as Medication-Assisted Treatment for opiate dependence, have been shown to substantially reduce the frequency of drug use, other risk behaviors, and new infections.[12] In 2011, the U.S. Surgeon General determined that syringe services programs reduce both drug abuse and the risk of HIV infection.[13]

Syringe services programs may also provide the overdose reversal medication naloxone. Drug overdose is the leading cause of injury-related death in the United States, killing more people every year than auto accidents. Opioids (both prescription painkillers and heroin) are responsible for most of these deaths. The death rate from prescription opioid-caused overdose nearly quadrupled from 1999 to 2013, while deaths from heroin overdose rose 270% between 2010 and 2013.[14] Most opioid overdose deaths can be prevented by the timely administration of naloxone. In the event of an overdose, witnesses such as injecting partners, friends and family, and first responders (e.g., law enforcement, Emergency Medical Services) should be trained to administer naloxone and have access to this life-saving medication. Syringe services programs have unique access to people at risk of overdose prevention, making them important points of naloxone distribution and training.

In the United States, public funding of syringe services programs has been limited due to a ban on the use of federal funding for syringe service programs, which was first enacted in 1988. In December 2009, the 111th Congress ended the nearly 20 year prohibition of using federal funds to support syringe service programs; however, in December 2011, the 112th Congress reinstated the ban through the Labor, Health and Human Services, and Education Appropriations bill included in the FY2012 Consolidated Appropriations Act (P.L.112-74). As long as the ban on federal funding to support syringe services programs is law, the responsibility of permitting, funding, and implementing such programs falls to the state and local level, which has resulted in a wide variation in syringe services program availability. Additional resources, as well as the removal of the ban on the use of federal funds to support syringe services programs, are needed to fully plan, implement, evaluate, and expand the inclusion of syringe services programs in comprehensive HIV and HCV prevention efforts and to address the health of people who inject drugs.

The cost savings of infections averted by syringe services programs are significant. Lifetime treatment of an HIV-positive person is estimated to cost $326,500 on average, whereas a sterile syringe costs less than a dollar.[15] An analysis conducted in 2015 calculated that the capacity of existing syringe services programs to provide a new syringe for each injection is estimated to be sufficient to meet only 3% of the need, and that expanding syringe services program coverage to meet even 10% of injections would avert nearly 500 new HIV infections annually.[16] Additional savings will be incurred by preventing the transmission of HCV and other blood-borne diseases, as well as supporting the overall health and well-being of people who inject drugs through linkage to substance use treatment, preventive medicine, and other health and supportive services offered by syringe services programs.

REFERENCES

1. Centers for Disease Control and Prevention. (2012). Integrated prevention services for HIV infection, viral hepatitis, sexually transmitted diseases, and tuberculosis for persons who use drugs illicitly: summary guidance from CDC and the U.S. Department of Health and Human Services. *Morbidity and Mortality Weekly Report, 61*(No. RR-5). Retrieved June 1, 2015, from http://www.cdc.gov/mmwr/preview/mmwrhtml/rr6105a1.htm.

2. Centers for Disease Control and Prevention. (2015). HIV in the United States: At a Glance. Retrieved June 1, 2015, from http://www.cdc.gov/hiv/pdf/statistics_basics_ataglance_factsheet.pdf.

3. Ibid.

4. Ibid.

5. Centers for Disease Control and Prevention. (2015). Increases in hepatitis C virus infection related to injection drug use among persons aged ≤30 years—Kentucky, Tennessee, Virginia, and West Virginia, 2006–2012. *Morbidity and Mortality Weekly Report, 64*(17). Retrieved June 1, 2015, from http://www.cdc.gov/MMWr/preview/mmwrhtml/mm6417a2.htm.

6. Centers for Disease Control and Prevention. Viral Hepatitis Surveillance, United States, 2013. (2013). Retrieved June 1, 2015, from http://www.cdc.gov/hepatitis/statistics/2013surveillance/index.htm.

7. National Commission on Acquired Immune Deficiency Syndrome. (1991). *The twin epidemics of substance use and HIV.* Retrieved June 22, 2015, from http://harmreduction.org/wp-content/uploads/2012/01/NationalCommissiononAIDS1991.

8. U.S. General Accounting Office. (1993). *Needle exchange programs: research suggests promise as an AIDS prevention strategy.* HRD-93-60. Retrieved June 25, 2015, from http://www.gao.gov/products/HRD-93-60.

9. Office of Technology Assessment, Congress of the United States. (1995) *The effectiveness of AIDS prevention efforts.* Retrieved June 22, 2015, from http://ota.fas.org/reports/9556.pdf.

10. National Research Council and Institute of Medicine. (1995). *Preventing HIV transmission: the role of sterile needles and bleach.* Retrieved June 22, 2015, from http://www.nap.edu/catalog/4975/preventing-hiv-transmission-the-role-of-sterile-needles-and-bleach.

11. Hagan, H., McGough, J.P., Thiede, H., Hopkins, S., Duchin, J., & Alexander, E.R. (2000). Reduced injection frequency and increased entry and retention in drug treatment associated with needle-exchange participation in Seattle drug injectors. *Journal of Substance Abuse Treatment, 19*, 247–252.

12. Metzger, D.S., Woody, G.E., & O'Brien, C.P. (2010). Drug treatment as HIV prevention: a research update. *Journal of Acquired Immune Deficiency Syndrome, 55*(Suppl 1), S32-6.

13. Health and Human Services Department. (2011). *Determination that a demonstration needle exchange program would be effective in reducing drug abuse and the risk of acquired immune deficiency syndrome infection among intravenous drug users (Federal Register Notice).* Retrieved June 1, 2015, from https://www.federalregister.gov/articles/2011/02/23/2011-3990/determination-that-a-demonstration-needle-exchange-program-would-be-effective-in-reducing-drug-abuse.

14. Davis, C. (2015). Naloxone for community opioid overdose reversal. Public Health Law Research. Retrieved June 25, 2015, http://phlr.org/product/naloxone-community-opioid-overdose-reversal.

15. amfAR, The Foundation for AIDS Research. (2015). Preventing HIV and Hepatitis C Among People Who Inject Drugs: Public Funding for Syringe Services Programs Makes the Difference. Retrieved June 25, 2015, from http://www.amfar.org/uploadedFiles/_amfarorg/On_the_Hill/BIMC_SSP_IB-WEB-VERSION_041315.pdf.

16. Nguyen, T.Q., Weir, B.W., Pinkerton, S.D., Des Jarlais, D.C., & Holtgrave, D. (2012, July). *Increasing investment in syringe exchange is cost-saving HIV prevention: modeling hypothetical syringe coverage levels in the United States.* Presented at the 19th International AIDS Conference, Washington, D.C.: Abstract no. MOAE0204. Retrieved June 25, 2015, from https://www.aids2014.org/Abstracts/A200746842.aspx.

Part IV

The Future

58. Some Good News on Opioid Epidemic

*Treatment Options Are Expanding**

WILLIAM GREENE *and* LISA J. MERLO

In the past two decades, the devastation associated with opioid addiction has escaped the relative confines of the inner city and extended to suburban and rural America. Due in large part to the proliferation of prescription pain relievers, rates of opioid abuse, addiction, overdose and related deaths have increased dramatically. This has affected families and communities that once felt immune to this crisis.

On August 1, an analysis of health care claims for treatment of opioid dependence showed a 3,000 percent increase from 2007 to 2014.

The knowledge that many are afflicted or affected has helped people understand the powerful psychological and physiological grip of addiction. As a result, stigma has decreased.

What was once relegated to the back burner of public concern has become a top public health priority.

We addiction experts also have gained better understanding of the illness, and we see reasons for hope.

Shifts in Public Policy

The Affordable Care Act and the Mental Health Parity and Addiction Equity Act combined to finally require insurance companies to cover treatment for patients suffering from addiction. Insurance companies can no longer deny treatment or significantly limit treatment for psychiatric disorders, including addiction, as they had in the past.

President Obama proposed $1.1 billion in funding to expand access to treatment for opioid addiction and overdose prevention.

In July, the House passed a bill that would further expand access to care for addiction and other mental health conditions.

---

*Originally published as William Greene and Lisa J. Merlo, "Some Good News on Opioid Epidemic: Treatment Options Are Expanding," *The Conversation*, https://theconversation.com/some-good-news-on-opioid-epidemic-treatment-options-are-expanding-61483 (August 9, 2016). Reprinted with permission of the publisher.

Then, on July 22, the president signed into law the Comprehensive Addiction and Recovery Act of 2016.

If adequately funded by Congress, the law will help to strengthen prevention, treatment and recovery efforts.

This improves treatment options for individuals in the criminal justice system, which may decrease rates of return to crime and prison. It also expands access to naloxone, a lifesaving drug that emergency medical workers and even family and friends, in certain cases, can administer to someone who has overdosed.

This stepped-up policy response is giving doctors the means to better treat people with opioid addiction. When combined with improvements in public understanding that addiction is a disease requiring treatment, we as a society are creating an environment that supports treatment. We believe this will save many thousands of lives.

A Societal Effort

Physicians are re-examining their own prescribing practices to decrease the likelihood of medication diversion or misuse and to minimize the development of iatrogenic addiction, or addiction that stems from medical treatment.

Law enforcement officials have worked to close down hundreds of "pill mills," or clinics purporting to serve patients with chronic pain disorders. In reality, they serve as primary access points for dealers selling prescription drugs on the black market.

In all states except Missouri, prescription drug monitoring programs have also helped to identify patients in need of intervention.

More patients have access to treatment than ever before, including many in the criminal justice system who participate in drug court diversionary programs. Such programs save taxpayer money and decrease recidivism.

Greater Understanding and Knowledge

The field of addiction medicine has matured and expanded, recently acquiring recognition as a dedicated medical specialty.

According to the American Society of Addiction Medicine, the disease of addiction is best understood as a single condition. There is no distinction made depending on the preferred drug(s) of abuse.

Addiction specialists conceptualize addiction as a bio-psycho-social-spiritual disease. They understand that continued use of psychoactive substances interferes with active participation in psychosocial treatment. Such usage prevents development of a personal program of recovery.

Therefore, successful treatment of opioid addiction begins with abstinence from all substances of abuse. Patients should not expect to quit using oxycodone, fentanyl or heroin but continue to drink alcohol or to smoke marijuana. The same holds true for treatment of addiction to alcohol, marijuana, cocaine or any other drug.

Some patients require medically supervised detoxification to abstain. Accessing the right treatment is crucial to success. Some will need a more intensive treatment setting. Even individuals who were unsuccessful maintaining abstinence with outpatient treatment may achieve recovery in a more intensive treatment setting.

Addiction, like other medical conditions with significant behavioral components, is a chronic condition. Relapse may occur. Thus, most patients need to learn skills that help them cope adaptively with stressors in their daily lives. Often, they need to address issues from their past that relate to substance abuse.

People with addiction may have other psychiatric conditions. They need to be treated for those, too. In many areas, publicly funded treatment programs are available for individuals lacking insurance or who cannot afford private treatment.

Support from Family and 12-Step Programs Helpful

Family members should encourage patients suffering from addiction to seek a professional evaluation. This will help determine the appropriate level of care, which could range from outpatient management to long-term residential treatment.

In addition, physicians and other treatment specialists highly encourage participation in a 12-step recovery program, such as Alcoholics Anonymous or Narcotics Anonymous. Such programs are free, and they offer many benefits. Research has documented significantly reduced risk of relapse with increased likelihood of successful outcome among patients treated for opioid addiction in this way.

Family members often benefit from 12-step programs, too. Al-Anon or Alateen can help them learn how best to support their loved one without enabling the addiction.

Medications Also Helpful

Patients with opioid use disorders may also benefit from medication assistance. Currently, four types of prescription medication are approved to assist with treatment of opioid addiction.

The opioid antagonist medication, naltrexone, is available as a daily oral pill or as a monthly intramuscular injection. It helps patients by decreasing cravings. It also blocks patients' ability to "get high," even if they use an opioid drug. Naltrexone has no abuse potential and can be safely used by most patients.

Second, the opioid partial agonist medication buprenorphine is available as an oral pill, dissolving tablet or filmstrip. It also reduces cravings and reduces and prevents withdrawal symptoms. It, too, blocks the ability to "get high."

Buprenorphine has some abuse potential, however. It should be used only under guidance and careful monitoring by a physician with sufficient expertise. In fact, doctors must receive a waiver to be allowed to prescribe buprenorphine.

Third, the opioid agonist medication methadone prevents withdrawal symptoms, reduces cravings and interferes with the ability to "get high" from other opioids.

Methadone also has abuse potential and risk of overdose if used inappropriately, however. As a result, methadone is typically dispensed in liquid form on a daily basis, and only from specialized methadone maintenance treatment clinics.

Finally, for individuals at high risk of relapse, new measures are in place to help prevent death in the event of accidental overdose. The opioid antagonist medication naloxone is now available in an automatic injector formulation for use by police, EMTs and other first responders. Naloxone has long been used by medical professionals in emergency rooms to reverse opioid overdose.

Naloxone is also available by prescription for patients with opioid addiction and their families to keep on hand as a safety precaution. In some states it is also available over the counter at certain pharmacies. It can be viewed much like an Epi-pen, which patients with severe allergies keep on hand for emergencies. A naloxone nasal spray is newly available, which may further facilitate access to this lifesaving medication.

These changes to public policy and advances in opioid treatment have greatly improved the prognosis for patients suffering from opioid addiction. Research and clinical evidence have demonstrated that long-term recovery is not only possible, but expected, following adequate treatment with appropriate follow-up care.

Now, more than ever, there is hope for healing from addiction.

59. Sterile Needles Can Stop the Spread of Disease in Prisons—Here's How*

JACK WALLACE

It's no secret that prisoners inject drugs. And because they don't have access to sterile needles, inmates not only share needles—they share infectious diseases as well.

The Australian Capital Territory (ACT) government is currently deciding whether to trial a program to distribute sterile needles and syringes to prisoners. But the Community and Public Sector Union (CPSU), which represents prison guards, is fighting the introduction of such a program, saying it doesn't want to facilitate illicit drug use and expose officers to potential needle stick injuries.

Spread of Infection

Hepatitis C is a virus that causes inflammation of the liver. It's present in the blood and is transmitted by blood-to-blood contact. Some people are able to clear the virus from their system but others can develop serious complications such as cirrhosis and liver cancer.

Hepatitis C is a significant public health issue, with more than 259,000 Australians estimated to be infected with the virus.

More than 40% of Victorian and New South Wales prisoners are infected with hepatitis C and the proportion may be higher in other jurisdictions.

Prisoners suffer poorer health than the general population and the common life experiences of inmates include sexual victimization, physical and emotional maltreatment, and suicide attempts by significant others.

Illicit Drug Use

Drug use occurs within prisons in spite of correctional authorities searching visitors and staff, testing prisoners for drugs, using sniffer dogs and, in some states and territories, offering drug substitution programs and detoxification.

---

*Originally published as Jack Wallace, "Sterile Needles Can Stop the Spread of Disease in Prisons—Here's How," *The Conversation*, https://theconversation.com/sterile-needles-can-stop-the-spread-of-disease-in-prisons-heres-how-3644 (October 17, 2011). Reprinted with permission of the publisher.

An evaluation of drug policy and services in the ACT's only full-time adult correctional center, Alexander Maconochie Centre, found almost one third of inmates reported having injected illicit drugs while in the center. The facility has been operating for less than two years.

Needles and syringes are shared within prisons in a process that one informant to the Regulating Hepatitis C report described as dangerous, unsterile and clandestine.

A 2009 survey of prisoner health noted that of 112 prisoners who reported injecting, only three used a new needle. This implies the other 109 prisoners were at risk of being infected with a blood borne virus such as hepatitis C or HIV.

Minimizing Harm

Unlike many other countries, Australia has a pragmatic approach to drug use. The government's blueprint for reducing the impact of drug use, the National Drug Strategy, wants to reduce the supply and demand of drugs but acknowledges that in spite of doing this, people will continue to use illegal drugs.

All levels of government support the National Drug Strategy's harm reduction interventions, including the distribution of sterile needles and syringes. But so far this hasn't translated to establishing a prison-based needle and syringe exchange program in any Australian state or territory.

Similar provisions are made in ACT legislation. The preamble to the ACT Corrections Management Act 2007 notes detainees should have access to health care that is equivalent to community standards and that conditions in detention should "promote the health and wellbeing of detainees."

There are various other regulatory instruments at a national, state and territory level that support the distribution of sterile needles and syringes, including statements from the Correctional Administrators from each state and territory who note "each prisoner is to have access to evidence based health services."

The Wrong Fight

There is substantial international evidence to support the safety and efficacy of needle and syringe programs in correctional settings.

A review of interventions to reduce the transmission of HIV in prisons, published in The Lancet, found prison needle exchange programs reduced the sharing of needles and syringes. The programs halted the spread of HIV and hepatitis (with no new cases found) and improved staff safety. There was also a reduction in overdoses.

The resistance to a prison needle exchange program in Australia reflects a culture within correctional services of being tough on prisoners.

Prison officers also have an uneasy history with injecting drug users since the death of prison officer Geoff Pearce, who was stabbed by a syringe filled with HIV-infected blood in Long Bay Gaol in 1990.

While some officers are breaking rank and calling for a trial needle exchange program, the CPSU seems unlikely to back down. A statement in its employment agreement with ACT custodial officers states that "for the safety of staff, no needle exchange program, however presented, shall be implemented without prior consultation."

The ACT Government is expected to make a decision by the end of the year about whether to trial a needle and syringe exchange program.

I hope it considers all the evidence and sees this decision for what it is—a human rights and health services issue that could reduce the spread of hepatitis C in the prison community and the wider population.

60. Meth vs. Opioids

*America Has Two Drug Epidemics,
but Focuses on One**

April Dembosky

Kim had been wine tasting with a friend in Sonoma, Calif. They got into an argument in the car that night and Kim thought someone was following them. She was utterly convinced. And she had to get away.

"I jumped out of the car and started running, and I literally ran a mile. I went through water, went up a tree," she said. "I was literally running for my life."

Kim was soaking wet when she walked into a woman's house, woke her from bed and asked for help. When the woman went to call the police, Kim left and found another woman's empty guesthouse to sleep in—Goldilocks-style.

"But then I woke up and stole her car," said Kim, who is 47 and now in recovery. (KHN is using her first name only because she has used illicit drugs.) Kim had been high on Xanax and methamphetamine. "I was crazy. Meth causes people to act completely insane."

While public health officials have focused on the opioid epidemic in recent years, another epidemic has been brewing quietly, but vigorously, behind the scenes. Methamphetamine use is surging in parts of the U.S., particularly the West, leaving first responders and addiction treatment providers struggling to handle a rising need.

Across the country, overdose deaths involving meth more than quadrupled from 2011 to 2017. Admissions to treatment facilities for meth are up 17%. Hospitalizations related to meth jumped by about 245% from 2008 to 2015. And throughout the West and Midwest, 70% of local law enforcement agencies say meth is their biggest drug threat.

But policymakers in Washington, D.C., haven't kept up, continuing to direct the bulk of funding and attention to opioids, said Steve Shoptaw, an addiction psychologist at UCLA in Los Angeles, where he hears one story after another about meth destroying people's lives.

"But when you're in D.C., where people are making decisions about how to deploy resources, those stories are very much muffled by the much louder story about the opioid epidemic," he said.

---

*Originally published as April Dembosky, "Meth vs. Opioids: America Has Two Drug Epidemics, but Focuses on One," *Kaiser Health News*, https://khn.org/news/meth-vs-opioids-america-has-two-drug-epidemics-but-focuses-on-one/ (May 7, 2019). Reprinted with permission of the publisher. Kaiser Health News is a nonprofit news service covering health issues. It is an editorially independent program of the Kaiser Family Foundation that is not affiliated with Kaiser Permanente. This story is part of a partnership that includes KQED, NPR and Kaiser Health News.

Even within drug treatment circles, there's a divide. Opioid addiction advocates are afraid their efforts to gain acceptance for measures like needle-exchange programs and safe injection sites will be threatened if meth advocates demand too much.

"The bottom line is, as Americans, we have just so much tolerance to deal with addiction," Shoptaw said. "And if the opioid users have taken that tolerance, then there's no more."

So, lawmakers in San Francisco are trying to get a grip on the toll meth is taking on their city's public health system on their own. The mayor recently established a task force to combat the epidemic.

"It's something we really have to interrupt," said Rafael Mandelman, a San Francisco district supervisor who will co-chair the task force. "Over time, this does lasting damage to people's brains. If they do not have an underlying medical condition at the start, by the end, they will."

Since 2011, emergency room visits related to meth in San Francisco have jumped 600% to 1,965 visits in 2016, the last year for which ER data is available. Admissions to the hospital are up 400% to 193, according to city public health data. And at San Francisco General Hospital, of 7,000 annual psychiatric emergency visits last year, 47% were people who were not necessarily mentally ill—they were high on meth.

"They can look so similar to someone that's experiencing chronic schizophrenia," said Dr. Anton Nigusse Bland, medical director of psychiatric emergency services at San Francisco General. "It's almost indistinguishable in that moment."

They have methamphetamine-induced psychosis.

"They're often paranoid, they're thinking someone might be trying to harm them," he said. "Their perceptions are all off."

If the person is extremely agitated, doctors might administer a sedative or even an antipsychotic medicine. Otherwise, the treatment is just waiting 12 to 16 hours for the meth to wear off. No more psychosis.

"Their thoughts are more organized, they're able to maintain adequate clothing. They're eating, they're communicating," Nigusse Bland said. "The improvement in the person is rather dramatic because it happens so quickly."

Trends in Drug Use Come in Waves

The trend in rising stimulant use is nationwide: cocaine on the East Coast, meth on the West Coast, said Dr. Daniel Ciccarone, a professor of medicine and substance use researcher at the University of California–San Francisco.

"It is an epidemic wave that's coming, that's already here," he said. "But it hasn't fully reached our public consciousness."

Drug preferences are generational, Ciccarone said. They change with the hairstyles and clothing choices, like bell-bottoms or leg warmers. It was heroin in the 1970s, cocaine and crack in the '80s. Then opiate pills. Then methamphetamine. Then heroin. And now meth again.

"The culture creates this notion of let's go up, let's not go down," Ciccarone said. "New people coming into drug use are saying, 'Whoa, I don't really want to do that. I hear it's deadly.'"

Kim has been with meth through two waves. When she got into speed in the 1990s, she was hanging out with bikers, going to clubs in San Francisco.

"Now what I see, in any neighborhood, you can find it. It's not the same as it used to be where it was kind of taboo," Kim said. "It's more socially accepted now."

Dying from Meth

A hint about who uses meth now comes from the data on deaths.

Meth is not as lethal as opioids: 47,600 people died of opioid-related overdoses in 2017 compared with 10,333 deaths involving meth. But the death rate for meth has been rising. Meth-related deaths in San Francisco doubled since 2011, another indication that more people are using meth and that today's supply is very potent, said the UCSF's Ciccarone.

Another hypothesis to explain the growth in meth-related overdoses is that meth users are aging. Most meth deaths are from a brain hemorrhage or a heart attack, which would be unusual for a 20-year-old.

"Because your tissue is so healthy at that age," said Dr. Phillip Coffin, a physician and the director of substance use research at the San Francisco Department of Public Health. "Whereas when you're 55 years old and using methamphetamine, you might be at higher risk for bursting a vessel and bleeding and dying from that."

Another explanation for the rising death rate is that meth has become contaminated. And that affects everyone, old and young. Last year, three young people in San Francisco died after smoking meth together. It turns out the meth had fentanyl in it. The synthetic opioid has been causing waves of heroin overdoses across the country, but now it's showing up mixed into cocaine and meth.

Most researchers believe the contamination happens accidentally, when a dealer uses the same equipment to bag fentanyl and later meth, Ciccarone said.

Relapses Are Common

Over her two decades of meth use, Kim has been through drug treatment more than a dozen times. Relapse is part of recovery, and among meth users, 60% will start using again within a year of finishing treatment. Unlike opioids, there are no medication treatments for meth addiction, which makes it particularly hard to treat.

In April, Kim completed a six-month residential treatment program for women in San Francisco called the Epiphany Center. She came directly from jail, after serving time for her housewarming-and-car-theft spree in Sonoma. She said that in the first 30 days all she could do was try to clear the chaos from her mind.

"You have to get used to sitting with yourself, which is essential for life, is to get along with your own self," she said.

Kim, who has four children, is hopeful that this round of treatment will stick. She is living in transitional housing now, has a job and has been accepted to a program at the University of California–Berkeley to finish her college degree.

"I've gone through 12 different programs and it's been for my children, for my mom, for the courts. I've never come to be there for myself," Kim said. "So it's like I've come to a place where it has to be for me."

61. Big Data for Big Disease*

H. Daniel Xu

Opiate drugs have taken a toll in the country. In 2016 alone, drug overdose killed over 60,000 Americans, of which 66 percent involved opioids. In fact, drug overdose surpassed motor vehicle as the leading cause for accidental deaths. In October 2017, President Donald Trump declared opioid epidemic as a public health emergency and called for increased efforts for drug overdose prevention measures. Data collection and analysis in public health has helped detect the crisis and has provided the public with the knowledge on what has happened and where it happened under the auspice of the Centers for Disease Control and Prevention (CDC). Drug overdose, or drug addiction, once stigmatized, has been generally seen as a disease after public health education programs. But that's not enough. The public needs a solution and demands to know "why it happened," "how it happened" and, more importantly, "how to stop it." Big data, characterized by its sheer volume, velocity and variety, holds enormous potential in finding and implementing solutions. However, successful application of big data strategy is yet to overcome significant challenges.

Admittedly, led by CDC, a considerable amount of data reporting and data analysis has already been used in routine disease surveillance and decision-making in resource allocation for public health. What's more, some states have already used the results of toxicology testing and the statistical analysis of opioid-related emergency department visits data for naloxone distribution among county emergency medical services. Meanwhile, the computing and modeling capacities required for processing big data have been developed and made more accessible to public organizations. For instance, SAS, Oracle and Microsoft have developed various types of powerful data analytics and data visualization tools that are applicable to public program management. However, there are still several major obstacles that prevent from formulating and implementing more effective and more responsive interventions through integrating and utilizing big data strategies.

The first obstacle is data quality. Nowadays, data is conveniently available in a digital age when all sorts of gadgets collect various kinds of data from citizens and businesses, ranging from payroll information to various social media posts, from prenatal care on birth certificates to causes of death on death certificates. Imagine the sheer amount of medical and financial data related to diagnostic procedures, drug information, insurance

---

*Originally published as Daniel Xu, "Big Data for Big Disease: Experiences from Applying Data-Driven Strategies to Combating the Opioid Epidemic," PA Times, https://patimes.org/big-data-for-big-disease-experiences-from-applying-data-driven-strategies-to-combating-the-opioid-epidemic/ (June 18, 2018). Reprinted with permission of the publisher and author.

claims, when over 1 million Medicaid recipients in Alabama who interact with health providers, program administrators, payers and insurers, on a daily, weekly or monthly basis. So, volume is not a major concern for big data in public health. However, the blessing of data volume becomes a deficit if the data are messy or replete with errors. The process of data collection/generating in the government system in many cases is a major concern due to human input errors or computer programming bugs. "Garbage in, garbage out" is the cliché. Investments have been made to ensure the quality of data, but there is still a significant gap between the automated data reporting and usable data in many areas.

The second barrier is fragmented data ownership and usage. To create a mega-sized data requires assembling and "linking" various data sources. However, data sharing is hindered by administrative and legal barriers. In an ideal world, all agencies and programs shared their data for collaborative projects or programs. But, just in the private sector, often times they operate in silos in data collection and analysis. In case of fighting opioid epidemic, the assessment, design and implementation of effective strategies require data from various departments at federal, state and local levels, including public health, mental health, Medicaid, law enforcement, courts and prisons, educational institutions, as well as non-governmental organizations such as hospitals, treatment and rehab services, medical and pharmacy associations, community-based and faith-based nonprofit organizations. In addition, the data from private health providers such as health insurance companies are also needed. Although there were some successes in sharing data through memorandums of understanding or other mechanisms among some agencies and organizations, it is yet to clear many more administrative and legal hurdles to obtain the necessary data from other agencies.

The third issue is data security and confidentiality. The Health Insurance Portability and Accountability Act (HIPPA) mandates the protection of patient privacy and data security to public and private health service agencies and organizations as a top priority, which makes the data linkage that is critical for many data sharing on some collaborative programs almost impossible, particularly when such linkage requires individual-level patient data. Even for some of the data collected by a single program, using personal identifiable information to track individual patients and create linkages may sometimes be prohibited in order to ensure equal and timely access to emergency care for drug overdose. A related concern is data security. The central question is "Are patient's private information in good hands?" The increased sharing of data, especially data containing identifiable personal information, potentially pose high risk of data breaches, as evidenced by the recent data breaches in both the public and private sectors.

The big data and data analytics potentially will create more and better opportunities to improve the efficiency and effectiveness to the programs targeted on the opioid epidemic. However, not until these prerequisites are met will the full potential of big data and data analytics be realized. To make the data-driven preventive programs more efficient and effective, increased data sharing is a must. More efforts are required to remove the administrative impediments and improve data quality at various levels and among various stakeholders while ensuring data security. The lessons learned from combating the opioid epidemic can be a good reference for the initiatives in many other public programs that are experiencing similar challenges in applying big data strategies.

62. Chittenden County's Hub and Spoke Model for Combatting Opioid Deaths*

Paul C. Prevey

In the United States, drug overdoses resulted in 702,568 deaths during the period between 1999 and 2017, with 399,230 (56.8%) involving opioids (Centers for Disease Control, Morbidity and Mortality Weekly Report, January 2019) As reflected in statistics tracked by every national and world health organization, the opioid crisis has been worsening over the course of nearly two decades. The development, marketing and expansive distribution of new synthetic opioids by pharmaceutical companies has fueled the opioid crisis across the country. Many of these highly potent and addictive drugs were designed to target people with both acute and chronic pain issues. Once addicted, these patients continue to pursue opioid prescriptions, and in many instances, transition to heroin and fentanyl-laced heroin. Burlington, Vermont, experienced a high rate of opioid overdose deaths for a city of its population (42,000). This paper evaluates the various evidence-based responses used to combat the surge in overdose-related deaths in Burlington and Chittenden County, Vermont.

Many communities such as Salem, Massachusetts, continue to struggle with the effects of the opioid crisis. Salem is nearly identical to Burlington, Vermont, in population number and demographic composition. Despite the similarities between the two communities, Salem, Massachusetts, recorded 20 overdose deaths in 2018 (Massachusetts Department of Public Health), compared to Chittenden County, Vermont, where Burlington is located. The entire county has a population of 164,000 people and reported 17 overdose deaths in 2018 (University of Vermont Health Network). In 2015, Burlington formed the CommunityStat program at the direction of Burlington's mayor. The police department, local health clinics and hospitals, Chittenden County's opioid alliance committee and Burlington's opioid policy director are all integral aspects of making the model work. The model uses accurate and timely data and information, effective tactics and strategies, rapid deployment of resources and relentless follow-up and assessment. The purpose of the program is to identify persons at risk and in crisis and respond immediately.

Across the country, communities of various sizes and demographics have been struggling with the rising death toll as a result of the crisis. Rural communities appear to be impacted more than larger urban areas as a result of disparities in the availability of

---

*Published with permission of the author.

public and private resources in the areas of prevention, treatment, recovery and stabilization services. Rural communities have been ravaged by the crisis more than urban areas as a result of several factors. Specifically, lifestyle choices, manual labor-intensive work which impacts physical health of rural individuals, limited medical services and the economic status of people living in those areas coupled with the overall, limited economic employment and business opportunities all created vulnerabilities, which do not exist to the same extent in more urban areas.

Specific elements of a comprehensive program were designed to provide services at a level that supports addicted persons in meaningful recovery and rehabilitation. The Vermont program is referred to as the Hub and Spoke model with assessment, medically assisted treatment (methadone, buprenorphine or vivitrol) being the hub and the spokes consisting of substance abuse treatment, mental health treatment, residential services, pain management, medical homes, family services and corrections (probation/parole). If successful, the target population's risk of overdosing and dying is substantially reduced. In theory, a successful and sustainable program would markedly reduce the number of overdose related deaths. Municipalities, in particular rural communities, would benefit from the research given that it highlights the effectiveness and usage of evidence-based programs and initiatives in reducing overdose deaths at a municipal-wide level.

The literature regarding the causes and development of the opioid crisis seems uniform in its presentation and breakdown of the devastating numbers of overdose deaths from 1999 to the present. The literature is also consistent in outlining the historical development of the opiate crisis, the role the pharmaceutical companies played and the fast and loose manner in which medical providers and pharmacists doled out potent opioid drugs. Many of the literary sources that delved into addressing the crisis cited specific regions, communities and states that are implementing policies, programs and initiatives that are making a difference in reducing the staggering number of overdose deaths that have been chronicled over the two past decades. The medical profession has also turned its focus toward developing policy changes regarding prescribing practices and exploring alternative forms of pain management. New, non-addictive drugs that address pain are being developed to prevent future addictions from occurring. It's clear from the literature that some areas of the country are having documented success with their efforts and approach to addressing the crisis, whereas, some areas continue to struggle due to an apparent unwillingness to explore and employ new strategies and approaches to the program. Data collection, tracking and program evaluations will need to be ongoing to determine sustained success in this area.

Conclusions

A review of the primary data collected, as well as secondary data, indicated that having a well-managed and sustained intervention effort does have an impact on overdoses and overdose fatalities. The programs in Burlington and Chittenden County, Vermont, have seen a remarkable decline in overdose deaths. Vermont now has the lowest overdose fatality rate in New England and is ranked below the national average. Approximately 2.6% of all adults between the ages of 18 and 64 state-wide in Vermont are connected to the Hub and Spoke and are receiving treatment. State officials anticipate expanding those resources to ensure complete access to treatment to all who are in need of them.

Prior to the formation of CommunityStat, the Chittenden County Opioid Alliance and the implementation of the Hub and Spoke model, treatment resources were limited and many people with opioid addictions were not being reached with evidence-based interventions. The impact of these newly developed and implemented initiatives and programs was felt because responses were immediate. Today, an overdose victim who is brought to the emergency room is immediately evaluated for medication-assisted treatment (methadone, buprenorphine or vivitrol). For those on medication-assisted treatment, they are connected immediately to the Hub and Spoke system. The Hub consists of treatment professionals focused on stabilizing the patient with the objective of eventually transitioning the patient to a Spoke where they can continue with ongoing treatment services with a physician, a nurse and social worker/substance abuse counselor. For individuals who are stable and participating in treatment, their risk of overdosing drops significantly compared to those who are not receiving treatment services through the Hub and Spoke.

Vermont, and Chittenden County in particular, have observed a decline in the number of overdoses and related deaths over the past 18 months. Last year, Chittenden County reported that its overdose fatalities were 50% fewer than in 2017. As of August 1, 2019, Chittenden County reported only seven overdose deaths, which is a decline from where their numbers were last year and the previous year.

The low number of overdoses and related deaths, support the theory, as well as the research hypothesis of this study, that implementing a well-crafted, evidence-based program at the rural municipal and county level has a positive impact on reducing overdose incidents and fatalities. Based upon the data gathered, this initiative was no small feat and required significant resources at the local, county and state level to build to scale an effective programming effort that encompasses every citizen affected by an opioid addiction. The data also indicates that public and private entities deliberately shift their approach to the solving the drug abuse problem from a criminal justice response to a major health-crisis, medical model response. In doing so, every person identified as having an opioid addiction is immediately evaluated and provided medication-assisted treatment as the first step toward a panoply of services designed to address and support sustained recovery. Many of the services offered extend beyond substance abuse treatment services but are connected to the individual's overall success, such as employment services, housing supports, mental health services, pain management and family and community supports.

By comparison, the data collected from Salem's Door Knock and Healthy Streets initiatives do not seem to yield similar results at this time. The Salem Police have partnered with the Healthy Streets program in identifying overdose victims who were revived through EMS interventions. The program funds efforts to provide harm reduction resources such as needle exchange, naloxone distribution and treatment placements and referrals. In 2018, Salem's overdose fatalities were higher than what officials in Vermont reported for Chittenden County. Salem, with a population of 43,000 residents, reported 20 overdose deaths, whereas Chittenden County, with a population of 164,000 residents, reported 17 overdose deaths. Data analyzed from key informants regarding Salem's efforts to reduce overdose and overdose deaths indicated that more resources are needed to have a meaningful and sustained impact. In comparison, Burlington and Chittenden County have dedicated significant resources toward developing and maintaining a multi-program system that works cohesively to ensure effective responses to those who are in the throes of addiction.

Vermont officials who work collaboratively in these programs expressed cautious optimism when looking at their efforts to combat the crisis in their communities. They are always monitoring changes in the drug culture in order to ascertain the need to adjust their program or approach. Currently, their program is designed to address those persons with opioid addictions and may not be effective in addressing other developing or shifting drugs of addiction. Program administrators acknowledge that many patients participating in their programs have a polysubstance abuse disorder with a primary addiction to opioids.

Recommendations

Burlington and Chittenden County have developed a model based upon evidenced-based programs that have proven their effectiveness. The policy and programming arm of Vermont's Department of Public Health is appropriately called Blueprint for Health.

Based upon the findings and conclusions, other communities should seriously examine what Burlington and Chittenden County did and are continuing to do to address the opioid crisis. Vermont now lauds the fact that their overdose rate has dropped to the lowest out of all the New England states, and is currently below the national average.

Massachusetts policy makers should review the key elements of Vermont's initiatives with a goal toward replicating its key provisions across the state. Adopting a mind-set shift in approaching the problem is foundationally necessary to begin addressing the crisis.

Massachusetts should move away from a criminal justice approach toward a public health-crisis, medical-model approach just as Vermont did. Significant resources are needed to support developing, implementing and sustaining programming efforts that are proving effective in addressing opioid addiction and reducing overdose deaths.

The medical model approach to the opioid crisis should continue to be studied in Vermont as pertains to long-term effectiveness and overall outcomes. The hypothesis that a comprehensive, evidence-based initiative can reduce overdoses and overdose deaths is supported by the literature, research and conclusions enumerated herein. However, studying these efforts long-term may bring to light more evidence that is instructive, clarifying and comprehensive.

Evidence-based treatment programming is at the core of Vermont's overall approach to addressing opioid addiction. Further study is needed to determine if improvements to current evidence-based programming is needed to enhance overall effectiveness. Additionally, further study of new and developing evidence-based measures should be conducted with an eye toward expanding available services in the Hub and Spoke system.

Lastly, the literature well documents and recounts how and why the opioid crisis developed over decades and which strategies are being employed to address those who are already victims of the epidemic. However, additional research should be done to explore evidence-based initiatives that are effective in the prevention of opioid addiction. Are there measures that can be implemented that will be effective in preventing individuals from developing an opioid addiction? Addressing the opioid crisis from both an intervention-treatment based perspective in conjunction with a preventative-based perspective may yield the best result in bringing an end to the opioid crisis.

Appendices

Appendix A

Glossary of Syringe Exchange and Opioid Terms, Abbreviations and Acronyms

Joaquin Jay Gonzalez III

Abstinence: Not using drugs or alcohol.

Acquired immune deficiency syndrome (AIDS): is the final stage of an HIV infection when the body is unable to fend off disease. A person with a healthy immune system has a T cell count between 500 and 1,600.

Addiction: A chronic, relapsing disorder characterized by compulsive (or difficult to control) drug seeking and use despite harmful consequences, as well as long-lasting changes in the brain. In the past, people who used drugs were called "addicts." Current appropriate terms are people who use drugs and drug users.

Affordable Care Act (ACA): Also known as, The Patient Protection and Affordable Care Act, or the Affordable Care Act, or Obamacare, is a United States federal statute enacted by the 111th United States Congress and signed into law by President Barack Obama on March 23, 2010. The ACA represents the U.S. healthcare system's most significant regulatory overhaul and expansion of coverage since the passage of Medicare and Medicaid in 1965

American Medical Association (AMA): is a powerful ally in patient care, giving strength to physician voices in courts and legislative bodies across the nation. The AMA is dedicated to driving medicine toward a more equitable future, removing obstacles that interfere with patient care and confronting the nation's greatest public health crises.

Amphetamine: A stimulant drug that acts on the central nervous system (CNS). Amphetamines are medications prescribed to treat attention deficit hyperactivity disorder (such as Adderall®) and narcolepsy.

Biomarkers: a measurable substance in an organism whose presence is indicative of some phenomenon such as disease, infection, or environmental exposure.

BPC Section 4145.5: a California law which requires SEPs and pharmacies that sell or provide nonprescription syringes to counsel consumers on safe disposal and also provide them with one or more of the following disposal options: (1) onsite disposal, (2) provision of sharps containers that meet applicable state and federal standards, and/or (3) provision of mail-back sharps containers.

BPC Section 4146: a California law which permits pharmacies to accept the return of needles and syringes from the public if contained in a sharps container, which is defined in HSC Section 117750 as "a rigid puncture-resistant container that, when sealed, is leak resistant and cannot be reopened without great difficulty."

Brainstem: A group of brain structures that process sensory information and control basic functions needed for survival such as breathing, heart rate, blood pressure, and arousal.

California Business and Professions Code (BPC) Section 4145.5(e): requires SEPs to counsel consumers on safe disposal and provide them with one or more of the following disposal options: (1) onsite disposal, (2) provision or sale of sharps containers that meet applicable state and federal standards, and/or (3) provision or sale of mail-back sharps containers.

California Health and Safety Code (HSC) Section 11364.7(a): establishes that no public entity, its agents, or employees shall be subject to criminal prosecution for distribution of syringes to participants in syringe exchange programs (SEPs) authorized by the public entity.

Centers for Disease Control and Prevention (CDC): is the U.S. federal agency that working 24/7 to protect America from health, safety and security threats, both foreign and in the U.S. Whether diseases start at home or abroad, are chronic or acute, curable or preventable, human error or deliberate attack, CDC fights disease and supports communities and citizens to do the same. CDC increases the health security of our nation. As the nation's health protection agency, CDC saves lives and protects people from health threats. To accomplish our mission, CDC conducts critical science and provides health information that protects our nation against expensive and dangerous health threats, and responds when these arise.

Client: A person who is accessing services through a syringe exchange program.

Cognitive-behavioral therapy (CBT): A form of psychotherapy that teaches people strategies to identify and correct problematic associations among thoughts, emotions, and behaviors in order to enhance self-control, stop drug use, and address a range of other problems that often co-occur with them.

Confidential Patient/Client Care Information: any individually identifiable information in possession or derived from a provider of health care, substance use treatment, and/or HIV/AIDS education services regarding a patient's/client's medical history, drug use history, mental, or physical condition or treatment, as well as the patients/clients and/or their family member's records, test results, conversations, treatment records, research records and financial information. Examples include, but are not limited to:

- Physical medical and psychiatric records including paper, photo, video, diagnostic and therapeutic reports, laboratory and pathology samples;
- Patient insurance and billing records;
- Mainframe and department based computerized patient data and alphanumeric radio
- pager messages;
- Visual observation of patients receiving medical care or accessing services; and
- Verbal information provided by or about a patient/client.

Dependence: A condition that can occur with the regular use of illicit or some prescription drugs, even if taken as prescribed. Dependence is characterized by withdrawal symptoms when drug use is stopped. A person can be dependent on a substance without being addicted, but dependence sometimes leads to addiction.

Detoxification: A process in which the body rids itself of a drug, or its metabolites. Medically assisted detoxification may be needed to help manage a person's withdrawal symptoms. Detoxification alone is not a treatment for substance use disorders, but this is often the first step in a drug treatment program.

Drug abuse: An older diagnostic term that defined use that is unsafe, use that leads a person to fail to fulfill responsibilities or gets them in legal trouble, or use that continues despite causing persistent interpersonal problems. This term is increasingly avoided by professionals because it can perpetuate stigma. Current appropriate terms include drug use (in the case of illicit substances), drug misuse (in the case of problematic use of legal drugs or prescription medications) and addiction (in the case of substance use disorder).

Drug Abuse Resistance Education (DARE): is an education program that seeks to prevent use of controlled drugs, membership in gangs, and violent behavior.

Drug Enforcement Agency (DEA): is a federal law enforcement agency under the U.S. Department of Justice, tasked with combating drug trafficking and distribution within the United States.

Fentanyl: is a powerful synthetic opioid analgesic that is similar to morphine but is 50 to 100 times more potent. It is a schedule II prescription drug, and it is typically used to treat patients with severe pain or to manage pain after surgery. It is also sometimes used to treat patients with chronic pain who are physically tolerant to other opioids.

Food and Drug Administration (FDA): is U.S federal agency responsible for protecting the public health by ensuring the safety, efficacy, and security of human and veterinary drugs, biological products, and medical devices; and by ensuring the safety of our nation's food supply, cosmetics, and products that emit radiation. FDA also has responsibility for regulating the manufacturing, marketing, and distribution of tobacco products to protect the public health and to reduce tobacco use by minors.

Harm Reduction: Practical strategies and ideas aimed at reducing negative consequences associated with drug use including, but not limited to, safer injection drug use, managed drug use, and abstinence. Strategies are aimed to meet users "where they are" in an effort to gain achievable results for each individual.

Hepatitis A Virus (HAV): A virus that can cause liver disease of varying severity and duration, which is acquired by ingesting the virus via contact with objects, food, or drink contaminated with fecal matter from an infected individual.

Hepatitis B Virus (HBV): A virus that can cause liver disease of varying severity and duration. It can be acute lasting only a few weeks, or can become a serious, lifelong illness. The hepatitis B virus is spread through contact with infected blood, semen, or other bodily fluids. Common routes of infection include birth (mother to child), sex with an infected partner, sharing personal items such as razors or toothbrushes with an infected individual, sharing needles or injection equipment, and exposure to blood from needle sticks. This virus can be prevented if a person receives the HBV vaccine.

Hepatitis C Virus (HCV): Hepatitis C virus causes liver disease of varying severity and duration. It can be acute, lasting only a few weeks, or can become a serious, lifelong illness. There is no vaccine or cure for HCV.

Heroin: is an opioid drug made from morphine, a natural substance taken from the seed pod of the various opium poppy plants grown in Southeast and Southwest Asia, Mexico, and Colombia. Heroin can be a white or brown powder, or a black sticky substance known as black tar heroin. Other common names for heroin include *big H, horse, hell dust,* and *smack*.

HSC Section 118286: a California law which prohibits individuals from discarding home-generated sharps waste in home or business recycling or waste containers. HSC Section 118286 also requires that home-generated sharps waste be transported only in a sharps container or other container approved by the applicable enforcement agency, which may be either the state (CalRecycle program) or a local government agency. Home-generated sharps waste may be managed at household hazardous waste facilities, at "home-generated sharps consolidation points," at the facilities of medical waste generators, or by the use of medical waste mail-back containers approved by the state.

Human Immunodeficiency Virus (HIV): The Human Immunodeficiency Virus attacks the body's immune system, specifically the CD4 cells (T cells), which help the immune system fight off infections. If left untreated, HIV can lead to the disease AIDS (Acquired Immunodeficiency Syndrome). No effective cure for HIV currently exists, but with proper treatment and medical care, HIV can be controlled.

Injection drug use (IDU): The act of administering drugs by injection. Blood-borne viruses, like HIV and hepatitis, can be transmitted via shared needles or other drug injection equipment.

Lancet: is used to poke the skin (usually on a finger or on your arm) to get a small drop of blood. You can adjust the depth setting to meet your particular needs. Thicker areas of skin, especially calloused areas, need a higher depth setting than thin or sensitive areas of skin. For maximum comfort, use a shallow depth that still allows you to get blood.

Medical Priority Dispatch System (MPDS): Also known as Advanced Medical Priority Dispatch System (AMPDS) is a unified system used to dispatch appropriate aid to medical emergencies including systematized caller interrogation and pre-arrival instructions.

Medication-assisted treatment (MAT): is the use of anti-craving medicine such as naltrexone (Vivitrol), buprenorphine (Suboxone) or methadone—along with comprehensive therapy and support—to help address issues related to opioid dependence, including withdrawal, cravings and relapse prevention.

Methadone: A long-acting opioid agonist medication used for the treatment of opioid addiction and pain. Methadone used for opioid addiction can only be dispensed by opioid treatment programs certified by SAMHSA and approved by the designated state authority.

Motivational Enhancement Therapy (MET): A counseling approach that uses motivational interviewing techniques to help individuals resolve any uncertainties they have about stopping their substance use. The therapy helps the person strengthen their own plan for change and engagement in treatment.

Naloxone: An opioid antagonist medication approved by the FDA to reverse an opioid overdose. It displaces opioid drugs (such as morphine or heroin) from their receptor and prevents further opioid receptor activation. Naloxone is a medication designed to rapidly reverse opioid overdose. It is an opioid antagonist—meaning that it binds to opioid receptors and can reverse and block the effects of other opioids. It can very quickly restore normal respiration to a person whose breathing has slowed or stopped as a result of overdosing with heroin or prescription opioid pain medications.

National Institute on Drug Abuse (NIDA): mission is to advance science on the causes and consequences of drug use and addiction and to apply that knowledge to improve individual and public health. This involves: (1) Strategically supporting and conducting basic and clinical research on drug use (including nicotine), its consequences, and the underlying neurobiological, behavioral, and social mechanisms involved and (2) Ensuring the effective translation, implementation, and dissemination of scientific research findings to improve the prevention and treatment of substance use disorders and enhance public awareness of addiction as a brain disorder.

National Institutes of Health (NIH): is a part of the U.S. Department of Health and Human Services, and is the nation's medical research agency—making important discoveries that improve health and save lives.

Needle stick injury: also known as syringe stick injury or injection stick injury, happens when the needle from a syringe used for injection accidentally pierces or punctures the skin.

Needle stick injury protocol: Policies and procedures that outline both immediate and subsequent remedial and prophylactic actions to take in the event of a needlestick injury.

Non-opioid analgesics: include nonsteroidal anti-inflammatory drugs (NSAIDs), selective COX-2 inhibitors, and acetaminophen. NSAIDs inhibit cyclooxygenases (COX-1 and COX-2), thereby disrupting the production of prostaglandin, an important mediator of pain and inflammation.

Nonpharmacological and noninvasive therapies: include physical therapy (massage, relaxation, gel pack), mind-body practices (yoga, tai chi, qigong), psychological therapies (cognitive-behavioral therapy, biofeedback, relaxation techniques, acceptance and commitment, pet therapy), and multidisciplinary rehabilitation.

Opiate Antagonist: A Food and Drug Administration-approved naloxone hydrochloride or similarly acting drug that is not a controlled substance, and is approved for the diagnosis or treatment of an opiate-related drug overdose.

Opioid Crisis: More than 130 people a day die from opioid-related drug overdoses. The misuse of and addiction to opioids—including prescription pain relievers, heroin, and synthetic opioids such as fentanyl—is a serious national crisis that affects public health as well as social and economic welfare. The CDC estimates that the total "economic burden" of prescription opioid misuse alone in the United States is $78.5 billion a year, including the costs of healthcare, lost productivity, addiction treatment, and criminal justice involvement

Opioid Epidemic: In the late 1990s, pharmaceutical companies reassured the medical community that patients would not become addicted to opioid pain relievers and healthcare providers began to prescribe them at greater rates. Increased prescription of opioid medications led to widespread misuse of both prescription and non-prescription opioids before it became clear that these medications could indeed be highly addictive. In 2017 HHS declared a public health emergency and announced a 5-Point Strategy to Combat the Opioid Crisis.

Opioid receptors: Proteins on the surface of neurons, or other cells, that are activated by endogenous opioids, such as endorphins, and opioid drugs, such as heroin. Opioid receptor subtypes include mu, kappa, and delta.

Opioid use disorder (OUD): can involve misuse of prescribed opioid medications, use of diverted opioid medications, or use of illicitly obtained heroin. OUD is typically a chronic, relapsing illness, associated with significantly increased rates of morbidity and mortality

Opioids: are a class of drugs that include the illegal drug heroin, synthetic opioids such as fentanyl, and pain relievers available legally by prescription, such as oxycodone (OxyContin®), hydrocodone (Vicodin®), codeine, morphine, and many others.

Overdose: An overdose occurs when a person uses enough of a drug to produce a life-threatening reaction or death.

Pain management: Paid is complex, so there are many treatment options—medications, therapies, and mind-body techniques, nonpharmacological or noninvasive.

Pharmacodynamics: The way a drug acts on the body. This includes the drug's interaction with its biological target and the resulting changes (such as activation or blocking of receptors), as well as the relationship between drug dosing and drug effects.

Post-exposure prophylaxis (PEP) for HIV: when people take antiretroviral medicines to prevent becoming infected after being potentially exposed to HIV. According to the CDC, PEP should be used within 72 hours after a recent possible exposure and only be used in emergency situations.

Pre-exposure prophylaxis (PrEP) for HIV: when people who are at significant risk for contracting HIV take a daily dose of HIV medications to prevent them from getting the infection. Research has shown that PrEP has been effective in reducing the risk of HIV infection in people who inject drugs.

Prescription drug misuse: The use of a medication in ways or amounts other than intended by a doctor, by someone other than for whom the medication is prescribed, or for the experience or feeling the medication causes. This term is used interchangeably with "nonmedical" use, a term employed by many national drug use surveys.

Prescription drug monitoring program (PDMP): is an electronic database that tracks controlled substance prescriptions. PDMPs can help identify patients who may be misusing prescription opioids or other prescription drugs and who may be at risk for overdose.

President's Commission on Combating Drug Addiction and the Opioid Crisis: Or, the Opioid and Drug Abuse Commission, was a commission that advised the Trump administration on combating the ongoing opioid epidemic claiming more than 30,000 American fatalities annually in the United States. The commission was chaired by New Jersey Governor Chris Christie. The commission disbanded in December 2017.

Program Participant: A person who is accessing services through a syringe exchange program.

Recall: as defined in 21 CFR 7.3(g) is "a firm's removal or correction of a marketed product that the Food and Drug Administration considers to be in violation of the laws it administers and against which the agency would initiate legal action, e.g., seizure. Recall does not include a market withdrawal or a stock recovery." If a firm conducts a recall to reduce a risk to health, the firm is required to submit a written report to the FDA with the information described in 21 CFR 806.10.

Receptor: A molecule located on the surface of a cell that recognizes specific chemicals (normally neurotransmitters, hormones, and similar endogenous substances) and transmits the chemical message into the cell.

Recovery: A process of change through which people with substance use disorders improve their health and wellness, live self-directed lives, and strive to reach their full potential.

Relapse: In drug addiction, relapse is the return to drug use after an attempt to stop. Relapse is a common occurrence in many chronic health disorders, including addiction, that requires frequent behavioral and/or pharmacologic adjustments to be treated effectively.

Remission: A medical term meaning that major disease symptoms are eliminated or diminished below a pre-determined harmful level.

Risk factors: Factors that increase the likelihood of beginning substance use, of regular and harmful use, and of other behavioral health problems associated with use.

Self-medication: The use of a substance to lessen the negative effects of stress, anxiety, or other mental disorders (or side effects of their pharmacotherapy) without the guidance of a health care provider. Self-medication may lead to addiction and other drug- or alcohol-related problems.

Sexually transmitted diseases (STD): Diseases that are most often—but not exclusively—spread by sexual intercourse, including HIV, chlamydia, genital herpes, genital warts, gonorrhea, some forms of hepatitis, syphilis, and trichomoniasis.

Sexually transmitted infection (STI): More than 30 different bacteria, viruses and parasites are known to be transmitted through sexual contact. Eight of these pathogens are linked to the greatest incidence of sexually transmitted disease. Of these 8 infections, 4 are currently curable: syphilis, gonorrhea, chlamydia and trichomoniasis. The other 4 are viral infections which are incurable: hepatitis B, herpes simplex virus (HSV or herpes), HIV, and human papillomavirus (HPV). Symptoms or disease due to the incurable viral infections can be reduced or modified through treatment.

Sharps waste: Used needles, syringes and lancets. Sharps waste from individuals is termed "home-generated sharps waste" by California law, and is not regulated as "medical waste," which is sharps and other waste generated on site by medical providers, and is subject to different laws and regulations.

Substance Abuse and Mental Health Services Administration (SAMHSA): is a branch of the U.S. Department of Health and Human Services whose mission is to reduce the impact of substance abuse and mental illness on America's communities.

Substance use disorder (SUD): A medical illness caused by disordered use of a substance or substances. According to the Fifth Edition of the Diagnostic and Statistical Manual of Mental Disorders (DSM-5), SUDs are characterized by clinically significant impairments in health, social function, and impaired control over substance use and are diagnosed through assessing cognitive, behavioral, and psychological symptoms. An SUD can range from mild to severe.

Supervised injection sites (SIS): or safe or supervised injection facilities, are medically supervised site designed to provide a clean and stress-free space in which persons are able to inject drugs intravenously and reduce nuisance from public drug use.

Syringe Exchange Operator: A syringe exchange operator is an entity engaging in the exchange of an individual's used syringe(s) for one or more new syringes, which are contained in sealed sterile packages. The entity must also provide individuals with verbal and written instructions on preventing the transmission of blood-borne diseases (including HIV/HCV) and options for obtaining substance-use treatment services, testing services, and an opiate antagonist.

Syringe exchange program: also known as syringe exchange service (SES) or needle exchange program (NEP) or injection exchange program (IEP) or safe injection service (SIS); a public service for people who inject drugs (PWID) providing them with new hypodermic needles and associated paraphernalia at reduced or no cost. Syringe exchange programs are one component of a comprehensive approach to reducing the spread of blood-borne diseases among people who inject drugs.

T cells: also called CD4 cells (T cells), which are needed to fight infections. HIV lowers the number of T cells in the immune system, making it harder for the body to fight off infections and disease.

Withdrawal: Symptoms that can occur after long-term use of a drug is reduced or stopped; these symptoms occur if tolerance to a substance has occurred, and vary according to substance. Withdrawal symptoms can include negative emotions such as stress, anxiety, or depression, as well as physical effects such as nausea, vomiting, muscle aches, and cramping, among others. Withdrawal symptoms often lead a person to use the substance again.

Abbreviations and Acronyms

ACA: Affordable Care Act
AMA: American Medical Association
AMPDS: Advanced Medical Priority Dispatch System
CDC: Centers for Disease Control and Prevention
DARE: Drug Abuse Resistance Education
DEA: Drug Enforcement Agency
EPA: Environmental Protection Agency
FDA: Food and Drug Administration
HAV: Hepatitis A virus
HBV: Hepatitis B virus
HCV: Hepatitis C virus
HHS: U.S. Department of Health and Human Services
HIV: Human Immunodeficiency Virus
IDU: Injection drug use
IEP: Injection Exchange Program
MAT: medication-assisted treatment
MET: Motivational Enhancement Therapy
MPDS: Medical Priority Dispatch System
NACCHO: National Association of County and City Health Officials
NEP: Needle exchange program
NIDA: National Institute on Drug Abuse

NIH: National Institutes of Health
OUD: Opioid use disorder
PDMP: Prescription Drug Monitoring Program
PEP: Post-exposure prophylaxis
PrEP: Pre-exposure prophylaxis
PWID: People who inject drugs
SAMHSA: Substance Abuse and Mental Health Services Administration
SEO: Syringe exchange operator
SEP: Syringe exchange program
SES: Syringe exchange service
SIS: Safe injection services, and Supervised injection site
SUD: Substance use disorder
STD: Sexually transmitted disease
STI: Sexually transmitted infection

References

California Department of Public Health (2018). *Guidelines for Syringe Exchange Programs*. Sacramento: California Department of Public Health, Office of AIDS.

Centers for Disease Control and Prevention, www.cdc.gov.

Food and Drug Administration. www.fda.gov.

National Institute on Drug Abuse, www.drugabuse.gov.

Utah Department of Public Health (2017). *Utah Syringe Exchange Program Handbook*. Salt Lake City: Utah DPH.

Appendix B

Syringe Exchange Programs (2019): North American Syringe Exchange Network*

CENTERS FOR DISEASE CONTROL AND PREVENTION

Syringe exchange programs provide free sterile syringes and collect used syringes from injection-drug users to reduce transmission of bloodborne pathogens, including human immunodeficiency virus (HIV), hepatitis B virus, and hepatitis C virus.

United States: 334

Rhode Island	1	Tennessee	3	Colorado	9
Missouri	1	Louisiana	4	Massachusetts	10
Hawaii	1	New Hampshire	4	Oregon	10
Oklahoma	1	Alaska	4	Connecticut	10
Arkansas	1	Montana	4	Indiana	12
Iowa	2	North Dakota	4	West Virginia	12
Puerto Rico	2	Maryland	4	Kentucky	13
Utah	2	Maine	5	Wisconsin	13
Georgia	2	Texas	6	Ohio	13
Virginia	3	New Jersey	6	Minnesota	18
District of Columbia	3	Arizona	6	North Carolina	26
South Carolina	3	Illinois	7	New York	27
Florida	3	Pennsylvania	7	Washington	29
Vermont	3	Michigan	8	California	32

Note: Total number of syringe exchange programs. The directory of syringe exchange programs is aggregated by self-reporting to the North American Syringe Exchange Network (NASEN) and is therefore unlikely to be a comprehensive and complete list of all syringe exchange programs. Does not include programs that do not distribute syringes. Syringe exchange programs wishing to be identified in the database should contact NASEN to be added to the file.

---

*Public document originally published as Centers for Disease Control and Prevention, "Syringe Exchange Programs (2019): North American Syringe Exchange Network," https://www.cdc.gov/ssp/syringe-services-programs-faq.html.

Appendix C

Adopting a Harm Reduction Policy for Substance Abuse, STD and HIV*

SAN FRANCISCO HEALTH COMMISSION
RESOLUTION NO. 10–00

WHEREAS, the San Francisco Department of Public Health seeks to reduce adverse health effects to individuals, to individuals' families and to the broader community through legal and compassionate interventions; and,

WHEREAS, the Harm Reduction model of health care offers multiple non-judgmental approaches to assist clients in their movement toward better health; and,

WHEREAS, the Harm Reduction model is client-centered and attempts to reach clients "where they are at," to assist them in making choices that lead toward better health; and,

WHEREAS, deaths in the City and County of San Francisco due to injection drug overdoses reached 180 in 1999, the third leading cause of lost years of life; and,

WHEREAS, existing research indicates that 90% of injection drug users who have injected for more than two years are infected with Hepatitis C, and 16% are infected with HIV; and,

WHEREAS, soft tissue infection associated with injection drug use is the leading diagnosis for admission at San Francisco General Hospital's Emergency Department, leading to 1,400 inpatient admissions in 1999 (costing $18 million), 70% of which were uninsured; and,

WHEREAS, needle exchange, a Harm Reduction program, has proven to decrease further HIV and Hepatitis C infections by providing clients with clean needles with which to inject; and,

WHEREAS, practicing safer sex reduces the likelihood of transmission of sexually transmitted diseases (STD), including HIV; and,

WHEREAS, abstinence-based programs are successful for some individuals, but not all; and,

WHEREAS, recovery from substance use, practicing safer sex and improving health status often take place in an incremental manner; and,

WHEREAS, the serious consequences of substance abuse and unsafe sex cause significant health problems for the residents of San Francisco and some harm reduction practices have been shown to mitigate these health effects, now, therefore, be it

RESOLVED that all Department of Public Health providers, including DPH contractors, who deliver substance abuse, STD, and HIV treatment and prevention services, and/or who serve drug users and abusers in their programs shall: (1) address in their program design and objectives how they will provide harm reduction treatment options, and (2) develop harm reduction guidelines.

I hereby certify that the foregoing resolution was adopted by the Health Commission at its meeting of September 5, 2000.

Sandy Ouye Mori, Executive Secretary to the Health Commission

---

*Public document originally published as San Francisco Health Commission, "Adopting a Harm Reduction Policy for Substance Abuse, STD and HIV," San Francisco Health Commission Resolution No. 10-00 https://www.sfdph.org/dph/hc/HCRes/Resolutions/2000Res/HCRes10-00.shtml.

Appendix D

Press Release: Mayor Mark Farrell Announces Innovative Program to Fight Opioid Crisis on San Francisco Streets

CITY AND COUNTY OF SAN FRANCISCO,
OFFICE OF THE MAYOR

San Francisco's first-in-the-nation program provides direct treatment to opioid users, helping to reduce cravings and withdrawal symptoms

San Francisco, CA, May 17, 2018—Mayor Mark Farrell announced that he will invest $6 million to create a dedicated drug addiction street team and bring opioid treatment directly to people experiencing addiction on San Francisco streets. The program will be a first-in-the-nation initiative to address the national drug and opioid crisis on our streets.

The investment will add 10 new clinicians to the Department of Public Health's Street Medicine Team, which provides the opioid treatment medicine buprenorphine directly to people suffering on the streets from heroin addiction.

Buprenorphine is a daily pill, or strip that dissolves in the mouth that reduces the cravings for opioids and the sickness that comes from withdrawal. It is effective in combatting addiction to heroin and other opioids, and reduces risk of overdose.

"The opioid crisis plaguing our country is alive and visible on the streets of San Francisco," said Mayor Farrell. "The status quo is simply unacceptable. I am creating this program to directly address drug addiction on our streets—to meet these individuals where they are and get them the help they need, and to ensure that our streets remain safe for all our residents."

With Mayor's Farrell $6 million investment, more than 250 patients will have access to buprenorphine, which is offered through the Low Barrier to Medications for Addiction Treatment (LBMAT) Program. LBMAT completed a successful one-year pilot in November 2017 of the distribution of buprenorphine.

Through the buprenorphine pilot program, homeless patients with opioid use disorders were engaged by peer outreach workers and offered assessment, education and same-day prescription for buprenorphine by the medical team. The patients received these services in a variety of locations, including at syringe access sites, navigation centers, or in streets and parks.

Mayor Farrell's budget investments double the size of the Street Medicine Team, which provides outreach, assessment, care and connections to services to homeless people with medical, psychiatric and substance use conditions, who have difficulty accessing health care services.

San Francisco has an estimated 22,500 active injection drug users, half of whom report using heroin. The Street Medicine LBMAT program is one part of the City's comprehensive response to the opioid epidemic. San Francisco's Health Department also provides methadone treatment on demand and citywide substance use services, including expanded access to buprenorphine for patients of the San Francisco Health Network. The LBMAT program's innovation puts outreach first, instead of waiting for people with addiction to seek care.

"The Street Medicine buprenorphine program is another important step to address the heroin, methamphetamine and fentanyl crisis afflicting drug users in our community," said Barbara Garcia, San Francisco Health Director. "Homeless people who use drugs are especially vulnerable, and our system of care needs to adapt. By going directly to them with compassionate outreach and expertise, we are able to help a group that we were missing by relying on a more traditional structure of clinic visits that does not work for everyone."

In addition to treatment options, harm reduction has been a long-standing and successful strategy in San Francisco to improve health and save lives. The City provides syringe access to clean needles to prevent the spread of HIV and hepatitis C, reducing new infections and transmissions. The naloxone (Narcan) program has kept overdose fatalities low for years by putting the power to reverse overdoses into the hands of people who use drugs and their friends and families, as well as first responders and physicians.

"We need to meet people where they are and make it easier for them to get care," said Dr. Barry Zevin, medical director of Street Medicine and Shelter Health. "These vulnerable and complex patients care about their health, but they have suffered from stigma that makes it difficult for them to access the health care system."

An important aspect of the LBMAT program is to involve patients in their own care. Once a patient is assessed and chooses to begin treatment, the provider works with the patient to develop a care plan that takes into account the patient's previous barriers to care and treatment. In addition to starting buprenorphine, treatment options may include transitioning to a methadone program, entering residential treatment and addressing other health needs to help the patient stabilize and remain in care.

The Street Medicine Team's LBMAT program fits into an overall strategy to expand access to buprenorphine for heroin and opioid users in San Francisco. That medication can now be started in the emergency room or as an inpatient at Zuckerberg San Francisco General Hospital, or at a primary care clinic in the San Francisco Health Network, a system of top-rated clinics, hospitals and programs operated by the Health Department.

Appendix E

Executive Summary: Secure and Responsible Drug Disposal Act of 2010[*]

FEDERAL REGISTER

A. Purpose of the Regulatory Action

On October 12, 2010, the Secure and Responsible Drug Disposal Act of 2010 (Disposal Act) was enacted (Pub. L. 111–273, 124 Stat. 2858). Before the Disposal Act, ultimate users who wanted to dispose of unused, unwanted, or expired pharmaceutical controlled substances had limited disposal options. The Controlled Substances Act (CSA) only permitted ultimate users to destroy those substances themselves (e.g., by flushing or discarding), surrender them to law enforcement, or seek assistance from the United States Drug Enforcement Administration (DEA). These restrictions resulted in the accumulation of pharmaceutical controlled substances in household medicine cabinets that were available for abuse, misuse, diversion, and accidental ingestion.

The Disposal Act amended the CSA to authorize ultimate users to deliver their pharmaceutical controlled substances to another person for the purpose of disposal in accordance with regulations promulgated by the Attorney General. 21 U.S.C. 822(g), 828(b)(3). This final rule implements regulations that expand the entities to which ultimate users may transfer unused, unwanted, or expired pharmaceutical controlled substances for the purpose of disposal, as well as the methods by which such pharmaceutical controlled substances may be collected. Specified entities may voluntarily administer any of the authorized collection methods in accordance with these regulations.

B. Summary of the Major Provisions of the Regulatory Action

The DEA is implementing new regulations for the disposal of pharmaceutical controlled substances by ultimate users in accordance with the Disposal Act. In drafting the implementing regulations, the DEA considered the public health and safety, ease and cost of program implementation, and participation by various communities. To this end, the DEA found that in order to properly address the disposal of controlled substances by ultimate users, it was necessary to conduct a comprehensive review of DEA policies and regulations related to each element of the disposal process, including the transfer, delivery, collection, destruction, return, and recall of controlled substances, by both registrants and non-registrants (i.e., ultimate users). The reverse distributor registration category, which is pertinent to the process of registrant disposal, was included in this comprehensive review. These regulations are incorporated into a new part 1317 on disposal. Definitions relating to the disposal of controlled substances are added to § 1300.05(b), including definitions for "employee," "law enforcement officer," "nonretrievable," and "on-site" and definitions relating to controlled substances generally are revised or added to § 1300.01.

---

[*]Public document originally published as U.S. Government Federal Register, "Executive Summary: Secure and Responsible Drug Disposal Act of 2010," https://www.federalregister.gov/documents/2014/09/09/2014-20926/disposal-of-controlled-substances.

The goal of this new part on disposal, consistent with Congress's goal in the Disposal Act, is to set parameters for controlled substance diversion prevention that will encourage public and private entities to develop a variety of methods for collecting and destroying pharmaceutical controlled substances in a secure, convenient, and responsible manner. Also, consistent with the Disposal Act's goal to decrease the amount of pharmaceutical controlled substances introduced into the environment, particularly into the water, these regulations provide individuals with various additional options to dispose of their unwanted or unused pharmaceutical controlled substances beyond discarding or flushing the substances. As a result of these regulations, the DEA hopes that the supply of unused pharmaceutical controlled substances in the home will decrease, thereby reducing the risk of diversion or harm.

Ultimate User Disposal

An ultimate user is defined by the CSA as a "person who has lawfully obtained, and who possesses, a controlled substance for his own use or for the use of a member of his household or for an animal owned by him or by a member of his household." 21 U.S.C. 802(27). This rule provides three voluntary options for ultimate user disposal: (1) take-back events, (2) mail-back programs, and (3) collection receptacles. Individuals lawfully entitled to dispose of an ultimate user decedent's property are authorized to dispose of the ultimate user's pharmaceutical controlled substances by utilizing any of the three disposal options. All of the collection methods are voluntary and no person is required to establish or operate a disposal program. The rule also does not require ultimate users to utilize any of these three methods for disposal of controlled substances. Although the three methods of disposal allowed by this rule seek to help protect the environment and prevent controlled substances from being diverted to illicit uses, this rule does not prohibit ultimate users from using existing lawful methods.

The DEA regulations provide specific language that will continue to allow Federal, State, tribal, and local law enforcement to maintain collection receptacles at the law enforcement's physical location; and either independently or in partnership with private entities or community groups, to voluntarily hold take-back events and administer mail-back programs. 21 CFR 1317.35. Thus, ultimate users will continue to be able to surrender their unwanted pharmaceutical controlled substances to law enforcement.

The DEA is also authorizing certain registrants (manufacturers, distributors, reverse distributors, narcotic treatment programs [NTPs], hospitals/clinics with an on-site pharmacy, and retail pharmacies) to be "collectors," with authorization to conduct mail-back programs. 21 CFR 1317.40 and 1317.70. All registrants that choose to establish mail-back programs must provide specific mail-back packages to the public, either at no cost or for a fee, 21 CFR 1317.70. Collectors that conduct mail-back programs must have and utilize an on-site method of destruction to destroy returned packages, 21 CFR 1317.05.

These DEA regulations authorize collectors to maintain collection receptacles at their registered location. 21 CFR 1317.40. Thus, ultimate users will be able to carry their unwanted pharmaceutical controlled substances to an authorized retail pharmacy or other authorized collector location and deposit those controlled substances in a secure container for disposal. Hospitals/clinics and retail pharmacies that are authorized to be collectors may also maintain collection receptacles at long-term care facilities (LTCFs). 21 CFR 1317.40. LTCFs may dispose of pharmaceutical controlled substances on behalf of an ultimate user who resides, or has resided, at that LTCF, 21 CFR 1317.80, through a collection receptacle that is maintained by an authorized hospital/clinic or retail pharmacy at that LTCF. 21 CFR 1317.40 and 1317.80. With this rule, the DEA allows all pharmaceutical controlled substances collected through take-back events, mail-back programs, and collection receptacles to be comingled with non-controlled substances, although such comingling is not required. 21CFR 1317.65, 1317.70, and 1317.75. Pharmaceutical controlled substances collected by collectors may not be individually counted or inventoried. 21 CFR 1317.75. This rule also imposes various registration, security, and recordkeeping requirements.

The DEA appreciates there is a cost to entities that choose voluntarily to provide these methods of collection and destruction. The DEA acknowledges that some State and local pharmaceutical disposal programs receive funding and other support from numerous sources, including conservation groups, local governments, State grants, and public and private donations. These expanded methods of disposal are expected to benefit the public by decreasing the supply of pharmaceutical controlled substances available for misuse, abuse, diversion, and accidental ingestion, and protect the environment from potentially harmful contaminants by providing alternate means of disposal for ultimate users. However, other advantages may accrue directly to those entities that opt to maintain a disposal program. For example, those authorized registrants that choose to maintain collection receptacles may be enhanced by the increased consumer presence at their registered locations and the goodwill that develops from providing a valuable community service. In addition, mail-back program collectors may partner with third parties to make mail-back packages available to the public. Those authorized registrants that choose to administer mail-back programs may gain from the opportunity to distribute to consumers promotional, educational, or other informational materials with the mail-back packages.

DEA Registrant Disposal

The DEA has deleted the existing rule related to registrant disposal, 21 CFR 1307.21, and incorporated similar requirements on proper disposal procedure and security in a new part 1317 on disposal. These changes provide consistent disposal procedures for each registrant category, regardless of geographic location. In addition, the DEA has modified DEA Form 41 and is explicitly requiring that form to be used to record the destruction of controlled substances that remain in the closed system of distribution and also to account for registrant destruction of pharmaceutical controlled substances collected from ultimate users and other non-registrants pursuant to the Disposal Act. As stated in the NPRM, a controlled substance dispensed for immediate administration pursuant to an order for medication in an institutional setting remains under the custody and control of that registered institution even if the substance is not fully exhausted (e.g., some of the substance remains in a vial, tube, transdermal patch, or syringe after administration but cannot or may not be further utilized, commonly referred to as "drug wastage" and "pharmaceutical wastage"). Such remaining substance must be properly recorded, stored, and destroyed in accordance with DEA regulations (e.g., § 1304.22[c]), and all applicable Federal, State, tribal, and local laws and regulations, although the destruction need not be recorded on a DEA Form 41.

Reverse Distributors

The DEA is providing regulations for entities that reverse distribute that are clear and consistent. Entities that reverse distribute are often the last registrant to possess controlled substances prior to destruction; however, the recordkeeping safeguards that exist when controlled substances are distributed between registrants are not present when these registrants destroy controlled substances. Because reverse distributors routinely acquire controlled substances for destruction from other registrants and may also be authorized as collectors, reverse distributors accumulate greater amounts of controlled substances that are destined for destruction in comparison to other registrants. The DEA is defining "reverse distribute"; revising the definition of "reverse distributor"; (21 CFR part 1300) outlining security (21 CFR part 1301), inventory, recordkeeping requirements, and other procedures that reverse distributors must follow to acquire controlled substances from registrants and to destroy such acquired substances. 21 CFR part 1304. The DEA also is clarifying that these security, inventory, and recordkeeping requirements apply to certain specified entities that reverse distribute but are not registered as reverse distributors. See, e.g., 21 CFR 1304.11(e)(3) ("each person registered or authorized to reverse distribute"). The DEA believes that these regulations will help all registrants that reverse distribute comply with the CSA in a manner that decreases the risk of the diversion of controlled substances during the disposal process.

Return and Recall

This rule removes the existing regulation on return and recall, 21 CFR 1307.12, and incorporates separate return and recall requirements for registrants and non-registrants into new §§ 1317.10 and 1317.85. This rule also imposes various recordkeeping requirements pertaining to controlled substances acquired for the purpose of return or recall in §§ 1304.22 and 1305.03. The DEA has simplified the requirements of § 1317.10(a) to more clearly describe the records that registrants must keep.

Methods of Destruction

Existing DEA regulations do not specify a standard to which controlled substances must be destroyed. With this final rule, the DEA is implementing a standard of destruction nonretrievable—for registrants that destroy controlled substances, and procedures for the destruction of controlled substances. 21 CFR 1300.05 ("non-retrievable"), 1317.90, and 1317.95. The DEA is not requiring a particular method of destruction, so long as the desired result is achieved. This standard is intended to allow public and private entities to develop a variety of destruction methods that are secure, convenient, and responsible, consistent with preventing the diversion of such substances. Destruction of controlled substances must also meet all other applicable Federal, State, tribal, and local laws and regulations. Once a controlled substance is rendered "non-retrievable," it is no longer subject to the requirements of the DEA regulations.

As explained above under "Compliance Date," this final rule supersedes all existing MOAs and MOUs that registrants may have pursuant to § 1307.21, including MOAs and MOUs pertinent to storage of controlled substances. The DEA retains in the new part 1317 the ability for practitioners to request assistance from the local Special Agent in Charge (SAC) regarding the disposal of controlled substances. 21 CFR 1317.05. Practitioners may request a new MOA or MOU pursuant to the new § 1317.05(a)(5).

C. Summary of the Changes in the Final Rule

The DEA carefully considered the 192 individually submitted comments received in response to the Notice of Proposed Rulemaking (NPRM) on the Disposal of Controlled Substances. 77 FR 75784, Dec. 21, 2012. The comment period closed on February 19, 2013.

All of the comments submitted, except two comments, are available for public inspection online at www.regulations.gov. Two comments are not posted (at the commenters' request) in order to protect confidential business information.

The DEA is making a number of significant changes after thorough consideration of the issues raised by the comments and the potential diversion risks associated with these changes. In response to concerns regarding ultimate users' ability to have convenient disposal options, the DEA is vastly expanding those entities that may be authorized as collectors, expanding the authority of those collectors to maintain collection receptacles at LCTFs, and relaxing some of the proposed security requirements related to storage and destruction of controlled substances.

Authorized Collector

In addition to manufacturers, distributors, reverse distributors, and retail pharmacies, the final rule also authorizes registered NTPs, as well as hospitals/clinics with an on-site pharmacy, to operate disposal programs. 21 CFR 1317.40. By permitting these additional registrant categories to be collectors, the DEA anticipates that ultimate users will now have even more locations where they can securely, safely, responsibly, and conveniently dispose of their unwanted pharmaceutical controlled substances.

In this final rule, the DEA is permitting those entities registered as NTPs to become authorized collectors to manage collection receptacles at their registered locations. As stated in the Disposal Act, "the nonmedical use of prescription drugs is a growing problem in the United States." Multiple commenters, including a national organization that represents NTPs, recommended that the DEA include NTPs as authorized collectors. The DEA recognizes the valuable role that NTPs have in helping those seeking substance abuse treatment. After considering the importance of providing secure, convenient, and responsible disposal options for those ultimate users currently receiving treatment for narcotic substance abuse or entering a narcotic treatment program, and the benefits of allowing NTPs to provide the opportunity to patients to dispose of unused controlled substances, the DEA is permitting NTPs to be collectors with certain enhanced security controls. 21 CFR 1317.75.

Due to the nature of the healthcare provided, NTPs face unique security challenges and heightened diversion risks and, as such, the final rule requires NTPs to securely place and maintain collection receptacles in a room that does not contain any other controlled substances and is securely locked with controlled access. 21 CFR 1317.75. The DEA understands that this security measure will require employees of the NTP to accompany the patient to the collection receptacle to facilitate the patient's disposal. See 21 CFR 1317.75. Additionally, as the Disposal Act and these regulations are intended to address the prescription drug abuse problem, NTPs and other collectors are not authorized to collect schedule I controlled substances. E.g., 21 CFR 1317.75. Collectors must be vigilant in ensuring that such illicit substances are not collected intentionally or inadvertently. E.g., 21 CFR 1317.70 and 1317.75.

After extensive review and careful deliberation, in this final rule, the DEA is also permitting registered hospitals/clinics with an on-site pharmacy to become authorized collectors to maintain collection receptacles inside their registered locations or at LTCFs, and to conduct mail-back programs. 21 CFR 1317.30, 1317.40, 1317.70, and 1317.80. In response to the NPRM, many commenters stated that collection receptacles located inside of hospitals would provide ultimate users with an opportunity to dispose of medication that may no longer be needed or may be expired. In determining whether to allow hospitals/clinics to become authorized collectors, the DEA carefully weighed the diversion risks with the convenience of authorizing such entities to be collectors. The DEA determined that the diversion risks require the DEA to limit those registered hospitals/clinics that may become collectors to those with onsite pharmacies, and also impose separate security conditions on the monitoring and location of collection receptacles inside hospitals/clinics that become authorized collectors. 21 CFR 1317.75.

The DEA is requiring these additional security measures in order to help protect against the diversion of collected controlled substances because hospitals/clinics are generally much larger and are open to a much larger general population than the other registrants authorized to be collectors; and, as discussed in the NPRM, hospitals/clinics do not operate under the same business model or with similar theft and loss prevention procedures as the other registrants authorized to become collectors. For example, the general public typically enters retail pharmacies for short durations in order to conduct retail business and retail pharmacies generally have open, clearly observable common areas with little opportunity to conceal an unlawful purpose. It would be unusual and suspicious for a person to spend an extended amount of time in a retail pharmacy without a known, specific purpose, triggering routine theft and loss prevention measures.

In contrast, hospitals are generally open 24 hours per day and allow for unsupervised public access for extended periods of time; they are much larger than retail pharmacies and many interactions occur behind closed doors without routine theft and loss prevention measures; and foot traffic generally is not routinely monitored for unlawful purposes. The DEA believes that limiting authorized collection activities to hospitals/clinics with an on-site pharmacy is necessary to help protect against diversion because these hospitals/clinics routinely handle a large volume of controlled substances that are dispensed to in-patients as well as to the public, and these entities are more experienced with security, theft and loss prevention procedures, and inventory, recordkeeping and reporting requirements than those hospitals/clinics without an on-site pharmacy.

For reasons discussed in the NPRM, this final rule generally requires that, when authorized collectors choose to install collection receptacles, those collection receptacles must be placed inside their registered locations in the immediate proximity of a designated area where controlled substances are stored and at which an employee is present. 21 CFR 1317.75; see also 1317.05. The DEA recognizes that hospitals/clinics with an on-site pharmacy can be unique in their design and it may be more effective to install collection receptacles at various locations within the hospital/

clinic, depending on factors such as security, convenience, and accessibility. As such, it would be challenging for authorized hospitals/clinics to adhere to the general rule to place collection receptacles in the immediate proximity of where controlled substances are stored and at which an employee is present. Accordingly, the DEA is requiring hospitals/clinics that are collectors to place collection receptacles in locations that are regularly monitored by employees. 21 CFR 1317.75. In addition, the DEA is prohibiting such collectors from placing collection receptacles in the proximity of any area where emergency or urgent care is provided. In the DEA's experience, the risk of diversion is particularly high in areas where emergency or urgent care is provided because of the often chaotic environment and the extended amounts of time persons spend in such areas.

This rule also makes clear that DEA registrants cannot use the collection receptacles to dispose of unused controlled substances in their inventory or stock. 21 CFR 1317.05 and 1317.75. Pharmaceutical controlled substances remain under the custody and control of the DEA registrant if they are dispensed by a practitioner for immediate administration at the practitioner's registered location (such as a hospital) pursuant to an order for medication. If that substance is not fully exhausted (e.g., some of the substance remains in a vial, tube, or syringe after administration but cannot or may not be further utilized), then the DEA registrant is obligated to destroy the remaining, unusable controlled substances, and record the destruction in accordance with § 1304.22(c). The DEA registrant shall not place such remaining, unusable controlled substance in a collection receptacle as a means of disposal. Hospital/clinic staff must also not dispose of any controlled substances in inventory or stock in a collection receptacle. The security requirements described above are the minimum required in order to detect and prevent diversion in the unique circumstances of NTPs and hospitals/clinics. These registrants should be vigilant in the execution of their responsibilities as registrants to ensure that collected controlled substances are not diverted to illicit use, and that they do not collect illicit substances. Finally, all registrants are reminded of the responsibility to report theft and significant loss of controlled substances within one business day of discovery.

Long-Term Care Facilities (LTCFs)

Significant changes are made in this final rule to help ensure that LTCFs have adequate disposal options. In addition to allowing retail pharmacies to manage and maintain collection receptacles at LTCFs, the DEA is also allowing hospitals/clinics with an on-site pharmacy to manage and maintain collection receptacles at LTCFs. The DEA hopes that expanding those authorized to collect at LTCFs will maximize disposal opportunities for LTCF residents. In addition, the DEA is alleviating two security requirements proposed to apply to collection receptacles located at LTCFs. First, the DEA is permitting authorized hospitals/clinics and retail pharmacies to store inner liners that have been sealed upon removal from a collection receptacle at LTCFs in a securely locked, substantially constructed cabinet or a securely locked room with controlled access for up to three business days until the liners can be transferred for destruction.

The DEA encourages collectors to schedule inner liner removals and installations to coincide with existing LTCF visits when possible, for example, arranging a routine system in which medication deliveries coincide with the removal and transfer of sealed inner liners for appropriate destruction, thereby making storage of sealed inner liners unnecessary. Collectors may not transfer sealed inner liners from LTCFs to their primary registered location (i.e., the hospital/clinic or retail pharmacy location). As echoed in the comments, the DEA remains concerned about the security risks of hospital/clinic and retail pharmacy employees transporting large quantities of collected substances, making them potential targets for drug seekers. Instead, collectors should deliver sealed inner liners to a reverse distributor or distributor's registered location by common or contract carrier pick-up or by reverse distributor or distributor pick-up at the LTCF, pursuant to § 1317.05(c)(2)(iv).

Second, the DEA relaxed the two-employee integrity requirement for inner liner installation, removal, storage, and transfer at LTCFs. Collectors will retain the option to authorize two of their own employees to install, remove, store, and transfer inner liners; however, the DEA is permitting collectors the option to designate a supervisor-level employee of the LTCF (e.g., a charge nurse, supervisor, or similar employee) to install, remove, store, or transfer inner liners with only one employee of the collector.

The DEA modified the above security requirements (storage and two-person integrity) to provide flexibility sufficient to encourage authorized hospitals/clinics and retail pharmacies to collect at LTCFs, while ensuring the minimum protections required to prevent diversion at LTCFs. The DEA hopes that the inclusion of certain hospitals/clinics as authorized to maintain collection receptacles at LTCFs, and the modifications described above will result in expanded safe and secure disposal options for LTCF residents. The DEA emphasizes that if LTCFs dispose of LTCF residents' controlled substances in collection receptacles, such activity must be in accordance with this regulation and all other applicable Federal, State, tribal and local laws and regulations, including environmental laws and regulations.

The DEA acknowledges that there may be some LTCFs that will not have a collection receptacle, and there will be instances where LTCF residents are incapable of disposing of their own unused or unwanted medication. As ultimate users, LTCF residents may use any of the disposal options afforded other ultimate users in this final rule (e.g., mail-back programs), in addition to the disposal options currently available to ultimate users (e.g., flushing or otherwise discarding) that will remain options even after this final rule is implemented. For example, an LTCF resident may request that LTCF personnel place the resident's unwanted medication in a mail-back package, seal the mail-back package, and deposit that package into the facility's outgoing mail system. 21 CFR 1317.70. LTCFs should be mindful however that the touchstone for this disposal method is the individual nature of the disposal activity; institutional facilities such as LTCFs should ensure that the individual patient is the disposer, and should be wary of establishing any protocols whereby the facility itself is engaging in collection activities. Simply providing the method of disposal (e.g., mail-back packages) does not implicate that concern.

Destruction

After careful and thorough consideration of comments received regarding the burdens associated with the proposed 14-day destruction requirement, the DEA is extending the time those registrants that reverse distribute have to destroy controlled substances to 30 days. 21 CFR 1317.15(d). The DEA anticipates that this extension will allow reverse distributors and distributors adequate time to collect and destroy controlled substances in a safe, convenient, and secure manner, while also preventing diversion and diversion opportunities.

Practitioner Physical Security

In this final rule, the DEA is not amending § 1301.75(b) pertaining to practitioner physical security and is instead adding a new paragraph (c) to clarify that practitioners shall only store sealed mail-back packages and inner liners containing collected substances at their registered location in a securely locked, substantially constructed cabinet or a securely locked room with controlled access. The DEA has made corresponding changes to §§ 1317.05(c)(1)(ii) and (c)(2)(ii). Part of this requirement was included in the proposed rule; however, after careful consideration of a number of comments, the DEA believes that the proposed requirement did not provide sufficient controls to protect against diversion and was impracticable. Pharmacies and institutional practitioners cannot store sealed inner liners or returned mail-back packages by dispersing them throughout the stock of noncontrolled substances. 21 CFR 1301.75(b) and (c).

Other Changes to the Final Rule

In addition to the changes described above, the DEA determined that the rule, as proposed, required other modifications, as generally described below. The DEA is also implementing additional technical modifications that will not have a substantive effect on this rule (e.g., relocating some sections in proposed part 1317 to other sections within title 21 of the CFR, re-phrasing some sections from the proposed rule to be simpler, clearer and easier to understand, and eliminating redundancy).

In the general definitions section of the DEA regulations, the DEA is amending § 1300.01(b) to be clear that the definitions that generally apply to most other parts of chapter II of title 21 of the CFR also apply to part 1317. In response to a number of comments, in § 1300.01(b) the DEA is amending the definition of "reverse distributor" to clarify that a reverse distributor is a person registered with the DEA as a reverse distributor.

Definitions were moved from § 1317.02 to § 1300.05 to provide consistency within the CFR pertaining to definitions. The DEA adds § 1300.05 "Definitions relating to the disposal of controlled substances," moves the terms "authorized employee," "law enforcement officer," and "non-retrievable" from part 1317 to § 1300.05(b), adds a definition of "on-site" to § 1300.05(b), and deletes the definitions of "for cause" and "inner liner" that were in proposed part 1317. The DEA also moves the definition of "collection" to § 1300.01(b). These changes are in response to comments or related to the movement of several other requirements from part 1317 to other parts, as discussed below.

In addition to moving them to § 1300.05(b), the DEA amends the definitions of "authorized employee" and "law enforcement officer." The DEA is omitting the word "authorized" from the definition of "authorized employee," and codifying the definition of "employee" in harmony with the general common law of agency. The DEA is modifying the definition of "law enforcement officer" in part 1317 to specifically include officers from law enforcement components of Federal agencies, and authorized police officers of the Veterans Health Administration and the Department of Defense. In addition, this rule clarifies who may qualify as a "law enforcement officer" for the purpose of disposal. The DEA is changing references to "law enforcement agencies" to "law enforcement" in order to include law enforcement components of Federal agencies.

Although the DEA defined "inner liner" in the NPRM, the final rule does not amend the CFR to add a definition for inner liner. As described below, inner liners used in the collection of controlled substances must meet the specifications outlined in § 1317.60. The DEA also is not amending the CFR to add a definition of "for cause," and instead is providing an explanation of "for cause" as it relates to the sections to which it applies.

The DEA added a definition of "on-site" to § 1300.05(b) to clarify that "on-site" means "located on or at the physical premises of the registrant's registered location" for purposes of destruction and registration as a collector. Specifically, a controlled substance is destroyed "onsite" when destruction occurs on the physical premises of the destroying registrant's registered location, and a hospital/clinic has an "on-site" pharmacy when it has a pharmacy located on the physical premises of the registrant's registered location.

Text was added to the registration table in § 1301.13 to reflect that distributors, as a coincident activity to distribution, may acquire controlled substances from collectors for the purpose of destruction. The registration table was updated so that it would be consistent with the regulations in the final rule, which authorize distributors to destroy controlled substances acquired from collectors.

The DEA received a number of comments indicating confusion regarding the procedures a registrant must follow to modify their DEA registration to become a collector. In order to clarify such requirements, the DEA is further revising § 1301.51. The additional revisions clarify the requirements by listing them independently of other types of registration modifications (e.g., change of name or address) and clearly indicating that any modifications may be made in writing by mail or online. 21 CFR part 1301. Also, the submission method has been modified from "letter" to "written request" to accurately encompass the various ways the modification request may be submitted (e.g., online), and the phrase "to be paid" was deleted from § 1301.51(c) for stylistic reasons. Similarly, the DEA is further revising § 1301.52 to clarify that any registrant who has been authorized as a collector and who desires to discontinue their collection of pharmaceutical controlled substances from ultimate users must notify the DEA.

The DEA is also streamlining certain registration and security procedures by moving certain requirements from part 1317, as proposed in the NPRM, to part 1301. Reverse distributor employee security requirements in proposed § 1317.20 were moved to § 1301.74(m) for ease of reference and consistency. Collector security requirements in proposed § 1317.45 were moved to § 1301.71(f) for clarity and consistency.

The DEA determined that inclusion of recordkeeping and reporting requirements in part 1317 may lead to confusion among registrants. As such, the DEA is moving all recordkeeping and reporting requirements from part 1317, as proposed in the NPRM, to part 1304—Records and Reports of DEA Registrants—in order to maintain consistency and consolidate all recordkeeping and reporting requirements into one part. In § 1304.03, "each" was changed to "every," and "who" was changed to "that" for stylistic reasons. In § 1304.11(e)(2), the first sentence, pertaining to an exception for reverse distributors, was removed and incorporated into § 1304.11(e)(3) of the final rule to accurately reflect the type of registrants to which the section applies.

The DEA is expanding the locations where a collector may maintain records in § 1304.04(a)(3). The text in § 1304.21(a) was updated to specifically include inner liners and mail-back packages, which were inadvertently overlooked in the NPRM. 21 CFR § 1304.21(c) was updated to include the general recordkeeping requirements for collection activities as outlined in the final rule. The recordkeeping requirements for disposal of controlled substances in 21 CFR § 1307.21 were moved to § 1304.21(e) and amended to include recordkeeping procedures for destruction. The title and introductory text in § 1304.22 were updated to accurately reflect their contents. Additionally, § 1304.22 was modified to include recordkeeping requirements for collected controlled substances. The second sentence in both § 1304.25(a)(9) and § 1304.25(b)(9), which required compliance with part 1317 when destroying narcotic controlled substances, were removed as superfluous. All disposal and destruction activities are clearly delineated in part 1317. Also, various Automation of Reports and Consolidated Ordering System (ARCOS) requirements are removed from part 1317, as proposed in the NPRM, and are consolidated and moved to § 1304.33. In addition, the title of § 1304.33 has been changed to add clarity, and the acronym "ARCOS" is clearly spelled out. The formatting for § 1304.33(f) was modified for ease of understanding, and "who" was changed to "that" in two locations for consistency.

The DEA is also amending § 1305.03 to add a new paragraph (f) to clarify that collectors are exempt from order form requirements for pharmaceutical controlled substances collected through mail-back programs and collection receptacles for the purpose of disposal. The title of § 1307.11 no longer references reverse distributors and has been changed to "Distribution by dispenser to another practitioner" because reverse distributor activities were moved to part 1317.

As discussed in the preamble to the NPRM and as mentioned in proposed § 1317.100, the DEA clarifies in § 1304.21 of this final rule that, in addition to any other recordkeeping requirements, all registrants that destroy or cause the destruction of a controlled substance must maintain a record of that destruction on a DEA Form 41. This requirement had been discussed in the preamble to the proposed rule, and in proposed § 1317.100 the DEA stated "any registered person that destroys or causes the destruction of a controlled substance shall maintain a record of destruction on a form issued by DEA." The DEA has determined that this requirement to keep such records on DEA Form 41 should be explicitly stated in the regulatory text, and not just the preamble, for registrants to clearly understand the requirements to which they are bound. As stated above, this requirement to record destruction activities on the DEA Form 41 does not apply to drug wastage or pharmaceutical wastage which must be properly recorded, stored, and destroyed in accordance with DEA regulations, and all applicable Federal, State, tribal, and local laws and regulations. 21 CFR part 1304.

The DEA is modifying proposed § 1317.70 to address the procedures that a collector must follow when ceasing operation of a mail-back program. This modification requires such collector to make reasonable efforts to notify the public of their intent to cease mail-back collection activities. 21 CFR 1317.70. Such collector must also establish an agreement with another collector authorized to conduct a mail-back program to receive all remaining packages and arrange for the forwarding of such packages to the second collector's registered location. These procedures will ensure that another authorized entity will be responsible for receiving and destroying any mail-back packages that were disseminated but not received back by the collector prior to the time that they ceased operation of their mail-back program.

Finally, the DEA is modifying proposed § 1317.75 for two purposes. The first modification clarifies that collected controlled and non-controlled substances can be comingled, but are not required to be comingled. 21 CFR 1317.75. As previously discussed, the second modification to this section allows certain LTCF employees, as designated by the collector authorized to maintain a collection receptacle at that LTCF, to install, seal, remove, store, and transfer for destruction the inner liners of the collection receptacle along with an employee of the collector. 21 CFR 1317.80. This modification allows greater flexibility for collectors authorized to maintain collection receptacles at LTCFs.

About the Contributors

Pauline **Bartolone** is a Sacramento correspondent for *California Healthline*.

Martha **Bebinger** covers health care and other general assignments for WBUR.

Geoff **Beckwith** is the executive director of the Massachusetts Municipal Association.

Brenda **Bond-Fortier** is an associate professor and chair of the Institute for Public Service at Suffolk University.

California Department of Public Health is the state department responsible for public health.

Emily B. **Campbell** is a visiting lecturer of sociology, College of the Holy Cross.

Centers for Disease Control and Prevention is the leading national public health institute of the United States.

City and County of San Francisco is the governing administrative division for the city-county of San Francisco, California.

April **Dembosky** is the health reporter for *The California Report* and KQED News.

Don C. **Des Jarlais** is a professor of epidemiology at New York University and a leader in the fields of AIDS and injecting drug use and has published extensively on these topics.

Jeannie D. **DiClementi** is an associate professor of psychology, Indiana University.

Amy **Driscoll** is a journalist with the *Miami Herald*.

Nabila **El-Bassel** is a professor of social work and director of Social Intervention Group, Columbia University.

Federal Register is the official daily journal of the United States Government.

Nina **Feldman** reports for WHYY in Philadelphia.

Audrey **Fraizer** is the managing editor, *Journal of Emergency Dispatch*, International Academies of Emergency Dispatch, Salt Lake City, Utah.

Joaquin Jay **Gonzalez** III is Mayor George Christopher Professor of Public Administration at the Edward S. Ageno School of Business of Golden Gate University.

Elana **Gordon** is a member of WHYY's health and science desk in Philadelphia and producer on the station's health and science show, *The Pulse*.

Anna **Gorman** is a senior correspondent with *Kaiser Health News* based in Los Angeles.

William **Greene** is an assistant professor, psychiatry, University of Florida.

Marty **Harding** is the director of training and consultation at the Hazelden Betty Ford Foundation.

Jaime Teeter **Householder** is a community activist and volunteer who served on the board of directors for Central Coast HIV/AIDS Services in Monterey County, California.

About the Contributors

International City/County Management Association is the leading organization of local government professionals dedicated to creating and sustaining thriving communities throughout the world.

Victoria **Knight** is a reporter with *Kaiser Health News*.

Shefali **Luthra** is a *Kaiser Health News* correspondent covering consumer issues in health care.

Sammy **Mack** covers health care policy for WLRN, South Florida's NPR news station.

Carolyn **McAllaster** is a clinical professor of law and director, AIDS/HIV and Cancer Legal Project, Duke University.

Mickey P. **McGee** is professor of public administration and director of the Doctor of Business Administration Program at the Edward S. Ageno School of Business of Golden Gate University.

Lisa J. **Merlo** is an associate professor, psychiatry, University of Florida.

National Association of County and City Health Officials is the Washington, D.C.–based organization representing more than 3,000 local public health departments in the United States.

National Institute on Drug Abuse is a federal government research institute whose mission is to lead the nation in bringing the power of science to bear on drug abuse and addiction.

New York State Department of Health is the state department responsible for public health.

Stephanie **O'Neill** reports for *Kaiser Health News* and *California Healthline*.

Paul C. **Prevey** is a retired senior U.S. probation officer and treatment specialist for the District of Massachusetts.

Susan **Reif** is a research associate, Center for Health Policy & Inequalities Research, Duke University.

Travis N. **Rieder** is a research scholar at the Berman Institute of Bioethics, Johns Hopkins University.

Carmen Heredia **Rodriguez** is a reporter for *Kaiser Health News*.

San Francisco Department of Public Health is the city agency that protects and promotes the health of all San Franciscans.

San Francisco Health Commission is the governing and policy-making body of the Department of Public Health.

Taylor **Sisk** is a free-lance writer, editor, and film/video producer based in Nashville, Tennessee.

Will **Stone** is a writer for *Kaiser Health News*.

Thomas J. **Stopka** is an assistant professor of public health and community medicine, Tufts University.

Jodi **Sutherland** is a clinical assistant professor, Binghamton University, State University of New York.

Sarah **Sweeney** is a professional social worker and graduate of Seattle University's master of public administration program.

Jenna **Tyler** is a graduate student enrolled in the criminal justice and public safety program at Indiana University–Purdue University Indianapolis.

U.S. Department of Health and Human Services is the federal government agency tasked with protecting the health of all Americans and providing essential human services.

U.S. Drug Enforcement Administration is the leading law enforcement agency responsible for preventing the distribution of illegal narcotics in the United States.

U.S. Environmental Protection Agency is an independent agency of the federal government for environmental protection.

U.S. Food and Drug Administration is a federal agency under the U.S. Department of Health and Human Services responsible for protecting and promoting public health.

Utah Department of Health is the state department responsible for public health.

Elissa **Velez** is a substance use services programs coordinator with the city and county of San Francisco and has more than a decade of experiences with HIV and substance use disorder treatment and prevention programs.

Jack **Wallace** is a research fellow, Australian Research Centre in Sex, Health and Society, La Trobe University.

Erin **Winstanley** is an associate professor of pharmacy, West Virginia University.

H. Daniel **Xu** is a research analyst at Alabama Department of Public Health.

Gerald **Young** is a senior research associate at the Center for State and Local Government Excellence.

Index

abstinence 243
Affordable Care Act (ACA) 40, 243
African American Community 61
Alabama 146, 251
American adult 211, 215
American cities 188
American Civil Liberties Union 1
American fatalities 248
American Foundation for AIDS Research 168
American history 19
American Indian or Alaskan Natives 211
American Journal of Epidemiology 150
American Medical Association (AMA) 208, 243, 249
American opioid crisis 19
American Pain 17
American Society of Addiction Medicine 182, 184, 226
amphetamine 243
Arizona 2, 25, 142–144, 251
Arizona Department of Health Services 144
Arkansas 178, 192, 251

biomarkers 243
Boston, MA 1
brainstem 244

California 3, 36–37, 68–69, 71–72, 118–124, 145, 150, 154, 158, 161, 164, 166, 171, 233–234, 243–244, 248, 250–251, 265–266
California Business and Professions Code 123, 244
California Department of Public Health 71, 118–121, 123, 161
California Health and Safety Code 122–124, 244
California Healthline 69
California Legal Code 122
California State Legislature 119
California State Sheriff's Association 69
California Syringe Exchange Program (CalSEP) 119–121
California's Office of AIDS 164
Centers for Disease Control and Prevention (CDC) 10, 16, 22, 32–35, 37, 41–44, 49–50, 53, 59–60, 64, 72, 83, 85–87, 92, 96–97, 102–111, 118, 130, 136–137, 152, 162, 167, 178, 191, 210, 214–215, 219–220, 235, 244, 247
cognitive-behavioral therapy (CBT) 244, 247
Colorado 113, 251
Congress 26, 36, 62, 188, 201–202, 211, 219–220, 226, 243, 256
Connecticut 251
Controlled Substances Act 75, 189, 255
crackhouse 188

Democratic 27, 59, 126
dependence 244

detoxification 244
District of Columbia 25, 40, 47, 76, 89, 176, 215, 251
Drug Abuse Resistance Education (DARE) 17
Drug Enforcement Administration (DEA) 3, 75
Duke University 49

Environmental Protection Agency 112
Environmental Protection Agency National Institute on Drug Abuse 3

fentanyl 1, 17, 46, 90, 96, 125, 143, 161, 173–174, 204, 212, 226, 237, 245, 247, 254
Florida 3, 17, 25, 49, 57–59, 61–62, 100, 125–127, 178–179, 251, 265–266
Florida Department of Health 59, 126
Florida International University 61
Food and Drug Administration (FDA) 3, 75, 77, 103, 112, 213, 216, 246, 247–250, 267

Georgia 25, 146, 251

harm reduction 18, 31–32, 36–38, 48, 56, 126, 132–133, 141, 143–147, 149, 151–152, 155–158, 160–161, 182, 187–188, 192, 196–198, 201, 210, 214, 218, 230, 239, 245, 252, 254
Hawaii 251
HBV 33–34, 78, 86, 105–108, 113, 140, 163, 167, 213–214, 245, 249
HCV 10, 32–34, 64, 78, 86–87, 97, 99, 106–108, 113, 133, 136–138, 140–141, 156, 160–161, 163, 166–167, 198, 213–214, 219–220, 245
hepatitis 1–3, 7–11, 25–26, 31–35, 38, 40–41, 48, 53, 57, 59–72, 77–78, 83–90, 92–93, 96–101, 105–111, 113, 119–121, 123–128, 130–137, 145–147, 152, 161, 163, 165–168, 191, 210, 214, 216, 218–221, 229–231, 245–246, 248–249, 251–252, 254
heroin 1, 11, 17, 22, 31, 37–38, 46, 54, 57–61, 63, 68–72, 75, 96, 115, 125, 127, 137, 142–143, 145–146, 149, 152, 155–156, 175, 179, 181–185, 192, 204, 212–213, 220, 226, 233–234, 237, 245–247, 253–254
HIV 1–4, 7–8, 10–12, 25–27, 31–44, 46, 48–54, 57–62, 65–66, 77–78, 83–94, 96, 99, 118–121, 123–131, 136–140, 143, 145–146, 149–154, 191–192, 194–203, 210, 213–214, 219–220, 243–249, 252, 254; HIV/AIDS 1, 32–33, 49, 62, 77, 85, 100, 121, 131, 136, 153–154, 163–164, 166–167, 169, 200–202, 216, 244, 265; epidemic 1–11; and hepatitis 1, 3–4, 7, 59–60, 62, 90, 99–101, 113, 119, 124–127, 161, 191, 221, 230, 246, 252, 254; testing 10–26; treatment and prevention 1, 252
Household Hazardous Waste Collection Sites 80

Idaho 25, 251
Illinois 150, 251

Indiana 3, 7, 27, 31, 26, 43–44, 128–130, 145, 214, 217, 251, 265–266
Indiana University 129
injection drug use 246
International City/County Management Association (ICMA) 175–177
Iowa 25, 251

Kentucky 17, 26, 42, 145, 178, 251
King County, WA 157

lancet 246
Lesbian, Gay, Bisexual and Transgender Health 133
long-term care facilities (LTCFs) 260
Louisiana 26, 49, 146, 251
Lowell, MA 3, 23, 172–174
Lowell Community Opioid Outreach Program 173
Lowell House 173
Lowell Opioid Overdose Project 172

Maine 251
Maryland 94, 251
Massachusetts 3, 8, 23, 42, 172–176, 178, 181–182, 185, 204–207, 214, 237, 240, 251
Massachusetts Ambulance Trip Reporting Information System (MATRIS) 173
Massachusetts Municipal Association 204
Medicaid 47
Medical Priority Dispatch System (MPDS) 246
medication-assisted treatment (MAT) 246
methadone 1, 17, 46, 48, 63, 66, 99, 106, 156, 161, 181–182, 204, 212, 227, 238–239, 246, 253–254
methamphetamine (meth) 1, 4, 36, 59, 71, 156, 232–234, 254
methicillin 99
methods of destruction 258
Miami-Dade County 59
Miami-Dade Infectious Disease Elimination Act (IDEA) 58
Michigan 251
Miller School of Medicine 58
Minnesota 178, 251
Mississippi 146, 251
Missouri 25, 226, 251
Montana 251
Monterey County 3
motivational enhancement therapy (MET) 246

Naloxone (Narcan) 3, 9, 11, 17, 47–48, 56, 69, 92, 94, 96–99, 105–106, 115–117, 140–142, 146–147, 157, 161, 173, 176, 179, 182, 185, 189–191, 198–200, 207, 210, 212–213, 218, 220, 226–228, 235, 239, 246–247, 254
National Academy of Medicine 13–14
National Academy of Science, Engineering, and Medicine 13
National Association of County and City Health Officials (NACCHO) 209–215, 218–220
National Council on Jewish Women 192
National Drug Control Policy 76
National Health Law Program 147
National HIV/AIDS 209Strategy 201
National HIV/AIDS Strategy and Viral Hepatitis Action Plan 136
National HIV Behavioral Surveillance System 11, 98
National HIV Prevention Conference 27
National HIV Testing Day 52
National Institute on Drug Abuse 3, 17, 31, 115, 170, 246
National Institutes of Health 120, 246
National Prescription Drug Take-Back 76
National Survey on Drug Use and Health 75
needle stick injury 246
New Hampshire 251
New Jersey 113, 248, 251
New York 3, 11–12, 94, 98, 101, 113, 131–134, 145–146, 150, 154, 175, 190, 214, 216, 251, 265
non-opioid analgesics 246
North American Syringe Exchange Network (NASEN) 34, 60, 90, 105, 251
North Carolina 3, 26, 99, 145–147, 191–192, 251
North Dakota 26, 251

Obama, Barack 83, 85, 105, 118, 243
Ohio 4, 18, 26, 37, 145, 170–171
Oklahoma 251
opiate antagonist 140, 198, 247, 249
opioid crisis 2, 4, 10, 13, 18–19, 23–24, 26, 54, 96, 101, 143, 154, 170, 172, 204–205, 207, 215–217, 237–238, 240, 247, 248, 253
opioid epidemic 1–5, 7–8, 12–20, 22, 24–26, 34, 46–47, 54–56, 63, 69, 97, 100, 142–143, 145, 175, 178–179, 191, 204, 209, 211–217, 225, 232, 235–236, 247–248, 253
opioid receptors 247
opioid use disorder (OUD) 1, 10, 17, 35, 46, 54, 56, 63, 99, 106, 176, 209–210, 213, 227, 247, 253
Oregon 251
overdose 2–3, 7–9, 11, 16–17, 19–20, 24, 38, 46–47, 54, 56, 58, 69–70, 75–76, 87, 89–90, 92–96, 98–99, 105–106, 108, 115–116, 119, 122–123, 126–127, 132, 136, 141–146, 150–152, 155–157, 161, 170–178, 180–182, 184–186, 188–189, 192, 198–202, 204, 207–208, 210–221, 225, 227, 232, 235–240, 246–247, 253–254

pain management 14, 22, 135, 238–239, 247
Pence, Mike 26, 59, 128
Pennsylvania 3, 117, 150, 188, 251
people who inject drugs (PWID) 1, 10, 63–64, 89, 105, 107, 118–119, 136, 155–158, 248
pharmacodynamics 247
Philadelphia, PA 6, 18, 69, 150, 186–190, 214
prayers 191
Presbyterian Church 192
prescription drug misuse 247
prescription drug monitoring program 247
President's Commission on Combating Drug Addiction and the Opioid Crisis 18, 248
Prevention Point Philadelphia 186
program participant 164, 166, 219, 248
prophylaxis 34, 87, 91, 99, 106, 108, 247, 250
Puerto Rico 113, 176, 251
Purdue University 129

Radiant Church 3, 191
recall 57, 70, 115, 145, 148, 248, 255, 257
receptor 115, 207, 246–248
recovery 14, 17, 20, 54, 56, 69–70, 103, 105, 130, 145, 173, 177, 183, 192, 205–207, 210, 212–213, 215, 226–228, 232, 234, 238–239, 248, 252
red states 3, 145
Rendell, Ed 188
Republican 25–27, 40, 57, 59, 125–126, 142, 145, 182
Rhode Island 113, 251
risk factors 33, 54, 60, 128, 167, 210, 212, 214, 219, 248

safehouse 188–190
San Francisco (City and County of San Francisco) 3–4, 12, 60, 62

San Francisco AIDS Foundation 194–203
Scott, Gov. Rick 58
Seattle, WA 157
Secure and Responsible Drug Disposal Act of 2010 (Disposal Act) 255
self-medication 248
Sessions, Jeff 145
sexually transmitted diseases (STD) 4, 66, 87, 99, 105–106, 108, 131, 133, 248, 252
sexually transmitted infections (STI) 133, 152, 248
sharps 77–82, 91, 103, 112–113, 118, 122–124, 127, 131–132, 138–139, 161–162, 165–166, 196, 243–245, 248
South Carolina 49, 146–147, 251
Stanford University 18
substance abuse 26, 44, 54, 72, 136, 138, 173, 175, 176–177, 205–208, 227, 238–239, 252, 259
Substance Abuse and Mental Health Services Administration (SAMHSA) 35, 90, 118, 138, 206, 248
substance use disorder (SUD) 1–2, 25, 32, 34–35, 48, 54–55, 86–88, 90, 92–93, 97, 99, 105–106, 108, 111, 156, 210, 213, 244, 246, 248
supervised injection sites (SIS) 70, 249
Syringe Exchange Certification Program 121
Syringe Exchange Operator 249
Syringe Exchange Programs and Safe Injection Services (Needle Exchange Programs) 1, 2, 4, 18, 25, 31–32, 42, 48, 50, 85, 92, 105, 118–119, 122–123, 128, 130, 135–136, 141, 143, 154, 163–164, 168–169, 191–192, 244, 249, 250–251
Syringe Service Programs (SSPs) 2, 11, 31–32, 63–64, 100, 105, 214, 219–220

T cells 33, 245, 249
Tennessee 26, 49, 146, 251
Texas 40, 49, 251
Trump, Donald 16, 39, 235

United Church of Christ 192
United Methodist Church, 192
United States 3, 7, 16–17, 23, 31, 46, 49–50, 53, 63, 69, 93, 136, 142, 157, 188, 204, 211, 244; cities 190; deaths 219; healthcare system 243; territories 76
U.S. Attorney General 145
U.S. Bureau of Justice Assistance Strategies for Policing Innovations 23
U.S. Centers for Disease Control and Prevention 1, 59, 64
U.S. Department of Health and Human Services 1, 3, 65, 83, 85, 111, 136, 206, 220, 246, 248–249, 266–267
U.S. Department of Justice 172
U.S. Surgeon General 55, 136, 143, 220
University of Buffalo 176
University of California 150, 154, 233, 234
University of Miami 57
University of Pennsylvania 150
University of Vermont Health Network 237
Utah 3, 135–141, 250–251, 265, 267
Utah Department of Health 137
Utah Syringe Exchange Program 135–142

Virginia 26, 251

Washington 27, 117, 157, 251
West Virginia 17–18, 26, 251
Wisconsin 171, 178, 251
Wisconsin Bureau of Working Families 171
Wisconsin Department of Children and Families 171
withdrawal 14, 116, 227, 244, 246, 249, 253
Worcester, MA 3, 175–177
World Health Organization (WHO) 53, 151, 237, 160

Yale University 58